Fungal Diseases

Guest Editors

KENNETH S. KNOX, MD
GEORGE A. SAROSI, MD, MACP

CLINICS IN CHEST MEDICINE

www.chestmed.theclinics.com

June 2009 • Volume 30 • Number 2

SAUNDERS an imprint of ELSEVIER, Inc.

W.B. SAUNDERS COMPANY
A Division of Elsevier Inc.

1600 John F. Kennedy Boulevard ● Suite 1800 ● Philadelphia, Pennsylvania 19103

http://www.theclinics.com

CLINICS IN CHEST MEDICINE Volume 30, Number 2
June 2009 ISSN 0272-5231, ISBN-13: 978-1-4377-0461-7, ISBN-10: 1-4377-0461-1

Editor: Sarah E. Barth
Developmental Editor: Donald Mumford

Clinics in Chest Medicine (ISSN 0272-5231) is published quarterly by Elsevier Inc., 360 Park Avenue South, New York, NY 10010-1710. Months of issue are March, June, September, and December. Business and Editorial Offices: 1600 John F. Kennedy Blvd., Suite 1800, Philadelphia, PA 19103-2899. Customer Service Office: 11830 Westline Industrial Drive, St. Louis, MO 63146. Periodicals postage paid at New York, NY and additional mailing offices. Subscription prices are $251.00 per year (domestic individuals), $400.00 per year (domestic institutions), $122.00 per year (domestic students/residents), $275.00 per year (Canadian individuals), $491.00 per year (Canadian institutions), $342.00 per year (international individuals), $491.00 per year (international institutions), and $171.00 per year (international and Canadian students/residents). International air speed delivery is included in all Clinics subscription prices. All prices are subject to change without notice. **POSTMASTER:** Send address changes to *Clinics in Chest Medicine,* 11830 Westline Industrial Drive, St. Louis, MO 63146. Customer Service (orders, claims, online, change of address): Elsevier Periodicals Customer Service, 11830 Westline Industrial Drive, St. Louis, MO 63146. Tel: 1-800-654-2452 (U.S. and Canada). Fax: 314-523-5170. E-mail: journalscustomerservice-usa@elsevier.com (for print support); journalsonlinesupport-usa@elsevier.com (for online support).

Reprints. For copies of 100 or more of articles in this publication, please contact the Commercial Reprints Department, Elsevier Inc., 360 Park Avenue South, New York, NY 10010-1710. Tel.: 212-633-3812; Fax: 212-462-1935; E-mail: reprints@elsevier.com.

Clinics in Chest Medicine is covered in *MEDLINE/PubMed (Index Medicus), Current Contents/Clinical Medicine, EMBASE/ Excerpta Medica, Science Citation Index,* and *ISI/BIOMED.*

Printed and bound by CPI Group (UK) Ltd, Croydon, CR0 4YY
Transferred to Digital Print 2011

Contributors

GUEST EDITORS

KENNETH S. KNOX, MD
Associate Professor of Medicine, Southern
Arizona VA Health Care System (SAVAHCS);
and University of Arizona College of Medicine,
Tucson, Arizona

GEORGE A. SAROSI, MD, MACP
Professor of Medicine, University of Minnesota
School of Medicine; and Staff Physician,
Minneapolis VA Medical Center, Minneapolis,
Minnesota

AUTHORS

NEIL M. AMPEL, MD
Professor of Medicine, University of Arizona,
Medical Service, SAVAHCS, Tucson, Arizona

ELIAS ANAISSIE, MD
Professor of Medicine; Vice Chair; and Director
of Supportive Care, Myeloma Institute for
Research and Therapy, University of Arkansas
for Medical Sciences, Little Rock, Arkansas

TAMRA M. ARNOLD, PharmD, BCPS
Clinical Pharmacy Specialist, Roudebush VA
Medical Center, Indianapolis, Indiana

MATTHEW J. BINNICKER, PhD
Assistant Professor, Laboratory Medicine and
Pathology, Mayo Clinic College of Medicine;
and Director, Infectious Diseases Serology
Laboratory, Division of Clinical Microbiology,
Mayo Clinic, Superior Drive Support Center,
Rochester, Minnesota

JOSE CADENA, MD
Department of Internal Medicine, Division
of Infectious Diseases, University of Texas
Health Science Center at San Antonio;
and South Texas Veterans Health Care
System, San Antonio, Texas

RABIH O. DAROUICHE, MD
VA Distinguished Service Professor, Michael A.
Debakey Veterans Affairs Medical Center; and
Director, Center for Prostheses Infection
Baylor College of Medicine, Houston, Texas

CHADI A. HAGE, MD
Assistant Professor of Medicine, Pulmonary-
Critical Care and Infectious Diseases, Indiana
University School of Medicine, Roudebush VA
Medical Center, Indianapolis, Indiana

SHAHID HUSAIN, MD, MS
Assistant Professor of Medicine; and Director,
Multiorgan Transplant Infectious Diseases,
University Health Network, University of
Toronto, Toronto, Ontario, Canada

SHAUNNA M. HUSTON, RN, BSc
Department of Medical Science, University
of Calgary, Calgary, Alberta, Canada

CAROL A. KAUFFMAN, MD
Chief, Infectious Diseases Division, Veterans
Affairs Ann Arbor Healthcare System; and
Professor of Internal Medicine, University of
Michigan Medical School, Ann Arbor, Michigan

KENNETH S. KNOX, MD
Associate Professor of Medicine, Southern
Arizona VA Health Care System (SAVAHCS);
and University of Arizona College of Medicine,
Tucson, Arizona

BRYAN J. KRAJICEK, MD
Instructor of Medicine, Division of Pulmonary
and Critical Care Medicine, Mayo Clinic,
Rochester, Minnesota

ANDREW H. LIMPER, MD
Professor of Medicine, Division of Pulmonary
and Critical Care Medicine, Mayo Clinic,
Rochester, Minnesota

JAMES A. McKINNELL, MD
Division of Infectious Diseases, University
of Alabama at Birmingham, Birmingham,
Alabama

LAURA MEINKE, MD
Assistant Professor of Clinical Medicine,
Division of Pulmonary and Critical Care
Medicine; and Arizona Respiratory Center,
University of Arizona College of Medicine,
Tucson, Arizona

CHRISTOPHER H. MODY, MD
Department of Microbiology and Infectious
Diseases; and Department of Internal Medicine,
University of Calgary, Calgary, Alberta, Canada

SUSANNA NAGGIE, MD
Infectious Disease Fellow, Division of
Infectious Diseases, Department of Internal
Medicine, Duke University Medical Center,
Durham, North Carolina

MARCIO NUCCI, MD
Associate Professor of Medicine; and Head
of the Mycology Laboratory, Department
of Internal Medicine, University Hospital,
Universidade Federal do Rio de Janeiro,
Rio de Janeiro, Brazil

PETER G. PAPPAS, MD
Division of Infectious Diseases, University
of Alabama at Birmingham, Birmingham,
Alabama

THOMAS F. PATTERSON, MD, FACP
Department of Internal Medicine, Division
of Infectious Diseases, University of Texas
Health Science Center at San Antonio; and
South Texas Veterans Health Care System,
San Antonio, Texas

JOHN R. PERFECT, MD
Professor of Medicine, Division of Infectious
Diseases, Department of Internal Medicine,
Duke University Medical Center, Durham,
North Carolina

BRENT P. RISCILI, MD
Pulmonary Critical Care Fellow, Division
of Pulmonary, Allergy, Critical Care, and Sleep
Medicine, The Ohio State University Medical
Center, Davis Heart and Lung Research
Institute, Columbus, Ohio

CATHERINE R. SEARS, MD
Pulmonary Critical Care Fellow, Indiana
University, Indianapolis, Indiana

CHARLES F. THOMAS, Jr, MD
Associate Professor of Medicine, Division of
Pulmonary and Critical Care Medicine, Mayo
Clinic, Rochester, Minnesota

GEORGE R. THOMPSON III, MD
Department of Internal Medicine, Division
of Infectious Diseases, University of Texas
Health Science Center at San Antonio; and
South Texas Veterans Health Care System,
San Antonio, Texas

NANCY L. WENGENACK, PhD
Associate Professor, Laboratory Medicine and
Pathology, Mayo Clinic College of Medicine;
and Director, Mycology and Mycobacteriology
Laboratory, Division of Clinical Microbiology,
Mayo Clinic, Rochester, Minnesota

L. JOSEPH WHEAT, MD
MiraVista Diagnostics and MiraBella
Technologies, Indianapolis, Indiana

KAREN L. WOOD, MD
Assistant Professor, Division of Pulmonary,
Allergy, Critical Care, and Sleep Medicine, The
Ohio State University Medical Center, Davis
Heart and Lung Research Institute, Columbus,
Ohio

Contents

from the use of empiric antifungal therapy, and on the investigation of novel approaches for the potential salvage of devices infected with *Candida* species.

Invasive fungal infections (IFIs) represent a major complication in recipients of hematopoietic stem cell transplantation and solid-organ transplantation. The incidence of IFIs in transplant recipients has increased over the past 20 years, and these infections continue to be associated with high morbidity and mortality. This article reviews the important concepts guiding the management of IFIs in transplant recipients, including epidemiologic trends, new risk factors, and a timetable of infections, pathogens, therapy, and prevention of these infections. An emphasis is given to invasive aspergillosis.

This article focuses on the unique clinical features of prevalent fungal infections and their management implications in lung transplant recipients. Topics include epidemiology, risk factors, clinical syndromes, non invasive diagnostic methods and antifungal prophylaxis. The article not only highlights the current state of knowledge in these areas but also points towards future direction of research to conquer fungal infections in lung transplants.

Aspergillus can cause several forms of pulmonary disease ranging from colonization to invasive aspergillosis and largely depends on the underlying lung and immune function of the host. This article reviews the clinical presentation, diagnosis, pathogenesis, and treatment of noninvasive forms of *Aspergillus* infection, including allergic bronchopulmonary aspergillosis (ABPA), aspergilloma, and chronic pulmonary aspergillosis (CPA). ABPA is caused by a hypersensitivity reaction to *Aspergillus* species and is most commonly seen in patients who have asthma or cystic fibrosis. Aspergillomas, or fungus balls, can develop in previous areas of cavitary lung disease, most commonly from tuberculosis. CPA has also been termed *semi-invasive aspergillosis* and usually occurs in patients who have underlying lung disease or mild immunosuppression.

Emerging fungi previously thought to be nonpathogenic are now recognized as playing a significant role in the increased incidence of invasive fungal disease. This change in the epidemiology of invasive fungal infections (IFIs) has occurred in the era of aggressive new therapies for hematopoietic stem cell and solid organ transplantation and malignancy, which have lead to profound immunosuppression for longer durations and has extended the survival of these critically ill patients. The significant morbidity and mortality associated with these infections is not only related to the host populations but to delayed recognition and diagnosis and high rates of resistance in some of these emerging pathogens to standard antifungal therapies.

Although a biopsy may need to be performed in complicated patients, bronchoalveolar lavage (BAL) is an important adjunct to the diagnosis of pulmonary and disseminated fungal infections. Culture is the gold standard for diagnosis in many instances, but cytologic and morphologic analysis is often diagnostic. Although newer molecular and antigen techniques may be applied to BAL samples, the role of such tests is yet to be defined for many pathogens.

Detection of galactomannan antigen in serum or bronchoalveolar lavage fluid is useful for diagnosis of invasive aspergillosis, but the current serologic tests are not useful. $(1 \rightarrow 3)$-ß-D-glucan can be detected in the serum of patients who have aspergillosis, candidiasis, and a few other mold infections, but false-positive results limit its reliability for diagnosis. None of these methods is useful for diagnosis of zygomycosis and certain other less common mold infections. This article focuses on the detection of antigen and ß-D-glucan for diagnosis of invasive aspergillosis and candidiasis.

The endemic mycoses are often overlooked in the evaluation of community-acquired pneumonia, and appropriate testing is not performed until the patient has failed to improve on antibacterial therapy. Antigen detection and fungal serology may be helpful in diagnosis of endemic mycoses as causes for pneumonia. Guidelines for recognition and evaluation of endemic mycoses as causes for community-acquired pneumonia are proposed. Performance of antigen testing on bronchial washings or lavage fluid may improve the sensitivity for diagnosis over microscopic examination and the speed of diagnosis over culture. This article focuses on antigen detection and serology for diagnosis of endemic mycoses. Of note is that isolation of the fungus by culture remains the only method for definitive diagnosis, and the only method for diagnosis in some patients.

This article summarizes the current state of the art in molecular diagnostic methods for the detection and identification of fungi as performed in the mycology laboratory. The advantages and limitations of current molecular testing methods are evaluated, with examples provided from the recent literature. Finally, commentary is provided on the future of molecular fungal diagnostics, including the potential role of multiplex detection assays, microarrays, and the molecular determination of antifungal resistance directly from clinical specimens.

Clinics in Chest Medicine

RELATED INTEREST

Infectious Disease Clinics March 2009 (Vol. 23, No. 1)
Staphylococcal Infections
R.J. Gorwitz and J.A. Jernigan, *Guest Editors*

Medical Clinics of North America November 2008 (Vol. 92, No. 6)
New and Emerging Infectious Diseases
M.E. Wilson, *Guest Editor*

Clinics in Geriatric Medicine August 2007 (Vol. 23, No. 3)
Infectious Disease
K. High, *Guest Editor*

THE CLINICS ARE NOW AVAILABLE ONLINE!

Access your subscription at:
www.theclinics.com

Preface

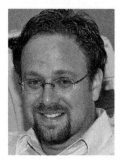 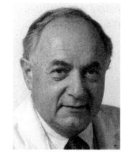

Kenneth S. Knox, MD   George A. Sarosi, MD, MACP

Guest Editors

Have you traveled anywhere recently? What medication did your rheumatologist start 3 months ago? What was your last CD4 count? When did you receive your last dose of chemotherapy? How old is that central line? The answers to these questions often point to a fungal pathogen as the cause of a new cough, unexplained fever, or persistent pulmonary infiltrates. A good history coupled with investigation into the immune status of the host is valuable to securing a diagnosis. Pathogens such as the endemic fungi and *Pneumocystis* often cause disease in patients with deficiencies in the T-cell–mediated arm of cellular immunity. In contrast, infections with *Aspergillus* spp and molds occur in individuals with quantitative or qualitative neutrophil defects. Because the diagnosis of fungal diseases can be elusive, study of these pathogens remains robust.

The study of fungal pathogenesis, diagnostics, and treatment has advanced rapidly over the past decade and is the topic of numerous studies and reviews. In this issue of *Clinics in Chest Medicine*, leading scientists and clinicians provide updates on individual pathogens as well as the field of fungal diagnostics and therapeutics.

Perhaps the most important advance in dealing with fungal diseases is the availability of new antifungal agents. Drs.Thompson, Cadena, and Patterson provide a comprehensive overview of currently available antifungal agents. In their review, important points regarding efficacy, adverse events, pharmacokinetics, and bioavailability are discussed.

The endemic fungi (*Histoplasma, Blastomyces,* and *Coccidioides*) and *Cryptococcus* can cause disease in immunocompetent individuals in whom uneventful recovery is the rule. However, in immunocompromised patients, particularly those with AIDS or those receiving anti-TNF agents, these infections are frequently severe and often have extrapulmonary dissemination requiring aggressive treatment.

Outside their usual endemic area, infections caused by these organisms may be difficult to diagnose and delays in therapy can be devastating. Dr. Kauffman reviews the classic presentation of histoplasmosis. Drs. McKinnell and Pappas provide new insight into the ecology and diagnosis of blastomycosis. Dr. Ampel provides a synopsis of the history and immunology of coccidioidomycosis and highlights the latest diagnostic and treatment strategies. Dr. Mody's group reviews the classification of cryptococcal disease and provides insight into the human immunological response. Drs. Krajicek, Thomas, and Limper discuss the genomics of *Pneumocystis* and recent advances in diagnostics.

The aforementioned pathogens often cause disease in patients with defects in T-cell–mediated immunity. A more recent clinical dilemma is the increased risk of fungal infections in patients receiving anticytokine therapy. Dr. Hage and colleagues provide new information regarding the impact of anti-TNF therapy and other "biologics" on fungal infection risk.

Candida blood stream invasion is common and Dr. Darouiche discusses the difficulties with diagnosis and treatment of *Candida* infections in the intensive care unit. Perhaps the most devastating fungal infections occur as a result of the high level

Clin Chest Med 30 (2009) xi–xii
doi:10.1016/j.ccm.2009.03.003

chestmed.theclinics.com

of immunosuppression needed posttransplantation. Drs. Nucci and Anaissie review the difficult problem of *Aspergillus* infection in the transplant recipient. Dr. Husain discusses the unique complications that often occur in lung transplant patients. Dr. Wood and colleagues provide an overview for management of allergic reactions, mycetomas, and other less invasive forms of fungal infections. Drs. Naggie and Perfect demystify mold infections.

A final area in which new information is available is the area of fungal diagnostics. Dr. Wheat discusses the utility of antigen and serologic testing for specific fungal diseases. However, not all pathogens are easily diagnosed by blood or serum testing. Dr. Meinke and I are interested in using bronchoalveolar lavage to improve the diagnosis of fungal infections. Perhaps newer antigen detection assays as described by Dr. Wheat, or advanced molecular techniques, as described by Drs. Binnicker and Wengenack, can be applied to blood, BAL, or even tissue biopsy to improve the future care of patients with fungal infections.

Kenneth S. Knox, MD
University of Arizona College of Medicine
Southern Arizona VA Health Care System
(SAVAHCS)
3601 S. 6th Avenue (1-11C)
Tucson, AZ 85723

George A. Sarosi, MD, MACP
University of Minnesota School of Medicine
Minneapolis VA Medical Center
Minneapolis, MN

E-mail addresses:
Kenneth.Knox2@va.gov (K.S. Knox)
georgesarosi@comcast.net (G.A. Sarosi)

Overview of Antifungal Agents

George R. Thompson III, MD, FACP[a,b,]*, Jose Cadena, MD[a,b],
Thomas F. Patterson, MD[a,b]

KEYWORDS

- Fungal infection • Invasive mycoses
- Triazoles • Echinocandins • Amphotericin • Flucytosine

The number of agents available to treat fungal infections has increased by 30% since the year 2000, yet still only 15 agents are currently approved for clinical use. The greater number of medications now available allows for therapeutic choices; however, differences in antifungal spectrum of activity, bioavailability, formulation, drug interactions, and side effects necessitates a detailed knowledge of each drug class.

POLYENES

Amphotericin B (AMB) and nystatin are the currently available polyenes, although differing safety profiles have limited nystatin to topical use.[1] The polyenes bind to ergosterol present within the fungal cell wall membrane. This process disrupts cell wall permeability by forming oligodendromes functioning as pores with the subsequent efflux of potassium and intracellular molecules causing fungal death.[2] There is also evidence that AMB acts as a proinflammatory agent and further serves to stimulate innate host immunity. This process involves the interaction of AMB with toll-like receptor 2 (TLR-2), the CD14 receptor, and by stimulating the release of cytokines, chemokines, and other immunologic mediators. It has been suggested that AMB may interact with host humoral immunity after the observation of synergistic activity of AMB and antibodies directed at heat shock protein 90 (hsp90), although further confirmatory data are needed.[2]

When AMB resistance occurs, it is generally attributed to reductions in ergosterol biosynthesis or the synthesis of alternative sterols with a reduced affinity for AMB. Resistance to AMB is common in *Aspergillus terreus*, *Scedosporium apiospermum*, *Scedosporium prolificans*, *Trichosporon* spp, and *Candida lusitaniae* (**Table 1**). Resistance has been reported with several other species, however.[3]

The peak serum level to mean inhibitory concentration (MIC) ratio is the best pharmacologic predictor of outcomes with polyene therapy. Drug levels are infrequently measured, nor are they necessary, and they are typically available only in the research setting.[4]

AMB is primarily used intravenously (IV) or through the inhalational route. In attempts to avoid the nephrotoxicity seen with amphotericin B deoxycholate (AmBd; Fungizone) several other formulations have been developed. The lipid preparations include: liposomal amphotericin B (L-AMB; Ambisome), amphotericin B lipid complex, (ABLC; Abelcet), and amphotericin B colloidal dispersion (ABCD; Amphotec, Amphocil). All currently available formulations are highly protein bound (>95%, primarily to albumin) and have long half-lives.

AMB exhibits poor cerebrospinal fluid levels (<5% of concurrent serum concentration); however, this agent remains the treatment of choice for cryptococcal meningitis.[5] Previous reports have described the use of intrathecal

[a] Department of Internal Medicine, Division of Infectious Diseases, University of Texas Health Science Center at San Antonio, 7703 Floyd Curl Drive, San Antonio, TX 78229, USA
[b] Department of Internal Medicine, Division of Infectious Diseases, South Texas Veterans Health Care System, 7400 Merton Minter Drive, San Antonio, TX 78229, USA
* Corresponding author. Department of Internal Medicine, Division of Infectious Diseases, University of Texas Health Science Center at San Antonio, 7703 Floyd Curl Drive, San Antonio, TX 78229.
E-mail address: thompsong2@uthscsa.edu (G.R. Thompson).

Clin Chest Med 30 (2009) 203–215
doi:10.1016/j.ccm.2009.02.001
0272-5231/09/$ – see front matter. Published by Elsevier Inc.

Table 1
Antifungal spectrum of activity against common molds and yeast

Organism	AMB	FLU	ITR	POS	VOR	ANI	MFG	CAS	5FC
Aspergillus fumigatus	+	−	+	+	+	+	+	+	−
A flavus	+/−	−	+	+	+	+	+	+	−
A terreus	−	−	+	+	+	+	+	+	−
A niger	+	−	+/−	+	+	+	+	+	−
A nidulans	+	−	+/−	+	+	+	+	+	−
Candida albicans	+	+	+	+	+	+	+	+	+
C glabrata	+	+/−	+/−	+	+	+	+	+	+
C krusei	+	−	+/−	+	+	+	+	+	+/−
C tropicalis	+	+	+	+	+	+	+	+	+
C parapsilosis	+	+	+	+	+/−	+/−	+/−	+	+
C guilliermondii	+	+	+	+	−	−	−	+	+
C lusitaniae	−	+	+	+	+	+	+	+	+
Cryptococcus spp	+	+	+	+	−	−	−	+	+
Blastomycoses	+	+	+	+	+	+/−	+/−	+/−	−
Histoplasmosis	+/−	+	+	+	+/−	+/−	+/−	−	−
Coccidioidomycosis	+	+	+	+	−	−	−	−	−
Fusarium spp	+/−	−	−	+	+	−	−	−	−
Phaeohyphomycoses[a]	−	+	+	+	+	+	+	−	−
Pichia spp	+	+	+/−	+	+	+	+	+	+
Saccharomyces spp	+	+	+	+	+	+	+	+	+
Scedosporium apiospermum	+/−	+	+	−	−	−	−	−	−
Scedosporium prolificans	−	+/−	+/−	−	−	−	−	−	−
Trichosporon spp	+/−	+	+	+	−	−	−	+	+
Zygomycetes	+/−	−	−	+	−	−	−	−	−

(+) implies antifungal activity against isolates, (−) implies no or limited activity against isolate, (+/−) implies variable activity against isolates.
  Abbreviations: AMB, amphotericin; ANI, anidulafungin; CAS, caspofungin; FLU, fluconazole; ITR, itraconazole; MFG, micafungin; POS, posaconazole; VOR, voriconazole; 5FC, flucytosine.
  [a] Infection requires debridement in almost all circumstances.
  Data from Refs.[6] and [95–97].

AMB in an attempt to circumvent the poor cerebrospinal fluid (CSF) penetration; however, this practice is seldom used because of the difficulty of administration, poor patient tolerability, and availability of alternative agents for use in the salvage setting of invasive mycoses. AMB also has low vitreous penetration (0%–38%) and intraocular injections may be required to achieve appropriate levels during therapy of deep ophthalmologic fungal infections, including candidal endopthalmitis.[6,7] The exact route of elimination of AMB is not known and despite the well-known nephrotoxicity, dosing need not be adjusted in patients who have a decreased glomerular filtration rate.

The broad antifungal spectrum and experience with the use of amphotericin B accounts for its continued use despite toxicity concerns. Liposomal amphotericin B remains the recommended antifungal during the treatment of neutropenic fever after an open-label, randomized international trial comparing L-AMB to voriconazole. Although fewer breakthrough infections (including those caused by *Aspergillus* spp) occurred in patients receiving voriconazole, predetermined noninferiority criteria were not reached.[8] Additionally, a recent meta-analysis suggested L-AMB may be associated with lower morality than AmBd during the empiric treatment of neutropenic fever.[9]

AMB was previously the preferred first-line agent during the treatment of invasive aspergillosis; however, a greater therapeutic response and survival have been demonstrated when voriconazole is administered in this setting—relegating AMB to second-line or salvage therapy during the treatment of invasive aspergillosis.[10] AMB does remain the agent of choice when the

Zygomycetes are encountered. In fact, a delay in the prescribing of an AMB formulation in patients infected with one of the Zygomycetes resulted in a twofold greater risk for death.[11] Discriminating between invasive zygomycoses and aspergillosis is difficult, but the differences in the choice of antifungal agents and outcomes mandate an aggressive diagnostic strategy and prompt initiation of antifungal agents.

Before the development of alternative agents, AMB was the recommended first-line agent for invasive candidal infections.[12] AMB in combination with flucytosine remains the drug of choice in the treatment of cryptococcal meningitis and in most cases a lipid formulation is preferred because of the decreased incidence of nephrotoxicity.[5] Severe infection caused by the endemic mycoses (ie, histoplasmosis, coccidioidomycosis, blastomycosis, and sporotrichosis) should be treated with an AMB formulation. Histoplasmosis remains the only infection for which a lipid formulation of AMB (L-AMB) has demonstrated greater efficacy than the conventional form.[13]

In attempts to avoid the potential nephrotoxicity of systemic administration and to deliver higher local concentrations, different formulations of AMB have been given by way of the inhalational route. The deoxycholate used to solubilize AMB acts as a detergent and may affect alveolar surfactant. Lipid preparations are thus preferred for inhalation delivery, although no decline in pulmonary lung function from AmBd has been documented. AmBd is often difficult to effectively administer in an aerosol form because of foaming caused by the solubilizing agent.[11,14–16] Aerosol delivery has been found effective in the prevention of pulmonary fungal infections in lung transplantation and in bone marrow transplant recipients, although data supporting its efficacy in other settings are limited.

Inhaled L-AMB has been found protective against development of invasive aspergillosis when given twice weekly to neutropenic patients who have cancer.[16] Inhalation delivery is also an attractive option in the treatment of lung transplant patients and a recent retrospective series reported nebulized ABLC provided effective prophylaxis against invasive aspergillosis in 98.3% of all patients.[14]

The recommended dose of IV AmBd is between 0.7 and 1 mg/kg and only recently have clinical data emerged evaluating higher doses of lipid formulations of AMB to potentially improve efficacy. The AmBiLoad trial evaluated the efficacy of higher initial doses of L-AMB (3 mg/kg versus 10 mg/kg) in the treatment of invasive aspergillosis. Treatment success rates were similar in both treatment arms although there was a greater incidence of nephrotoxicity in those receiving the higher dose of L-AmB.[17] In severe and life-threatening disease it is the authors' experience that escalating doses of lipid formulations of AMB may be indicated when alternative agents are not available or have been found ineffective.

AmBd infusion is associated with infusion-related reactions, such as fever, chills, rigors, myalgias, bronchospasm, nausea and vomiting, tachycardia, tachypnea, and hypertension.[12] These events are less likely to occur when one of the lipid formulations is used; however, ABCD has been associated with the development of dyspnea and hypoxia and L-AMB has been associated with back pain during infusion.[6] Amphotericin B has been associated with acute kidney injury and nephrotoxicity in many studies and is a well-known potential complication of therapy occurring in up to 30% of patients. This toxicity is believed secondary to vascular smooth muscle dysfunction with resultant vasoconstriction and ischemia.[18] For this reason most advocate ensuring adequate volume status before administration. Lipid preparations of AMB have a lower incidence of renal toxicity, and studies have shown that when AmBd is replaced by a lipid formulation after the development of creatinine elevation, renal function stabilizes or improves in a significant proportion of patients.[19]

The avoidance of AmBd and use of a lipid formulation has been met with skepticism by some because of the vast price difference in compounds. The reduction in hospital days when toxicity is avoided, however, has proven the lipid formulations more cost effective than AmBd.[19]

TRIAZOLES

The triazoles also exert their effects within the fungal cell membrane. The inhibition of cytochrome P450 (CYP)-dependent 14-α-demethylase prevents the conversion of lanosterol to ergosterol. This mechanism results in the accumulation of toxic methylsterols and resultant inhibition of fungal cell growth and replication (**Fig. 1**). This class of agents has demonstrated species- and strain-dependent fungistatic or fungicidal activity in vitro and the area under the curve (AUC) to MIC ratio is the primary predictor of drug efficacy.

The indirect immunomodulatory effects are poorly understood because of the complex interaction of triazoles and phagocytic cells. Evidence suggests that ergosterol depletion increases fungal cell vulnerability to phagocytic oxidative damage[20] and voriconazole has been shown to

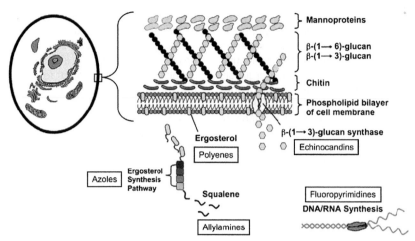

Fig. 1. Targets of systemic antifungal agents.

induce the expression of TLR2, nuclear factor-κB, and tumor necrosis factor-α.[2]

Azoles differ in their affinity for the 14-α-demethylase enzyme and this difference is largely responsible for their varying antifungal potency and spectrum of activity. Cross-inhibition of several human CYP-dependent enzymes (3A4, 2C9, and 2C19) is responsible for most of the clinical side effects and drug interaction profiles that have been described with this class. Itraconazole and posaconazole act primarily as inhibitors of 3A4 and 2C9 with little effect on 2C19. Voriconazole acts as both an inhibitor and a substrate on all three isoenzymes providing ample opportunity for drug–drug interactions because of this frequently shared metabolic pathway.

Comprehensive lists of triazole drug interactions can be found elsewhere. Briefly, caution should be used when these agents are concurrently administered with: most HMG-CoA reductase inhibitors, benzodiazepines, phenytoin, carbamazepine, cyclosporine, tacrolimus, sirolimus, methylprednisolone, buspirone, alfentanil, the dihydropyridine calcium channel blockers verapamil and diltiazem, the sulfonylureas, rifampin, rifabutin, vincristine, busulphan, docetaxel, trimetrexate, and the protease inhibitors ritonavir, indinavir, and saquinavir.[21–27]

The triazoles have also been associated with QTc prolongation[28] and coadministration with other agents known to have similar effects (cisapride, terfenadine, astemizole, mizolastine, dofetilide, quinidine, and pimozide, amongst others) should be avoided.[29–31] The triazoles are additionally embryotoxic and teratogenic and are secreted into breast milk, and thus administration should be avoided during pregnancy or while lactating.[28,32,33]

Fluconazole

Fluconazole (Diflucan) remains one of the most frequently prescribed triazoles because of its excellent bioavailability, tolerability, and side-effect profile. More than 80% of ingested drug is found in the circulation, and 60% to 70% is excreted unchanged in the urine. Oral absorption remains unchanged in patients receiving acid-suppressive therapy (proton pump inhibitors, H2-blockers). Only 10% of fluconazole is protein bound.[34]

Fluconazole also exhibits excellent tissue penetration. CSF levels are 70% of matched serum levels, and levels reported in saliva, sputum, and other sites are well within therapeutic ranges. The half-life is 27 to 34 hours in the presence of normal renal function allowing once-daily dosing. In patients who have a reduced creatinine clearance the normal dose should be reduced by 50%. Fluconazole serum levels are rarely necessary. Currently 50-, 100-, 150-, and 200-mg tablets are available and IV formulations exist in 200- or 400-mg doses.

Fluconazole is active against most *Candida* spp with the exception of *C krusei* and *C glabrata* isolates. If a *C glabrata* isolate is found susceptible to fluconazole higher doses (12 mg/kg/d) should be used.[7,35] There is no appreciable activity against *Aspergillus*, *Fusarium*, *Pseudoallescheria*, or the Zygomycetes.

Although fluconazole has substantially fewer drug–drug interactions than other triazole compounds, caution remains necessary because of increases in the serum levels of phenytoin, glipizide, glyburide, warfarin, rifabutin, and cyclosporine. Fluconazole levels are reduced in the presence of rifampin.

Fluconazole is well tolerated by most patients, even if chronic therapy is necessary.[36] Headache, alopecia, and anorexia are the side effects most common (10%) with transaminase elevation in less than 10%.

Fluconazole remains the drug of choice in the treatment of oropharyngeal candidiasis (OPC) (100 mg/d for 7–14 days).[7] Newer data suggest a one-time dose of 750 mg for the treatment of OPC with equivalent relapse rates to standard therapy.[37] Patients who have frequent relapse should remain on chronic suppressive fluconazole until immune reconstitution has been documented.

Fluconazole has also been used for prophylaxis in those at high risk for invasive fungal infections. Initiation of 400 mg/d of fluconazole for the first 75 days after bone marrow transplantation has been found effective in reducing cases of candidemia.[38] Preemptive therapy within ICUs remains controversial. The high incidence of invasive candidiasis within this setting (1%–2% of all patients) makes prophylaxis an attractive option; however, the largest randomized, multicenter, blinded clinical trial comparing empiric fluconazole therapy in ICU patients with several risk factors for invasive candidiasis to placebo showed no clear benefit to fluconazole therapy.[39]

After induction therapy with AMB and flucytosine, fluconazole is used for suppression of cryptococcosis. An initial dose of 400 mg for 10 weeks followed by 200 mg weekly pending immune reconstitution has been recommended.[5] Although recent data has accrued regarding the use of high-dose fluconazole monotherapy during the induction course of cryptococcal meningitis, this practice should be used only in resource-limited settings and not when AMB is available.[40]

Fluconazole is also useful for infections caused by *Coccidioides immitis*. In cases of meningitis or disseminated infection high-dose fluconazole (up to 2 g daily) is often necessary.[41]

Itraconazole

Itraconazole is currently available as capsules and as an oral solution suspended in hydroxypropyl-β-cyclodextrin (HPCD). Unfortunately, the IV preparation of itraconazole is no longer commercially available. Itraconazole capsules depend on an acidic environment for maximal absorption, and the concomitant administration of H_2-receptor antagonists, proton pump inhibitors, or antacids causes erratic and unpredictable drug absorption; it is thus recommended that itraconazole capsules be taken with food or a cola beverage.[42,43]

Itraconazole solution allows for greater oral bioavailability and the AUC and peak

concentrations are both increased by 30% when itraconazole solution is taken in the fasting state.[44,45] The cyclodextrin carrier has minimal absorption and no systemic side effects have been attributed to its use in the oral formulation.[46] With once-daily dosing, steady state is reached in 7 to 14 days, although oral loading (200 mg three times daily for 3 days) allows for more rapid attainment of therapeutic serum levels.[47] Itraconazole is also highly protein bound with less than 1% available as free drug and has a relatively high volume of distribution.

Itraconazole is extensively metabolized by the liver and its major metabolite, hydroxy-itraconazole, does possess antifungal activity similar to that of the parent drug. Despite similar antifungal efficacy, hydroxyl-itraconazole is not measured during serum drug level determination by high performance liquid chromatography, although the active metabolite is detected by bioassay.[48]

The development of newer and more effective antifungal agents (ie, voriconazole) has relegated itraconazole to second-line therapy during the treatment of invasive aspergillosis. Itraconazole is thus licensed in the United States only for salvage therapy of invasive aspergillosis (IA).[10] Itraconazole does, however, remain the drug of choice for those who have mild to moderate infection caused by histoplasmosis and is the mainstay of secondary prophylaxis in patients who have HIV with a history of histoplasmosis before immune reconstitution with antiretrovirals.[49] Itraconazole is also approved for allergic bronchopulmonary aspergillosis.[10]

The recommended dosage of oral itraconazole in adults is 400 mg/d (capsules) and 2.5 mg/kg twice daily (HPCD solution).[10] Steady-state levels can be more rapidly attained, however, when administered as 200 mg three times daily for 3 days and then 200 mg twice daily for the duration of therapy. Considerable concern remains regarding adequate oral absorption and oral itraconazole is not recommended in seriously ill patients or patients who have life-threatening disease. Dose adjustment is not indicated when the oral formulation of itraconazole is used in patients who have renal insufficiency or those receiving hemodialysis/continuous ambulatory peritoneal dialysis. The half-life of itraconazole is prolonged in patients who have hepatic dysfunction and drug dose adjustment, liver function testing, and drug interactions need to be carefully assessed.[50]

Itraconazole is usually well tolerated and although adverse reactions have been observed in up to 39% of patients no fatalities and only rare toxicity requiring discontinuation of therapy were reported. The most frequent side effects include: nausea and vomiting (<10%), hypertriglyceridemia (9%), hypokalemia (6%), liver enzyme elevations (5%), skin rashes/pruritus (2%), headache and dizziness (<2%), and pedal edema (1%).[51] Gastrointestinal intolerance (46%) is exceedingly common with the oral HPCD solution at doses greater than 400 mg/d with vomiting the most frequent complaint.[52] The myocardial depressant effects of itraconazole are also well known and cases of congestive heart failure have been reported.[53]

Posaconazole

Posaconazole is a lipophilic second-generation antifungal triazole with a similar molecular structure to that of itraconazole. The spectrum of activity of posaconazole includes agents of the Zygomycetes, and it has improved activity against *Aspergillus* spp compared with itraconazole.[54]

Posaconazole is insoluble in water and no IV formulation has yet been developed. It is thus administered as a cherry-flavored suspension using polysorbate 80 as the emulsifying agent.[55] Optimal dosing of posaconazole is obtained when given as two to four divided doses administered with food or a liquid nutritional supplement.[56,57] Although initial studies suggested that changes in gastric acidity do not affect posaconazole absorption subsequent work has shown H_2-receptor antagonists and proton pump inhibitors may decrease posaconazole serum levels and if possible coadministration should be avoided.[32,55,58,59]

Posaconazole has demonstrated dose-dependent pharmacokinetics with saturable absorption greater than 800 mg/d; thus oral loading is not possible and steady state is typically achieved after 7 to 10 days of therapy.[60] This prolonged time required to reach steady-state levels may affect the use of posaconazole as primary therapy for invasive fungal infections. This agent also has a large volume of distribution despite its high protein binding and a half-life of approximately 24 hours.

Peak serum concentrations have shown considerable interpatient variability for reasons that remain unclear. Some have proposed genetic polymorphisms within P-glycoprotein to play a role because posaconazole is both a substrate and inhibitor, but this remains unproven.[61] Glucuronidation plays a minor role in posaconazole metabolism and single nucleotide polymorphisms within UGT (uridine diphosphate-glucuronyl transferase) have also been proposed to account for these differences but confirmatory studies are lacking.[62] This unpredictable variation in serum posaconazole levels has heightened interest and the necessity of therapeutic drug monitoring (TDM).

Posaconazole is hepatically metabolized and undergoes minimal glucuronidation. Renal clearance plays a minor role in the clearance of posaconazole, which is predominantly eliminated fecally.

Oral posaconazole has proved effective in the prevention of proven or probable invasive aspergillosis in neutropenic patients who have acute myelogenous leukemia and in hematopoietic stem cell transplant recipients who have graft versus host disease.[63,64] The efficacy and safety of posaconazole in the treatment of invasive fungal infections has also been assessed, and although this study predates the development of echinocandins and voriconazole the statistically significant success rate of posaconazole compared with other agents allows for its use during salvage therapy.[65]

Currently, 200 mg three times daily is recommended for prophylaxis, and 800 mg divided in two or four doses is recommended in the salvage setting. For patients not tolerating food, a liquid nutritional supplement has been recommended to increase absorption.[61] Pediatric dosing schedules have yet to be established.[10] Dose adjustment by age, sex, race, and hepatic or renal insufficiency is not necessary given the minimal glucuronidation and renal clearance of posaconazole.[66]

Posaconazole is usually well tolerated and infrequently requires discontinuation because of adverse events. The most frequent side effects of posaconazole therapy are gastrointestinal (14%), with transaminase elevation and hyperbilirubinemia occurring in 3%.[64] In one trial, however, more serious adverse events were reported in patients treated with posaconazole than with fluconazole. Three cardiac events were reported among those possibly related to posaconazole treatment, including decreased ejection fraction, QTc prolongation, and torsades de pointes.[63] For most patients posaconazole is well tolerated and even long-term therapy (>6 months) is frequently without toxicity.[67]

Posaconazole is not significantly metabolized through the cytochrome P450 system and serum levels are unlikely to be increased by concomitant administration of P450 inhibitors.

Voriconazole

Voriconazole is a low molecular weight water-soluble second-generation triazole with a chemical structure similar to fluconazole. Voriconazole exhibits a broad spectrum of activity against molds with the exception of the Zygomycetes.[68]

Voriconazole is available in oral and IV formulations. Similar to itraconazole, the IV form depends on sulfobutyl ether β–cyclodextrin for solubility.[68] When 3 to 6 mg/kg of daily voriconazole is administered, steady-state levels are reached in 5 to 6 days. If IV loading is given, however, steady state can be reached within 1 day.[69] The oral formulation obtains steady-state levels within 24 hours if appropriate loading is administered; however, fatty foods have been found to reduce bioavailability by 80%.[70]

Although voriconazole in children has demonstrated linear pharmacokinetics, in adults nonlinear metabolism is observed, likely secondary to saturable metabolic enzymes required for drug clearance.[69] Interpatient serum concentration differences have been attributed to polymorphisms within CYP2C19, the major metabolic pathway for voriconazole.[68] Up to 20% of non-Indian Asians have low CYP2C19 activity and voriconazole serum levels are thus up to four times higher than those found in white or black populations in which the "poor metabolizer" status is uncommon.[71] The unpredictability of patient enzymatic activity has generated an increased interest in the routine use of voriconazole serum level determination.

For IV administration 6 mg/kg twice daily on day one, followed by 4 mg/kg IV twice daily for the duration of therapy is recommended. The oral dosages in adults are also weight based. For those weighing greater than 40 kg, 400 mg twice daily on day one, followed by 200 mg twice daily until completion of therapy is suggested, whereas those weighing less than 40 kg should receive 200 mg twice daily for one day followed by 100 mg twice daily.[68] Pediatric patients are known to hypermetabolize voriconazole and for this reason an IV dose of 7 mg/kg twice daily and oral dosing of 200 mg twice daily without loading is recommended.[33] In patients who have liver dysfunction standard loading doses should be given, but the maintenance dose reduced by 50%. The safety of voriconazole use in severe liver disease remains uncertain. No dosage adjustment is required if oral drug is given to patients who have renal insufficiency. The presence of a cyclodextrin vehicle within the IV formulation has caused concerns about vehicle accumulation in renal insufficiency or dialysis dependence and IV administration is best avoided in patients who have a creatinine clearance less than 50 mL.[68]

Voriconazole is typically well tolerated, and the side-effect profile is similar to other triazoles with few exceptions. Most of those experiencing a reported adverse reaction to voriconazole describe abnormal vision (up to 23%) that is transient, infusion related, and without sequelae. This unique effect typically occurs 30 minutes after infusion and abates 30 minutes after onset.

Other well-known effects of voriconazole therapy include skin rash and transaminase elevation.[72] Baseline evaluation of hepatic function has been recommended before and during treatment, and rare cases of hepatic failure during voriconazole use have been reported.[73] Elevated voriconazole serum levels have been attributed to most side effects encountered in clinical practice, and higher levels (>5.5 mg/L), although associated with favorable outcomes, have also been suggested to be responsible for the uncommon potential side effects of encephalopathy or hallucinations.[74–76]

Voriconazole has become the drug of choice for most cases of invasive aspergillosis based on recent data comparing voriconazole to conventional amphotericin B, followed by other antifungal therapy in patients who have invasive aspergillosis.[77] Voriconazole has also been evaluated in the treatment of neutropenic fever. Although voriconazole did not meet predetermined noninferiority criteria, there were significantly fewer breakthrough infections (including those caused by *Aspergillus* spp) in patients receiving voriconazole.[8]

Voriconazole has also been evaluated for use during infection caused by *Fusarium* and *Scedosporium* spp. A retrospective series evaluated its use in these infections and reported a favorable response in 63% of patients treated with voriconazole.[33]

Therapeutic Drug Monitoring

Commercial assays are available for monitoring the serum concentrations of all currently available triazoles; however, at this time existing guidelines recommend only itraconazole TDM.[49,78,79] Itraconazole levels are typically drawn after steady state is reached to ensure therapeutic levels (>1 μg/mL) have been obtained. Fluconazole levels are infrequently monitored because of the excellent bioavailability of this agent. Clinical circumstances may dictate drug monitoring when therapeutic levels are uncertain (ie, concurrent use of rifampin, rifampicin, and so forth).

The newer triazoles, posaconazole and voriconazole, have received increased attention because of their erratic absorption (posaconazole) or concerns for toxicity and the interpatient variability of serum levels (voriconazole). No guidelines exist for posaconazole TDM; however, past evidence supports a relationship between posaconazole serum drug level and efficacy.[80] TDM should also be considered when drug interactions are of concern, such as the aforementioned potential for acid-suppressive agents to reduce absorption. Although goal levels remain to be determined, most advocate trough concentrations 0.5 μg/mL or greater when given for antifungal prophylaxis. The interpatient variability of voriconazole also warrants consideration of TDM during use. Low concentrations (<1 mg/L) are more common in those receiving oral therapy and failure rates have been associated with low serum drug levels.[72] Conversely, levels greater than 5.5 mg/L have been associated with encephalopathy without an improvement in efficacy.[74] The frequency with which to monitor these newer triazoles remains to be determined.

ECHINOCANDINS

Echinocandins (caspofungin, micafungin, anidulafungin) are synthetic compounds that inhibit the synthesis of β-1,3 glucan, by inhibiting the activity of glucan synthase. This mechanism impairs cell wall integrity and leads to osmotic lysis.[81] Their clinical use is primarily limited to *Candida* spp and *Aspergillus* spp and they lack activity against the Zygomycetes, *Cryptococcus* spp, and other clinically important molds (see **Table 1**). Although activity is observed against all *Candida* spp, the MICs are elevated (>1 μg/mL) when *Candida parapsilosis* and *Candida guilliermondii* are encountered and susceptibility differences between the different agents in this class are minimal.[82] Echinocandins also have immunomodulatory effects. By exposing β-glucan by the disruption of fungal cell wall mannoproteins, additional antigens are exposed for antibody deposition and fungal recognition by the host immune system.[83]

Echinocandin efficacy is predicted by peak to MIC ratios, and optimal fungicidal activity is obtained when peak concentrations exceed MICs by 5- to 10-fold.[6] TDM of echinocandins is seldom required, however, and not routinely recommended. Echinocandin resistance is uncommon but may develop during therapy.[84]

Multiple in vitro studies have confirmed a paradoxical effect of the echinocandins. In this circumstance, above a certain concentration of drug decreased antifungal activity is observed. The exact mechanism responsible for this phenomenon has not been fully elucidated and the clinical significance remains uncertain.[85]

Echinocandins have poor oral absorption and current agents are available only in the IV formulation. Echinocandins are highly protein bound

(anidulafungin 84%, caspofungin 97%, and micafungin 99%) and have a half-life of 26, 30, and 15 hours, respectively. Their vitreal and CSF penetration is negligible and this point is of clinical significance during the treatment of candidemia if endophthalmitis is also observed.

Caspofungin was the first available agent of this class, and is metabolized by both hepatic hydrolysis and N-acetylation. Inactive metabolites are subsequently eliminated in the urine. Severe hepatic dysfunction thus mandates caspofungin dose reduction.[6] Caspofungin has several drug interactions with agents metabolized through the cytochrome P450 system and serum levels are reduced in the presence of rifampin and may increase levels of sirolimus, nifedipine, and cyclosporine.[6] Micafungin is metabolized by nonoxidative metabolism within the liver and anidulafungin undergoes nonenzymatic degradation within the kidney. Both agents are eliminated in stool. These agents therefore do not require dosage adjustment with hepatic impairment.[6]

The side-effect profile of the echinocandins is minimal and these agents are typically well tolerated. An infusion-related reaction has been described if rapid administration is given, with tachycardia, hypotension, or thrombophlebitis.

Clinical Use

The increased incidence of triazole-resistant *Candida* spp and the fungicidal activity of the echinocandins (caspofungin, micafungin, anidulafungin) has prompted some authorities to recommend these agents as first-line therapy for invasive candidiasis. Additionally, their proven efficacy, infrequency of side effects, and favorable drug interaction profiles make them attractive options over other available antifungals.[12,86–88]

Comparative trials have found the echinocandins equally efficacious and better tolerated than AMB in the treatment of candidemia.[12] In one such trial, caspofungin (70 mg loading dose followed by 50 mg daily) was compared to amphotericin B deoxycholate (0.6–1 mg/kg) in the treatment of invasive candidiasis. Although *C albicans* was more common in the AMB arm, modified intention to treat revealed similar survival in each group, with a trend toward increased survival and a statistically significant decrease in drug side effects in those receiving caspofungin.[12]

Similarly, micafungin (100 mg IV daily) has been compared to L-AMB 3 mg/kg IV daily in an international, double-blind trial. In this study assigning patients to 14 days of IV treatment, successful treatment was equivalent in each group. There were fewer treatment-related adverse events, including those that were serious or led to treatment discontinuation, with micafungin than there were with liposomal amphotericin.[86]

Only one comparative trial of different echinocandins has been performed in invasive candidiasis. In this trial patients were enrolled to one of three treatment groups: micafungin 100 mg IV daily, micafungin 150 mg IV daily, or caspofungin 70 mg IV loading dose followed by 50 mg IV daily. Intention to treat analysis found no differences in response to therapy, treatment or microbiologic failure, or all-cause mortality.[88] Although this trial found that higher doses of an echinocandin may not equate to a greater therapeutic response, no increase in toxicity was seen with higher doses, and dose escalation can thus be safely used in unusual circumstances or in obesity.

Anidulafungin has been compared with fluconazole for the treatment of invasive candidiasis. At the end of IV therapy, treatment was successful in 75.6% of patients treated with anidulafungin, as compared with 60.2% of those treated with fluconazole. Despite a greater response rate and a lower rate of death from all causes in the anidulafungin group, however, predetermined criteria for statistical superiority were not reached and only noninferior status granted.[87]

It is common practice from the results of these trials for local resistance patterns and the severity of infection to be taken into account and echinocandins are frequently used as first-line therapy. After clinical improvement is obtained or the absence of fluconazole resistance documented, therapy is often changed to a triazole, such as fluconazole. As noted previously, CNS and intraocular infections should not be treated with echinocandin monotherapy because of their poor penetration into these sites.

Although clinical trials have been primarily limited to patients who have candidemia, observational data have shown efficacy in candidal osteomyelitis, peritoneal infections, and abdominal abscesses.[89] Additional retrospective data have also shown a potential role for the echinocandins in infective endocarditis caused by Candida spp.[90]

The echinocandins have also been found efficacious in the treatment of invasive aspergillosis, although they are fungistatic against this agent. The growing number of patients who are at risk for this infection has prompted a greater interest in the use of other agents that may be of clinical use against this devastating infection. The known toxicity of AMB and its different formulations and the potential for voriconazole-induced drug–drug interactions or toxicity has also increased interest in the echinocandins for use during treatment of IA.[91]

Caspofungin as a potential first-line agent has been evaluated only in limited settings and although acceptable responses have been observed, data are not sufficient to recommend caspofungin for first-line use during the treatment of IA.[10] Patients who are unresponsive or intolerant to voriconazole may benefit from a change to caspofungin.[91] In vitro studies and limited clinical data have also shown the potential role for combination therapy (an echinocandin plus AMB or an azole) and prospective studies are ongoing.

ANTIMETABOLITES
Flucytosine

Flucytosine (5FC; Ancobon) is deaminated to 5-fluorouracil by fungal cytosine deaminase. 5-fluorouracil is further converted to 5-fluorodeoxyuridylic acid, which interferes with DNA synthesis. Mammalian cells lack cytosine deaminase allowing for a selective inhibition of fungal organisms (see **Fig. 1**).[92] This agent may be either fungistatic or fungicidal depending on fungal species and strain.

Activity has been observed against most fungal pathogens, including Candida, Cryptococcus, Cladosporium, Phialophora, and Saccharomyces spp. Aspergillus spp, the Zygomycetes, dermatophytes, and the endemic mycoses are all resistant to 5FC (see **Table 1**). Additionally, resistance commonly develops when 5FC is used as monotherapy even in susceptible organisms and it should not be used as such except during the treatment of chromoblastomycoses or during the treatment of localized candidal infections when alternative agents are unavailable or contraindicated.

5FC has excellent oral bioavailability with greater than 80% to 90% absorption. Peak serum levels occur 1 to 2 hours after ingestion (30–45 μg/mL) of a single dose. The volume of distribution of 5FC is 0.6 to 0.9, yet bone, peritoneal, and synovial fluid 5FC levels have been demonstrated and urinary levels are several-fold higher than concurrent serum levels. Greater than 95% of 5FC is eliminated unchanged in the urine. 5FC is typically administered by mouth at 100 or 150 mg/kg/d divided in four doses.

Side effects of therapy include rash, diarrhea, hepatic transaminase elevation, and bone marrow suppression. The marrow suppressive effects are more common if blood levels exceed 100 to 125 μg/mL.[93] In the presence of prolonged therapy (>7 days) or with alterations in renal function serum drug monitoring is recommended. Other less common side effects, such as abdominal pain or diarrhea, are frequently indirect markers of elevated flucytosine levels and therapy is typically stopped in these circumstances. 5FC is terato-genic and should not be administered during pregnancy.

5FC is primarily used only in the treatment of cryptococcus (combined with AMB) and chromo-blastomycosis. Despite concerns for additive toxicity the synergistic effects of dual therapy in cryptococcus allow for more rapid CSF clearance.[94]

SUMMARY

The incidence of infection with invasive mycoses continues to increase with the increasing immuno-suppressed patient population. The recently expanded antifungal armamentarium offers the potential for more effective and less toxic therapy and these agents offer distinct pharmacologic profiles and indications for use.

REFERENCES

1. Ellis D. Amphotericin B: spectrum and resistance. J Antimicrob Chemother 2002;49(Suppl 1):7–10.
2. Ben-Ami R, Lewis RE, Kontoyiannis DP. Immuno-compromised hosts: immunopharmacology of modern antifungals. Clin Infect Dis 2008;47(2): 226–35.
3. Rex JH, Pfaller MA. Has antifungal susceptibility testing come of age? Clin Infect Dis 2002;35(8): 982–9.
4. Andes D. In vivo pharmacodynamics of antifungal drugs in treatment of candidiasis. Antimicrob Agents Chemother 2003;47(4):1179–86.
5. Saag MS, Graybill RJ, Larsen RA, et al. Practice guidelines for the management of cryptococcal disease. Infectious Diseases Society of America. Clin Infect Dis 2000;30(4):710–8.
6. Dodds Ashley Es LR, Lewis JS, Martin C, Andes D. Pharmacology of systemic antifungal agents. Clin Infect Dis 2006;43(s1):S28–39.
7. Pappas PG, Rex JH, Sobel JD, et al. Guidelines for treatment of candidiasis. Clin Infect Dis 2004;38(2): 161–89.
8. Walsh TJ, Pappas P, Winston DJ, et al. Voriconazole compared with liposomal amphotericin B for empir-ical antifungal therapy in patients with neutropenia and persistent fever. N Engl J Med 2002;346(4): 225–34.
9. Goldberg E, Gafter-Gvili A, Robenshtok E, et al. Empirical antifungal therapy for patients with neutro-penia and persistent fever: systematic review and meta-analysis. Eur J Cancer 2008;44(15):2192–203.
10. Walsh TJ, Anaissie EJ, Denning DW, et al. Treatment of aspergillosis: clinical practice guidelines of the Infectious Diseases Society of America. Clin Infect Dis 2008;46(3):327–60.

11. Chamilos G, Lewis RE, Kontoyiannis DP. Delaying amphotericin B-based frontline therapy significantly increases mortality among patients with hematologic malignancy who have zygomycosis. Clin Infect Dis 2008;47(4):503–9.
12. Mora-Duarte J, Betts R, Rotstein C, et al. Compar-ison of caspofungin and amphotericin B for inva-sive candidiasis. N Engl J Med 2002;347(25): 2020–9.
13. Johnson PC, Wheat LJ, Cloud GA, et al. Safety and efficacy of liposomal amphotericin B compared with conventional amphotericin B for induction therapy of histoplasmosis in patients with AIDS. Ann Intern Med 2002;137(2):105–9.
14. Borro JM, Sole A, de la Torre M, et al. Efficiency and safety of inhaled amphotericin B lipid complex (Abelcet) in the prophylaxis of invasive fungal infec-tions following lung transplantation. Transplant Proc 2008;40(9):3090–3.
15. Slobbe L, Boersma E, Rijnders BJ. Tolerability of prophylactic aerosolized liposomal amphotericin-B and impact on pulmonary function: data from a randomized placebo-controlled trial. Pulm Phar-macol Ther 2008;21(6):855–9.
16. Rijnders BJ, Cornelissen JJ, Slobbe L, et al. Aerosol-ized liposomal amphotericin B for the prevention of invasive pulmonary aspergillosis during prolonged neutropenia: a randomized, placebo-controlled trial. Clin Infect Dis 2008;46(9):1401–8.
17. Cornely OA, Maertens J, Bresnik M, et al. Liposomal amphotericin B as initial therapy for invasive mold infection: a randomized trial comparing a high-loading dose regimen with standard dosing (AmBi-Load trial). Clin Infect Dis 2007;44(10):1289–97.
18. Saliba F, Dupont B. Renal impairment and amphoter-icin B formulations in patients with invasive fungal infections. Med Mycol 2008;46(2):97–112.
19. Kleinberg M. What is the current and future status of conventional amphotericin B? Int J Antimicrob Agents 2006;27(Suppl 1):12–6.
20. Shimokawa O, Nakayama H. Increased sensitivity of Candida albicans cells accumulating 14 alpha-methylated sterols to active oxygen: possible rele-vance to in vivo efficacies of azole antifungal agents. Antimicrob Agents Chemother 1992;36(8):1626–9.
21. Kramer MR, Marshall SE, Denning DW, et al. Cyclo-sporine and itraconazole interaction in heart and lung transplant recipients. Ann Intern Med 1990; 113(4):327–9.
22. Varis T, Kaukonen KM, Kivisto KT, et al. Plasma concentrations and effects of oral methylpredniso-lone are considerably increased by itraconazole. Clin Pharmacol Ther 1998;64(4):363–8.
23. Tucker RM, Denning DW, Hanson LH, et al. Interac-tion of azoles with rifampin, phenytoin, and carba-mazepine: in vitro and clinical observations. Clin Infect Dis 1992;14(1):165–74.

24. Kivisto KT, Lamberg TS, Kantola T, et al. Plasma buspirone concentrations are greatly increased by erythromycin and itraconazole. Clin Pharmacol Ther 1997;62(3):348–54.

25. Engels FK, Ten Tije AJ, Baker SD, et al. Effect of cytochrome P450 3A4 inhibition on the pharmacokinetics of docetaxel. Clin Pharmacol Ther 2004;75(5): 448–54.

26. Grub S, Bryson H, Goggin T, et al. The interaction of saquinavir (soft gelatin capsule) with ketoconazole, erythromycin and rifampicin: comparison of the effect in healthy volunteers and in HIV-infected patients. Eur J Clin Pharmacol 2001;57(2):115–21.

27. Jeng MR, Feusner J. Itraconazole-enhanced vincristine neurotoxicity in a child with acute lymphoblastic leukemia. Pediatr Hematol Oncol 2001;18(2): 137–42.

28. Itraconazole [package insert]. (Sempera) product monograph. Janssen-Cilag GmbH N, Germany, 2003.

29. Kaukonen KM, Olkkola KT, Neuvonen PJ. Itraconazole increases plasma concentrations of quinidine. Clin Pharmacol Ther 1997;62(5):510–7.

30. Lefebvre RA, Van Peer A, Woestenborghs R. Influence of itraconazole on the pharmacokinetics and electrocardiographic effects of astemizole. Br J Clin Pharmacol 1997;43(3):319–22.

31. Honig PK, Wortham DC, Hull R, et al. Itraconazole affects single-dose terfenadine pharmacokinetics and cardiac repolarization pharmacodynamics. J Clin Pharmacol 1993;33(12):1201–6.

32. Posaconazole [package insert]. Kenilworth NSC.

33. Voriconazole (V-fend) [package insert]. Summary of Product Characteristics SAahemou.

34. DeMuria D, Forrest A, Rich J, et al. Pharmacokinetics and bioavailability of fluconazole in patients with AIDS. Antimicrob Agents Chemother 1993; 37(10):2187–92.

35. Baddley JW, Patel M, Bhavnani SM, et al. Association of fluconazole pharmacodynamics with mortality in patients with candidemia. Antimicrob Agents Chemother 2008;52(9):3022–8.

36. Stevens DA, Diaz M, Negroni R, et al. Safety evaluation of chronic fluconazole therapy. Fluconazole Pan-American Study Group. Chemotherapy 1997; 43(5):371–7.

37. Hamza OJ, Matee MI, Bruggemann RJ, et al. Single-dose fluconazole versus standard 2-week therapy for oropharyngeal candidiasis in HIV-infected patients: a randomized, double-blind, double-dummy trial. Clin Infect Dis 2008;47(10): 1270–6.

38. Slavin MA, Osborne B, Adams R, et al. Efficacy and safety of fluconazole prophylaxis for fungal infections after marrow transplantation—a prospective, randomized, double-blind study. J Infect Dis 1995; 171(6):1545–52.

39. Schuster MG, Edwards JE Jr, Sobel JD, et al. Empirical fluconazole versus placebo for intensive care unit patients: a randomized trial. Ann Intern Med 2008;149(2):83–90.

40. Longley N, Muzoora C, Taseera K, et al. Dose response effect of high-dose fluconazole for HIV-associated cryptococcal meningitis in southwestern Uganda. Clin Infect Dis 2008;47(12):1556–61.

41. Johnson RH, Einstein HE. Coccidioidal meningitis. Clin Infect Dis 2006;42(1):103–7.

42. Jaruratanasirikul S, Kleepkaew A. Influence of an acidic beverage (Coca-Cola) on the absorption of itraconazole. Eur J Clin Pharmacol 1997;52(3): 235–7.

43. Lange D, Pavao JH, Wu J, et al. Effect of a cola beverage on the bioavailability of itraconazole in the presence of H2 blockers. J Clin Pharmacol 1997;37(6):535–40.

44. Barone JA, Moskovitz BL, Guarnieri J, et al. Enhanced bioavailability of itraconazole in hydroxypropyl-beta-cyclodextrin solution versus capsules in healthy volunteers. Antimicrob Agents Chemother 1998;42(7):1862–5.

45. Van de Velde VJ, Van Peer AP, Heykants JJ, et al. Effect of food on the pharmacokinetics of a new hydroxypropyl-beta-cyclodextrin formulation of itraconazole. Pharmacotherapy 1996;16(3):424–8.

46. Stevens DA. Itraconazole in cyclodextrin solution. Pharmacotherapy 1999;19(5):603–11.

47. Como JA, Dismukes WE. Oral azole drugs as systemic antifungal therapy. N Engl J Med 1994; 330(4):263–72.

48. Warnock DW, Turner A, Burke J. Comparison of high performance liquid chromatographic and microbiological methods for determination of itraconazole. J Antimicrob Chemother 1988;21(1):93–100.

49. Wheat LJ, Freifeld AG, Kleiman MB, et al. Clinical practice guidelines for the management of patients with histoplasmosis: 2007 update by the Infectious Diseases Society of America. Clin Infect Dis 2007; 45(7):807–25.

50. De Beule K, Van Gestel J. Pharmacology of itraconazole. Drugs 2001;61(Suppl 1):27–37.

51. Tucker RM, Haq Y, Denning DW, et al. Adverse events associated with itraconazole in 189 patients on chronic therapy. J Antimicrob Chemother 1990; 26(4):561–6.

52. Glasmacher A, Hahn C, Molitor E, et al. Itraconazole through concentrations in antifungal prophylaxis with six different dosing regimens using hydroxypropyl-beta-cyclodextrin oral solution or coated-pellet capsules. Mycoses 1999;42(11–12):591–600.

53. Ahmad SR, Singer SJ, Leissa BG. Congestive heart failure associated with itraconazole. Lancet 2001; 357(9270):1766–7.

54. Manavathu EK, Cutright JL, Loebenberg D, et al. A comparative study of the in vitro susceptibilities of

clinical and laboratory-selected resistant isolates of Aspergillus spp. to amphotericin B, itraconazole, voriconazole and posaconazole (SCH 56592). J Antimicrob Chemother 2000;46(2):229–34.

55. Nagappan V, Deresinski S. Reviews of anti-infective agents: posaconazole: a broad-spectrum triazole antifungal agent. Clin Infect Dis 2007;45(12):1610–7.

56. Courtney R, Wexler D, Radwanski E, et al. Effect of food on the relative bioavailability of two oral formulations of posaconazole in healthy adults. Br J Clin Pharmacol 2004;57(2):218–22.

57. Ezzet F, Wexler D, Courtney R, et al. Oral bioavailability of posaconazole in fasted healthy subjects: comparison between three regimens and basis for clinical dosage recommendations. Clin Pharm 2005;44(2):211–20.

58. Jain R, Pottinger P. The effect of gastric acid on the absorption of posaconazole. Clin Infect Dis 2008; 46(10):1627–8 [author reply].

59. Krishna G, MA, Ma L, et al. Effect of gastric pH, dosing regimen and prandial state, food and meal timing relative to dose, and gastrointestinal motility on absorption and pharmacokinetics of the antifungal posaconazole [abstract]. In: 18th European Congress of Clinical Microbiology and Infectious Diseases. Barcelona. p. 1264.

60. Courtney R, Pai S, Laughlin M, et al. Pharmacokinetics, safety, and tolerability of oral posaconazole administered in single and multiple doses in healthy adults. Antimicrob Agents Chemother 2003;47(9): 2788–95.

61. Sansone-Parsons A, Krishna G, Calzetta A, et al. Effect of a nutritional supplement on posaconazole pharmacokinetics following oral administration to healthy volunteers. Antimicrob Agents Chemother 2006;50(5):1881–3.

62. Meletiadis J, Chanock S, Walsh TJ. Human pharmacogenomic variations and their implications for antifungal efficacy. Clin Microbiol Rev 2006;19(4): 763–87.

63. Cornely OA, Maertens J, Winston DJ, et al. Posaconazole vs. fluconazole or itraconazole prophylaxis in patients with neutropenia. N Engl J Med 2007; 356(4):348–59.

64. Ullmann AJ, Lipton JH, Vesole DH, et al. Posaconazole or fluconazole for prophylaxis in severe graft-versus-host disease. N Engl J Med 2007;356(4): 335–47.

65. Walsh TJ, Raad I, Patterson TF, et al. Treatment of invasive aspergillosis with posaconazole in patients who are refractory to or intolerant of conventional therapy: an externally controlled trial. Clin Infect Dis 2007;44(1):2–12.

66. Courtney R, Sansone A, Smith W, et al. Posaconazole pharmacokinetics, safety, and tolerability in subjects with varying degrees of chronic renal disease. J Clin Pharmacol 2005;45(2):185–92.

67. Raad II, Graybill JR, Bustamante AB, et al. Safety of long-term oral posaconazole use in the treatment of refractory invasive fungal infections. Clin Infect Dis 2006;42(12):1726–34.

68. Johnson LB, Kauffman CA. Voriconazole: a new triazole antifungal agent. Clin Infect Dis 2003;36(5):630–7.

69. Purkins L, Wood N, Ghahramani P, et al. Pharmacokinetics and safety of voriconazole following intravenous- to oral-dose escalation regimens. Antimicrob Agents Chemother 2002;46(8):2546–53.

70. Lazarus HM, Blumer JL, Yanovich S, et al. Safety and pharmacokinetics of oral voriconazole in patients at risk of fungal infection: a dose escalation study. J Clin Pharmacol 2002;42(4):395–402.

71. Ikeda Y, Umemura K, Kondo K, et al. Pharmacokinetics of voriconazole and cytochrome P450 2C19 genetic status. Clin Pharmacol Ther 2004;75(6):587–8.

72. Denning DW, Ribaud P, Milpied N, et al. Efficacy and safety of voriconazole in the treatment of acute invasive aspergillosis. Clin Infect Dis 2002;34(5):563–71.

73. Scherpbier HJ, Hilhorst MI, Kuijpers TW. Liver failure in a child receiving highly active antiretroviral therapy and voriconazole. Clin Infect Dis 2003; 37(6):828–30.

74. Pascual A, Calandra T, Bolay S, et al. Voriconazole therapeutic drug monitoring in patients with invasive mycoses improves efficacy and safety outcomes. Clin Infect Dis 2008;46(2):201–11.

75. Lewis RE. What is the "therapeutic range" for voriconazole? Clin Infect Dis 2008;46(2):212–4.

76. Zonios DI, Gea-Banacloche J, Childs R, et al. Hallucinations during voriconazole therapy. Clin Infect Dis 2008;47(1):e7–10.

77. Herbrecht R, Denning DW, Patterson TF, et al. Voriconazole versus amphotericin B for primary therapy of invasive aspergillosis. N Engl J Med 2002;347(6): 408–15.

78. Chapman SW, Bradsher RW Jr, Campbell GD Jr, et al. Practice guidelines for the management of patients with blastomycosis. Infectious Diseases Society of America. Clin Infect Dis 2000;30(4):679–83.

79. Kauffman CA, Hajjeh R, Chapman SW. Practice guidelines for the management of patients with sporotrichosis. For the Mycoses Study Group. Infectious Diseases Society of America. Clin Infect Dis 2000;30(4):684–7.

80. Goodwin ML, Drew RH. Antifungal serum concentration monitoring: an update. J Antimicrob Chemother 2008;61(1):17–25.

81. Cappelletty D, Eiselstein-McKitrick K. The echinocandins. Pharmacotherapy 2007;27(3):369–88.

82. Pfaller MA, Diekema DJ, Ostrosky-Zeichner L, et al. Correlation of MIC with outcome for Candida species tested against caspofungin, anidulafungin, and micafungin: analysis and proposal for interpretive MIC breakpoints. J Clin Microbiol 2008;46(8): 2620–9.

83. Lamaris GA, Lewis RE, Chamilos G, et al. Caspofungin-mediated beta-glucan unmasking and enhancement of human polymorphonuclear neutrophil activity against Aspergillus and non-Aspergillus hyphae. J Infect Dis 2008;198(2):186–92.

84. Thompson GR 3rd, Wiederhold NP, Vallor AC, et al. Development of caspofungin resistance following prolonged therapy for invasive candidiasis secondary to Candida glabrata infection. Antimicrob Agents Chemother 2008;52(10):3783–5.

85. Wiederhold NP. Attenuation of echinocandin activity at elevated concentrations: a review of the paradoxical effect. Curr Opin Infect Dis 2007;20(6):574–8.

86. Kuse ER, Chetchotisakd P, da Cunha CA, et al. Micafungin versus liposomal amphotericin B for candidaemia and invasive candidosis: a phase III randomised double-blind trial. Lancet 2007;369(9572):1519–27.

87. Reboli AC, Rotstein C, Pappas PG, et al. Anidulafungin versus fluconazole for invasive candidiasis. N Engl J Med 2007;356(24):2472–82.

88. Pappas PG, Rotstein CM, Betts RF, et al. Micafungin versus caspofungin for treatment of candidemia and other forms of invasive candidiasis. Clin Infect Dis 2007;45(7):883–93.

89. Cornely OA, Lasso M, Betts R, et al. Caspofungin for the treatment of less common forms of invasive candidiasis. J Antimicrob Chemother 2007;60(2):363–9.

90. Baddley JW, Benjamin DK Jr, Patel M, et al. Candida infective endocarditis. Eur J Clin Microbiol Infect Dis 2008;27(7):519–29.

91. Heinz WJ, Einsele H. Caspofungin for treatment of invasive aspergillus infections. Mycoses 2008; 51(Suppl 1):47–57.

92. Polak A, Scholer HJ. Mode of action of 5-fluorocytosine and mechanisms of resistance. Chemotherapy 1975;21(3–4):113–30.

93. Stamm AM, Diasio RB, Dismukes WE, et al. Toxicity of amphotericin B plus flucytosine in 194 patients with cryptococcal meningitis. Am J Med 1987; 83(2):236–42.

94. Brouwer AE, Rajanuwong A, Chierakul W, et al. Combination antifungal therapies for HIV-associated cryptococcal meningitis: a randomised trial. Lancet 2004;363(9423):1764–7.

95. Enache-Angoulvant A, Hennequin C. Invasive Saccharomyces infection: a comprehensive review. Clin Infect Dis 2005;41(11):1559–68.

96. da Matta VL, de Souza Carvalho Melhem M, Colombo AL, et al. Antifungal drug susceptibility profile of Pichia anomala isolates from patients presenting with nosocomial fungemia. Antimicrob Agents Chemother 2007;51(4):1573–6.

97. Paphitou NI, Ostrosky-Zeichner L, Paetznick VL, et al. In vitro antifungal susceptibilities of Trichosporon species. Antimicrob Agents Chemother 2002;46(4):1144–6.

Histoplasmosis

Carol A. Kauffman, MD

KEYWORDS

- Histoplasmosis • Endemic mycoses
- *Histoplasma capsulatum*
- Pulmonary histoplasmosis • Disseminated histoplasmosis

Histoplasmosis is the most common endemic mycosis causing human infection. Large outbreaks have been ascribed to histoplasmosis, but most infections are sporadic. Similar to the other fungi in this category, initial exposure to *Histoplasma capsulatum* is by way of the respiratory tract, but once inhaled into the alveoli, the organism readily spreads in macrophages throughout the reticuloendothelial system. The ability to contain infection is almost entirely mediated by cell-mediated immunity. In most patients, infection is associated with no symptoms or with only mild pulmonary symptoms. People who have either intrinsic or secondary defects in cell-mediated immunity, however, are at risk for development of severe disseminated histoplasmosis. As new and increasingly more immunosuppressive therapeutic regimens have been developed, the risks for the development of severe disseminated histoplasmosis have likewise increased. Compared with a decade ago, improvements in diagnostic tests have made it feasible to more quickly establish a diagnosis of histoplasmosis, thus allowing appropriate antifungal therapy to be started promptly. Treatment guidelines have been updated recently and are reviewed for the various forms of histoplasmosis.

EPIDEMIOLOGY AND PATHOGENESIS

H capsulatum is a dimorphic fungus that exists as a mold in the environment and as a yeast in tissues at 37 °C. The endemic area includes the Ohio and Mississippi River valleys, Central and South America, and microfoci in the Eastern United States, southern Europe, Africa, and southeastern Asia. The organism grows profusely in soil that is rich in the droppings from birds and bats.[1] Old abandoned buildings and caves often contain high concentrations of *H capsulatum*. Most cases are sporadic, but outbreaks involving a few people to hundreds of individuals have implicated demolition of buildings, moving soil, cleaning of bridge structures, and spelunking as the point source for dispersal of the organism.[2] The largest outbreak occurred in an urban setting and led to infection in more than a hundred thousand people who passively acquired infection because they happened to live downwind from a demolition site.[3]

The microconidia formed in the mold phase of *H capsulatum* are easily aerosolized, inhaled into the lungs, and then phagocytized by alveolar macrophages. Inside the macrophage, the organism converts to the yeast phase, survives within the macrophage for the first few weeks, and disseminates widely throughout the reticuloendothelial system. Within several weeks, when specific cell-mediated immunity against *H capsulatum* develops, sensitized T cells activate the macrophages, which then are able to kill the organism.[4] If cell-mediated immunity is deficient because of immunosuppressive drugs or underlying illnesses, the organisms remain viable within macrophages and cause progressive infection.[5,6]

The severity of disease is determined by the number of conidia that are inhaled and the immune response of the host. In the vast majority of individuals, infection is asymptomatic or manifested only by mild, nonspecific symptoms. Healthy individuals who are exposed to a large inoculum of conidia, however, such as might occur with spelunking in a heavily contaminated cave or removing heavy encrustations of bird or bat droppings, can develop severe pulmonary infection.[7] In a severely immunocompromised host, even a small inoculum can cause severe pulmonary infection or progress to disseminated histoplasmosis.

Division of Infectious Diseases, Veterans Affairs Ann Arbor Healthcare System, Department of Internal Medicine, University of Michigan Medical School, 2215 Fuller Road, Ann Arbor, MI 48105, USA
E-mail address: ckauff@umich.edu

Clin Chest Med 30 (2009) 217–225
doi:10.1016/j.ccm.2009.02.002
0272-5231/09/$ – see front matter. Published by Elsevier Inc.

The major risk factors that portend an increased risk for disseminated infection with *H capsulatum* are exposure to the organism as an infant before cell-mediated immunity is adequate to handle intracellular pathogens,[8] AIDS with CD4 cells less than 150/μL,[6,9] corticosteroids and other immunosuppressive agents given for various conditions,[1,10,11] hematologic malignancies,[5] and solid organ transplantation.[11,12] In comparison with solid organ transplantation, histoplasmosis complicating stem cell transplantation is uncommon.[11] With increasing use of tumor necrosis factor (TNF) antagonists, this form of therapy has emerged as a major risk factor for histoplasmosis.[13–15] Not surprisingly, this cytokine is of integral importance in the cell-mediated immune response to histoplasmosis,[16] and blockade, as occurs with etanercept (Enbrel), infliximab (Remicade), and adalimumab (Humira), results in widely disseminated histoplasmosis.[13–15]

Because it is an intracellular pathogen, *H capsulatum* has the ability to remain viable in tissues for years in a latent state. If cell-mediated immunity wanes because of illness, organ transplantation, or immunosuppressive drugs, the organism can reactivate and cause disease.[1] This reactivation can occur years after the initial exposure and outside of the endemic area, making the diagnosis more difficult. Given its ability to remain latent in tissues, *H capsulatum* has been transmitted with donated organs.[11,17]

CLINICAL MANIFESTATIONS
Pulmonary Histoplasmosis

The predominant clinical manifestation of histoplasmosis is pneumonia, but most patients have either no symptoms or mild pulmonary complaints that are not severe enough to seek medical care. Most cases of acute pulmonary histoplasmosis are thus not identified as such, and the patient gets well without specific treatment. Those who do see a physician are usually believed to have an atypical pneumonia, are treated with antibiotics active against organisms such as *Mycoplasma* or *Legionella*, and a diagnosis of fungal infection is not entertained. The chest radiograph, if ordered, usually shows patchy infiltrates (**Fig. 1**). The presence of hilar or mediastinal lymphadenopathy should raise the suspicion for fungal pneumonia.[18,19]

Patients who do develop severe pneumonia because of an intense exposure or because they are immunosuppressed develop symptoms that include chills, high fevers, dyspnea, chest pain, and cough. They often appear quite ill, are hypoxemic, and the clinical course can progress quickly

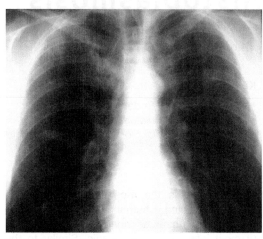

Fig. 1. Chest radiograph of a young man who developed acute pulmonary histoplasmosis. There are patchy infiltrates in the right mid-lung and left upper lung fields. (*Courtesy of* P. Pernicano, University of Michigan, Ann Arbor, MI.)

to acute respiratory distress syndrome (ARDS). Diffuse reticulonodular infiltrates are noted on chest radiographs and CT scans (**Fig. 2**).

An entirely different group of individuals at risk for pulmonary histoplasmosis are those individuals who develop chronic cavitary pulmonary histoplasmosis. These patients almost always are older, have underlying emphysema, and present with a chronic illness that mimics reactivation pulmonary tuberculosis in its clinical manifestations and radiographic findings.[20] Patients have fever, fatigue, anorexia, weight loss, cough productive of purulent sputum, and hemoptysis. Chest radiographs and CT scans demonstrate unilateral or bilateral upper lobe infiltrates and cavities, and often show extensive fibrosis in the lower lung fields (**Fig. 3**).

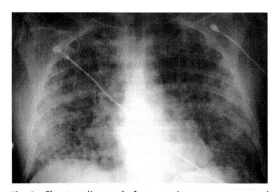

Fig. 2. Chest radiograph from an immunosuppressed patient who had histoplasmosis. The diffuse infiltrates had worsened over a few days as the patient developed ARDS. (*Courtesy of* P. Pernicano, University of Michigan, Ann Arbor, MI.)

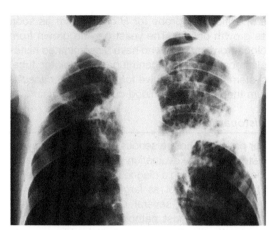

Fig. 3. Chest radiograph showing extensive upper lobe cavitary infiltrates in an elderly gentleman who had chronic pulmonary histoplasmosis.

Complications of Pulmonary Histoplasmosis

Granulomatous mediastinitis (or mediastinal granuloma) is an uncommon complication of acute pulmonary histoplasmosis.[18,21,22] For most patients who have acute histoplasmosis, hilar and mediastinal lymphadenopathy resolve within a few months after the pneumonia resolves. A small proportion of patients have persistently enlarged nodes that sometimes coalesce into a large encapsulated lesion that may caseate (**Fig. 4**). The mass can impinge on other structures, causing symptoms. Compression of a bronchus can result in intermittent obstruction and recurrent pneumonia. Impingement on the esophagus can lead to a traction diverticulum or a tracheoesophageal fistula. Spontaneous drainage of the involved nodes into adjacent soft tissues of the neck is also seen.

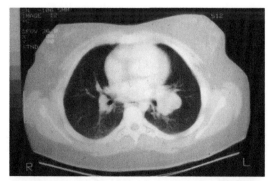

Fig. 4. CT scan of a young woman who had persistent left hilar and mediastinal lymphadenopathy more than a year after an episode of acute atypical pneumonia later discovered to be due to histoplasmosis.

The vast majority of patients who have granulomatous mediastinitis have no symptoms, and the presence of abnormal nodes is noted only when a chest radiograph or CT scan, done for another problem, reveals lymphadenopathy. Lymphadenopathy is best evaluated by CT scans that often show calcium deposits and areas of necrosis. Mediastinoscopy and biopsy reveal caseous material, which may contain a few yeast-like organisms typical for *H capsulatum*, but it is unusual to grow the organism from this material.

Fibrosing mediastinitis (or mediastinal fibrosis) is, thankfully, a rare complication of pulmonary histoplasmosis. Patients who have granulomatous mediastinitis do not progress to fibrosing mediastinitis; these syndromes seem to be due to two separate pathophysiologic processes. In patients who have fibrosing mediastinitis, the response to infection with *H capsulatum* is that of excessive fibrosis.[22–24] The exuberant fibrous tissue entraps the great vessels causing respiratory distress, heart failure, pulmonary emboli, and superior vena cava syndrome; constriction of the bronchi can occur, resulting in dyspnea, cough, wheezing, and hemoptysis. In many patients, the process is restricted to one side, and this portends a much better prognosis than when pulmonary vessels from both lungs are involved.[18,25] The extent of obstruction of pulmonary arteries and veins is best visualized using CT scans and angiographic procedures. The organism is rarely seen on biopsy of involved tissue, and there is no evidence for ongoing infection in this syndrome.

Pericarditis is another complication of acute pulmonary histoplasmosis.[26,27] Pericardial effusions, often seen with accompanying pleural effusions, reflect an inflammatory response to pulmonary infection; *H capsulatum* has rarely been isolated from pericardial fluid, and the syndrome is almost always self-limited. The pericardial fluid is exudative and usually bloody, resembling that seen with tuberculous pericarditis. Although symptoms generally resolve after several months, relapses can occur. Surgical drainage is required only if tamponade is imminent, and constrictive pericarditis has been reported only rarely.

Disseminated Histoplasmosis

Hematogenous dissemination is common in the early stages of infection with *H capsulatum*, but almost all people in whom this occurs remain asymptomatic. Symptomatic acute disseminated infection occurs almost entirely in those who are immunosuppressed.[5,6,8–15,17]

The most common manifestations are chills, fever, malaise, anorexia, and weight loss.[28] Those who have gastrointestinal tract involvement usually complain of diarrhea and abdominal pain. More severely ill patients have sepsis syndrome with ARDS, disseminated intravascular coagulation, and acute adrenal insufficiency. Mucous membrane ulcers, skin lesions, and hepatosplenomegaly are common. Gastrointestinal involvement is reflected in diffuse ulcerations of the mucosa and sometimes malabsorption. Pancytopenia is frequently noted; liver enzymes, especially alkaline phosphatase, are elevated; and the serum ferritin levels can be extremely high.[29] In some patients, pulmonary involvement is not a major component, but in others extensive pneumonia is present. Hemophagocytic syndrome has been noted with disseminated histoplasmosis in immunosuppressed patients.[30,31]

Chronic progressive disseminated histoplasmosis occurs mostly in middle-aged to elderly men who have no known immunosuppression but who are unable to contain the organism.[1,10,28] The illness is chronic and characterized by fever, night sweats, weight loss, and fatigue. On physical examination, patients appear chronically ill and often have painful ulcerations in the oral cavity, and hepatosplenomegaly is found. The symptoms and signs of adrenal insufficiency occur with adrenal gland destruction. Increased erythrocyte sedimentation rate, pancytopenia, elevated alkaline phosphatase, and diffuse pulmonary infiltrates reflect widespread involvement. This form of histoplasmosis, although chronic, is fatal if not treated.

Central nervous system histoplasmosis is uncommon. It can occur as a component of acute disseminated histoplasmosis in immunosuppressed patients, and it also occurs as isolated chronic meningitis without other signs of disseminated infection.[32,33] The symptoms are headache, behavioral changes, and sometimes focal neurologic deficits. Signs of increased intracranial pressure may be prominent. The most common presentation is that of chronic lymphocytic meningitis, but focal lesions also can occur in the brain and the spinal cord and are best seen with MRI techniques.

DIAGNOSIS
Culture

Growth of the mold phase of *H capsulatum* from involved tissue is the definitive diagnostic test for histoplasmosis, but it may take 4 to 6 weeks for growth to appear.[1,34] The tuberculate macroconidia are characteristic of *H capsulatum*, but identification should be verified with the use of a specific DNA probe for *H capsulatum* as soon as growth occurs. The yeast can be grown from blood from patients who have disseminated histoplasmosis; the lysis-centrifugation (Isolator tube) system is more sensitive for detecting *H capsulatum* than automated blood culture systems.[35]

Histopathology

For patients who are seriously ill, tissue biopsy for histopathologic evaluation for fungi is a rapid means to establish a diagnosis of histoplasmosis.[1] The yeasts are not as large or as distinctive as those seen with several of the other endemic mycoses, but most pathologists should be able to identify the 2- to 4-μm oval budding yeasts typical of *H capsulatum* on methenamine silver or periodic acid-Schiff staining of tissues (**Fig. 5**). In patients who have severe acute disseminated histoplasmosis, yeasts can sometimes be seen inside white blood cells on the peripheral blood smear.

Antibody Assays

Measurement of antibodies against *H capsulatum* is accomplished by complement fixation (CF) and immunodiffusion (ID) assays.[1,34] Whenever possible, serum should be sent to fungal reference laboratories knowledgeable in the performance of these assays. Antibody tests are most useful for diagnosis in patients who are not immunosuppressed and for those who are not severely ill so that there is time to wait for the results. In those who have marked immunosuppression, one cannot rely on the development of antibody as a diagnostic tool.[36,37] For patients who have chronic cavitary pulmonary histoplasmosis and chronic progressive disseminated histoplasmosis, however, antibody tests are useful. Both CF and ID

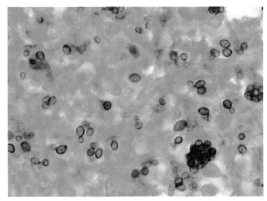

Fig. 5. Biopsy sample of lung tissue stained with methenamine silver stain showing many 2- to 4-μm oval budding yeasts typical of *H capsulatum*.

tests are usually positive in these patients. Antibody tests also are helpful in those who have acute pulmonary histoplasmosis; in this type of histoplasmosis, a fourfold change in CF titer or the appearance of an M band on ID is diagnostic.[1,34]

The ID test is slightly more specific than the CF test; false-positive CF tests occur in patients who have lymphoma, tuberculosis, sarcoidosis, and other fungal infections. Both assays have a sensitivity of about 80%. Because CF antibodies can persist for years after infection, a single low CF titer means little other than that the patient was at some time exposed to H capsulatum.

For patients who have fibrosing mediastinitis or granulomatous mediastinitis, antibody tests are often negative or may be positive at a low titer that could also reflect a false-positive CF test. Serology is not adequate to rule out tumors or other granulomatous processes in patients who have isolated mediastinal lymphadenopathy.

Antigen Detection

Increasingly, detection of circulating H capsulatum polysaccharide antigen by an enzyme immunoassay (EIA) in urine, serum, and other body fluids is used for the rapid diagnosis of disseminated histoplasmosis.[34,38–40] There are now several commercial antigen assays available, and it seems that there may be differences in sensitivity among these different assays.[41,42] Almost all of the data reported on the use of this test have been with the use of the MiraVista Laboratory assay.[39]

Urine, rather than serum, is preferred for testing because of enhanced sensitivity. The sensitivity of the urine assay for the diagnosis of disseminated histoplasmosis is approximately 90% among patients who have AIDS;[34] there are no studies that have specifically evaluated the assay in a large number patients who did not have AIDS. The urine antigen test seems less useful for pulmonary histoplasmosis, probably because of a lower burden of organisms than in disseminated histoplasmosis. The one exception is acute pulmonary histoplasmosis, in which it has been noted that up to 75% of patients can have a positive urine Histoplasma antigen test. The antigen assay is not useful in patients who have granulomatous or fibrosing mediastinitis or other focal forms of pulmonary histoplasmosis.

False-positive reactions occur in other endemic fungal infections, including coccidioidomycosis, blastomycosis, paracoccidioidomycosis, and penicilliosis.[43] The major differential diagnosis is obviously between histoplasmosis and blastomycosis because the endemic areas overlap. Additionally, false-positive reactions occur in patients who have histoplasmosis when their urine is tested with an EIA assay for Blastomyces dermatitidis.[44] These two fungi share similar galactomannans in their cell walls.

The serum Aspergillus galactomannan EIA also has been noted to be falsely positive in patients who have disseminated histoplasmosis and who have high concentrations of circulating Histoplasma antigen.[45] Patients who have aspergillosis, however, do not have false-positive Histoplasma antigen tests, probably because the level of circulating Aspergillus galactomannan is relatively low.

The usefulness of the Histoplasma EIA for detection of antigen in bronchoalveolar lavage fluid and cerebrospinal fluid is not yet defined. There are a few reports of its use in patients who have AIDS.[33,46]

It is recommended that urine Histoplasma antigen levels be used as a guide to follow the course of a patient's illness.[34,36] The levels decrease after initiation of antifungal therapy and increase with a relapse of infection. It should be noted, however, that some patients seem to have persistence of low levels of antigenuria, even though they are clinically well; thus, urine antigen levels cannot be the sole parameter used to define the response to therapy. The clinical response is most important, and laboratory parameters should be used in that context.

Molecular-Based Methods

The role of polymerase chain reaction (PCR)–based methods for the diagnosis of histoplasmosis has not been defined. Only a small number of patients have been reported, and there are no standardized methods established for the use of PCR for detecting H capsulatum.[47,48]

TREATMENT
General

Guidelines for the management of histoplasmosis recently have been revised by the Infectious Diseases Society of America (IDSA).[49] Treatment recommendations revolve around the use of itraconazole for mild to moderate infection and an amphotericin B formulation for severe infection. Many clinicians now use lipid formulations of amphotericin B, either amphotericin B lipid complex (Abelcet) or liposomal amphotericin B (AmBisome) because they are less nephrotoxic than amphotericin B deoxycholate. Indeed, the new guidelines recommend lipid formulations rather than amphotericin B deoxycholate for most indications.[49]

Several trials have shown the efficacy of itraconazole for the treatment of nonmeningeal histoplasmosis.[50,51] Fluconazole is considered a second-line agent because primary response rates are lower and relapse rates are higher when compared with itraconazole.[52,53] Ketoconazole is rarely used any more because it is more toxic and less effective than itraconazole. Voriconazole and posaconazole also are considered second-line agents because there are no treatment trials using these agents; the published reports reflect clinical anecdotes.[12,54–57] There is one report of voriconazole resistance developing among strains of *H capsulatum* that had become resistant to fluconazole while AIDS patients were being treated with fluconazole for disseminated histoplasmosis.[58] The generalizability of this finding is not known. The echinocandins are not active and should not be used for the treatment of histoplasmosis.

A loading dose of itraconazole, 200 mg three times daily for 3 days, should be given so that appropriate serum levels can be achieved more quickly. Either the capsule formulation that requires both food and stomach acid for absorption or the oral solution that is given on an empty stomach can be used. It is recommended that serum itraconazole levels be monitored to ensure adequate absorption; a serum concentration greater than 1 μg/mL is recommended.[49] The appropriate time to obtain levels is about 2 weeks after treatment is started. The half-life of itraconazole is long so that the levels can be obtained at random times and do not have to be keyed to the timing of the medication.

Pulmonary Histoplasmosis

Treatment is rarely needed for patients who have acute pulmonary histoplasmosis because this infection is almost always self-limited. If the patient is symptomatic for more than 4 weeks, however, therapy with itraconazole 200 mg once or twice daily for 6 to 12 weeks should be given.

Patients who have severe acute pulmonary infection should be treated with a lipid formulation of amphotericin B. This group includes most patients who are immunosuppressed. When a favorable clinical response to amphotericin B has occurred and the patient is stable, treatment can be changed to oral itraconazole, 200 mg twice daily.[49] Itraconazole should be continued for at least a year in patients who have severe histoplasmosis. A short course of methylprednisolone, 0.5 to 1 mg/kg, may be useful in patients who have ARDS, but there are no specific studies to prove this.[49]

Patients who have the chronic cavitary form of pulmonary histoplasmosis must be treated with an antifungal agent.[20,49] For most patients, amphotericin B is not needed, and treatment with itraconazole, 200 mg twice daily, is appropriate. Therapy should continue for at least 1 year. Many of these patients have a poor outcome because of severe underlying emphysema and the progressive fibrosis that occurs with this form of histoplasmosis.

Complications of Pulmonary Histoplasmosis

In general, patients who have complications after acute pulmonary histoplasmosis do not need to be treated with antifungal agents. There are patients who have granulomatous mediastinitis who present relatively soon after the acute illness and who have continuing infection in the nodes, however. These patients might benefit from a 6- to 12-week course of 200 to 400 mg itraconazole daily.[49]

Fibrosing mediastinitis does not respond to antifungal therapy. Because of the dismal outcome for patients who have bilateral involvement of the great vessels, however, most patients have received several months of therapy with itraconazole, on the chance that this might help.

Pericarditis is treated with nonsteroidal anti-inflammatory agents or, rarely, corticosteroids for severe cases. Itraconazole is recommended only if corticosteroids are given to ensure that dissemination does not occur.

Disseminated Histoplasmosis

All patients who have disseminated histoplasmosis should be treated with an antifungal agent.[49] Patients who have only mild to moderate illness can be treated with oral itraconazole, 200 mg twice daily.[49–51] Most patients who have the chronic progressive disseminated form of histoplasmosis present in this manner and can be treated with itraconazole. It is essential that serum levels of itraconazole be measured in patients who have disseminated infection to ensure the best chance for efficacy.

Patients who have moderately severe to severe disseminated infection should be treated initially with liposomal amphotericin B, 3 mg/kg daily.[49] This group includes most immunosuppressed patients. A randomized, double-blind, controlled trial in patients who had AIDS who had severe disseminated histoplasmosis showed that liposomal amphotericin B led to more prompt resolution of fever and improved survival when compared with amphotericin B deoxycholate.[59] As the patient's condition improves, step-down treatment with oral itraconazole, 200 mg twice daily, can be initiated and then continued for a total of 12 months. A retrospective analysis of the length of time that patients who had AIDS remained funge-mic and had persistent antigenuria when treated with either itraconazole or liposomal amphotericin B showed that those patients who had received liposomal amphotericin B had more rapid clear-ance of both fungemia and *Histoplasma* antigenuria than those who had received itraconazole.[60]

Patients who have central nervous system histo-plasmosis constitute a difficult management problem; they may or may not have evidence of disseminated histoplasmosis at the time of presentation with meningitis. The recommenda-tions are to treat with higher-dose liposomal amphotericin B, 5 mg/kg daily for at least 4 to 6 weeks and then to change to an oral azole for at least 1 year and until all symptoms have resolved and cerebrospinal fluid (CSF) changes have reverted to normal.[49] The azole that is most effec-tive for long-term therapy of *Histoplasma* menin-gitis is not known. Itraconazole and fluconazole have been used, the former having greater activity against *H capsulatum* and the latter achieving much higher CSF levels.[33] Voriconazole and posa-conazole have also been used successfully.[12,57] The number of reported cases receiving any of these azoles is small, however. The IDSA guide-lines recommend itraconazole at a dosage of 200 mg two or three times daily.[49]

PREVENTION

It is difficult to prevent exposure to a ubiquitous pathogen, but some high-risk activities can be performed safely if protective measures are taken. Recommendations from the National Institute for Occupational Safety and Health and the National Center for Infectious Diseases give explicit infor-mation to protect workers who must participate in high-risk activities, such as demolishing old buildings or digging in areas known to be heavily contaminated with *H capsulatum*.[61] Workers should wear respirators, and water sprays should be used during demolition work to decrease dust and the chance of aerosolizing conidia. Immuno-compromised individuals should not indulge in spelunking or undertake renovation projects that involve soil or buildings that could be contami-nated with *H capsulatum*.

Itraconazole, 200 mg daily, has been shown in a randomized controlled trial to prevent the devel-opment of histoplasmosis in patients who have AIDS who have CD4 less than 150/μL.[62] Prophy-laxis is only feasible in highly endemic areas that have documented rates greater than10 cases/ 100 patient-years. Histoplasmosis is much less common now in patients who have AIDS with the widespread use of effective antiretroviral therapy.

Those patients who do present with disseminated histoplasmosis are either unaware that they have HIV infection or they have not followed through with antiretroviral treatment that had been prescribed for them.

Of great interest is the issue of whether patients who are about to receive a transplant or begin treatment with TNF antagonists or other immuno-suppressive agents should receive prophylaxis against histoplasmosis. There are few data and no firm recommendations in this regard. One study has noted a negligible risk for developing histo-plasmosis in a cohort of recipients who were from a highly endemic area and who were followed for a mean of 16 months after stem cell or solid organ transplantation.[63] The risk may be even higher for those receiving TNF antagonists than those receiving a transplant. Treatment of all people from the endemic area who are to receive TNF antagonists is not appropriate given the side effects, drug interactions (including those with several other immunosuppressive agents), and cost of itraconazole; one should use prophylaxis only in those at highest risk. Clearly, if a patient has had a recent documented infection with *H capsulatum,* prophylaxis should be strongly considered. For other patients, however, there are no established markers to aid in defining those at risk. Antigenuria is not helpful because it is an indicator of active infection requiring therapy, not prophylaxis. Some centers obtain *Histoplasma* antibody studies, and consider giving prophylaxis to those who have a positive CF antibody titer. If itraconazole is prescribed, the duration of prophy-laxis is unknown. Unfortunately, there are unlikely to be studies aimed at defining the risks and the appropriateness of antifungal prophylaxis in these situations. Most importantly, physicians should alert their patients who are taking TNF antagonists to the dangers of environmental exposure to *H capsulatum* and the symptoms that might indicate infection.

REFERENCES

1. Kauffman CA. Histoplasmosis: a clinical and labora-tory update. Clin Microbiol Rev 2007;20:115–32.
2. Cano M, Hajjeh RA. The epidemiology of histoplas-mosis: a review. Semin Respir Infect 2001;16: 109–18.
3. Wheat LJ, Wass J, Norton J, et al. Cavitary histoplas-mosis occurring during two large urban outbreaks: analysis of clinical, epidemiologic, roentgeno-graphic, and laboratory features. Medicine (Balti-more) 1984;63:201–9.
4. Newman SL. Cell-mediated immunity to *Histoplasma capsulatum*. Semin Respir Infect 2001;16:102–8.

5. Kauffman CA. Endemic mycoses in patients with hematologic malignancies. Semin Respir Infect 2002;17:106–12.

6. McKinsey DS, Spiegel RA, Hutwagner L, et al. Prospective study of histoplasmosis in patients infected with human immunodeficiency virus: incidence, risk factors, and pathophysiology. Clin Infect Dis 1997;24:1195–203.

7. Jones TF, Swinger GL, Craig AS, et al. Acute pulmonary histoplasmosis in bridge workers: a persistent problem. Am J Med 1999;106:480–2.

8. Odio CM, Navarrete M, Carrillo JM, et al. Disseminated histoplasmosis in infants. Pediatr Infect Dis J 1999;18:1065–8.

9. Couppie P, Sobesky M, Aznar C, et al. Histoplasmosis and acquired immunodeficiency syndrome: a study of prognostic factors. Clin Infect Dis 2004; 38:134–8.

10. Assi MA, Sandid MS, Baddour LM, et al. Systemic histoplasmosis. A 15-year retrospective institutional review of 111 patients. Medicine (Baltimore) 2007; 86:162–9.

11. Kauffman CA. Endemic mycoses after hematopoietic stem cell or solid organ transplantation. In: Bowden RA, Ljungman P, Paya CV, editors. Transplant infections. 2nd edition. Philadelphia: Lippincott Williams & Wilkins; 2003. p. 524–34.

12. Freifeld AG, Iwen PC, Lesiak BL, et al. Histoplasmosis in solid organ transplant recipients at a large midwestern university transplant center. Transpl Infect Dis 2005;7:109–15.

13. Crum NF, Lederman ER, Wallace MR. Infections associated with tumor necrosis factor–alpha antagonists. Medicine (Baltimore) 2005;84:291–302.

14. Wood KL, Hage CA, Knox KS, et al. Histoplasmosis after treatment with anti-TNF-(alpha) therapy. Am J Respir Crit Care Med 2003;167:1279–82.

15. Lee J-H, Slifman NR, Gershon SK, et al. Life-threatening histoplasmosis complicating immunotherapy with tumor necrosis factor α antagonists infliximab and etanercept. Arthritis Rheum 2002; 46:2565–70.

16. Deepe GS Jr. Modulation of infection with *Histoplasma capsulatum* by inhibition of tumor necrosis factor-α factor activity. Clin Infect Dis 2005;41:S204–7.

17. Limaye AP, Connolly PA, Sagar M, et al. Transmission of *Histoplasma capsulatum* by organ transplantation. N Engl J Med 2000;343:1163–6.

18. Wheat LJ, Conces D, Allen SD, et al. Pulmonary histoplasmosis syndromes: recognition, diagnosis, and management. Semin Respir Crit Care Med 2004;25:129–44.

19. Gurney JW, Conces DJ. Pulmonary histoplasmosis. Radiology 1996;199:297–306.

20. Goodwin RA Jr, Owens FT, Snell JD, et al. Chronic pulmonary histoplasmosis. Medicine (Baltimore) 1976;55:413–52.

21. Landay MJ, Rollins NK. Mediastinal histoplasmosis granuloma: evaluation with CT. Radiology 1989; 172:657–9.

22. Parish JM, Rosenow EC III. Mediastinal granuloma and mediastinal fibrosis. Semin Respir Crit Care Med 2002;23:135–43.

23. Loyd JE, Tillman BF, Atkinson JB, et al. Mediastinal fibrosis complicating histoplasmosis. Medicine (Baltimore) 1988;67:295–310.

24. Davis A, Pierson D, Loyd JE. Mediastinal fibrosis. Semin Respir Infect 2001;16:119–30.

25. Doyle TP, Loyd JE, Robbins IM. Percutaneous pulmonary artery and vein stenting: a novel treatment for mediastinal fibrosis. Am J Respir Crit Care Med 2001;164:657–60.

26. Picardi JL, Kauffman CA, Schwarz J, et al. Pericarditis caused by *Histoplasma capsulatum*. Am J Cardiol 1976;37:82–8.

27. Wheat LJ, Stein L, Corya BC, et al. Pericarditis as a manifestation of histoplasmosis during two large urban outbreaks. Medicine (Baltimore) 1983;62: 110–9.

28. Goodwin RA Jr, Shapiro JL, Thurman GH, et al. Disseminated histoplasmosis: clinical and pathologic correlations. Medicine (Baltimore) 1980;59: 1–33.

29. Kirn DH, Fredericks D, McCutchan JA, et al. Serum ferritin levels correlate with disease activity in patients with AIDS and disseminated histoplasmosis. Clin Infect Dis 1995;21:1048–9.

30. Rouphael NG, Talati NJ, Vaughan C, et al. Infections associated with haemophagocytic syndrome. Lancet Infect Dis 2007;7:814–22.

31. Masri K, Mahon N, Rosario A, et al. Reactive hemophagocytic syndrome associated with disseminated histoplasmosis in a heart transplant recipient. J Heart Lung Transplant 2003;22:487–91.

32. Schestatsky P, Chedid MF, Amaral OB, et al. Isolated central nervous system histoplasmosis in immunocompetent hosts: a series of 11 cases. Scand J Infect Dis 2006;38:43–8.

33. Wheat LJ, Musial CE, Jenny-Avital E. Diagnosis and management of central nervous system histoplasmosis. Clin Infect Dis 2005;40:844–52.

34. Wheat LJ. Improvements in diagnosis of histoplasmosis. Expert Opin Biol Ther 2006;6:1207–21.

35. Fuller DD, Davis TE Jr, Denys GA, et al. Evaluation of BACTEC MYCO/F lytic medium for recovery of mycobacteria, fungi, and bacteria from blood. J Clin Microbiol 2001;39:2933–6.

36. Wheat LJ. Antigen detection, serology, and molecular diagnosis of invasive mycoses in the immunocompromised host. Transpl Infect Dis 2006;8: 128–39.

37. Kauffman CA. Diagnosis of histoplasmosis in immunosuppressed patients. Curr Opin Infect Dis 2008; 21:421–5.

38. Wheat LJ, Connolly-Stringfield P, Kohler RB, et al. *Histoplasma capsulatum* polysaccharide antigen detection in the diagnosis and management of disseminated histoplasmosis in patients with acquired immunodeficiency syndrome. Am J Med 1989;89:396–400.

39. Wheat LJ, Garringer T, Brizendine E, et al. Diagnosis of histoplasmosis by antigen detection based upon experience at the histoplasmosis reference laboratory. Diagn Microbiol Infect Dis 2002;43:29–37.

40. Connolly PA, Durkin MM, LeMonte AM, et al. Improvement in the detection of Histoplasma antigen by a quantitative immunoassay. Clin Vaccine Immunol 2007;14:1587–91.

41. LeMonte A, Egan L, Connolly P, et al. Evaluation of the IMMY ALPHA Histoplasma antigen enzyme immunoassay for diagnosis of histoplasmosis marked by antigenuria. Clin Vaccine Immunol 2007;14:802–3.

42. Cloud JL, Bauman SK, Pelfrey JM, et al. Biased report on the IMMY ALPHA Histoplasma antigen enzyme immunoassay for diagnosis of histoplasmosis. Clin Vaccine Immunol 2007;14:1389–91.

43. Wheat J, Wheat H, Connolly P, et al. Cross-reactivity in *Histoplasma capsulatum* variety capsulatum antigen assays of urine samples from patients with endemic mycoses. Clin Infect Dis 1997;24:1169–71.

44. Durkin M, Witt J, Lemonte A, et al. Antigen assay with the potential to aid in diagnosis of blastomycosis. J Clin Microbiol 2004;42:4873–5.

45. Wheat LJ, Hackett E, Durkin M, et al. Histoplasmosis-associated cross-reactivity in the BioRad platelia *Aspergillus* enzyme immunoassay. Clin Vaccine Immunol 2007;14:638–40.

46. Wheat LJ, Connolly-Stringfield P, Williams B, et al. Diagnosis of histoplasmosis in patients with the acquired immunodeficiency syndrome by detection of *Histoplasma capsulatum* polysaccharide antigen in bronchoalveolar lavage fluid. Am Rev Respir Dis 1992;145:1421–4.

47. Bialek R, Ernst F, Dietz K, et al. Comparison of staining methods and a nested PCR assay to detect *Histoplasma capsulatum* in tissue sections. Am J Clin Pathol 2002;117:597–603.

48. Bracca A, Tosello ME, Girardini JE, et al. Molecular detection of *Histoplasma capsulatum* var *capsulatum* in human clinical samples. J Clin Microbiol 2003;41:1753–5.

49. Wheat LJ, Freifeld AG, Kleiman MB, et al. Clinical practice guidelines for the management of patients with histoplasmosis: 2007 update by the Infectious Diseases Society of America. Clin Infect Dis 2007; 45:807–17.

50. Dismukes WE, Bradsher RW Jr, Cloud GC, et al. Itraconazole therapy for blastomycosis and histoplasmosis. Am J Med 1992;93:489–97.

51. Wheat J, Hafner R, Korzun AH, et al. Itraconazole treatment of disseminated histoplasmosis in patients with the acquired immunodeficiency syndrome. Am J Med 1995;98:336–42.

52. McKinsey DS, Kauffman CA, Pappas PG, et al. Fluconazole therapy for histoplasmosis. Clin Infect Dis 1996;23:996–1001.

53. Wheat J, Mawhinney S, Hafner R, et al. Treatment of histoplasmosis with fluconazole in patients with acquired immunodeficiency syndrome. Am J Med 1997;103:223–32.

54. Nath DS, Kandaswamy R, Gruessner R, et al. Fungal infections in transplant recipients receiving alemtuzumab. Transplant Proc 2005;37:934–6.

55. Restrepo A, Tobon A, Clark B, et al. Salvage treatment of histoplasmosis with posaconazole. J Infect 2007;54:319–27.

56. Clark B, Foster R, Tunbridge A, et al. A case of disseminated histoplasmosis successfully treated with the investigational drug posaconazole. J Infect 2005;51:e177–80.

57. Pitisuttithum P, Negroni R, Graybill JR, et al. Activity of posaconazole in the treatment of central nervous system fungal infections. J Antimicrob Chemother 2005;56:745–55.

58. Wheat LJ, Connolly P, Smedema M, et al. Activity of newer triazoles against *Histoplasma capsulatum* from patients with AIDS who failed fluconazole. J Antimicrob Chemother 2006;57:1235–9.

59. Johnson PC, Wheat LJ, Cloud GA, et al. Safety and efficacy of liposomal amphotericin B compared with conventional amphotericin B for induction therapy of histoplasmosis in patients with AIDS. Ann Intern Med 2002;137:105–9.

60. Wheat LJ, Cloud G, Johnson PC, et al. Clearance of fungal burden during treatment of disseminated histoplasmosis with liposomal amphotericin B versus itraconazole. Antimicrobial Agents Chemother 2001;45:2354–7.

61. Lenhart SW, Schafer MP, Singal M, et al. Histoplasmosis: protecting workers at risk. DHHS (NIOSH) Publication No. 97–146, 1997.

62. McKinsey DS, Wheat LJ, Cloud GA, et al. Itraconazole prophylaxis for fungal infections in patients with advanced human immunodeficiency virus infection: randomized, placebo-controlled, double-blind study. Clin Infect Dis 1999;28:1049–56.

63. Vail GM, Young RS, Wheat LJ, et al. Incidence of histoplasmosis following allogeneic bone marrow transplant or solid organ transplant in a hyperendemic area. Transpl Infect Dis 2002;4:148–51.

Blastomycosis: New Insights into Diagnosis, Prevention, and Treatment

James A. McKinnell, MD*, Peter G. Pappas, MD

KEYWORDS

- Blastomycosis • Blastomyces dermatitidis
- Antifungal agents/therapeutic use • Vaccine
- Endemic mycosis • Blastomyces adhesion 1

The basic science and clinical understanding of infection with *Blastomyces dermatitidis* has been a field of constant evolution and continued revision of hypotheses. In his original description of the disease in 1894, Thomas C. Gilchrist first suggested that blastomycosis was caused by a protozoan.[1] Shortly thereafter, Gilchrist disproved his own theory when he and Stokes recovered a fungal organism from the tissue of a patient.[2,3] Quantum advancements were made with the discovery that *B dermatitidis* caused systemic infection[4] and studies indicating that human inoculation usually occurs by way of the lungs with secondary dissemination.[5] Since these early studies, continued research has documented varied clinical manifestations of blastomycosis, explored epidemiology, described important pathogenesis, and led to breakthrough discoveries in specific antifungal therapy. Although many of these breakthrough studies have important implications for clinical care, they have not received significant attention in clinical literature.

Although comprehensive exploration of *B dermatitidis* research is outside the scope of this article, it highlights some areas in which recent progress has the potential for significant impact on the clinical care of patients. Specifically, this article examines the application of modern technology to epidemiologic studies, the development of novel vaccine candidates, emerging populations at risk for the disease, rapid diagnostic tools,

and the application of novel antifungal agents in the treatment of blastomycosis.

EPIDEMIOLOGY AND ECOLOGY

Attempts to define the epidemiology and ecology of *B dermatitidis* have proved more challenging than other endemic mycoses, but newly developed techniques and technologies for ecologic studies may soon lead to significant advancements in the field. Unlike histoplasmosis or coccidioidomycosis, there are no reliable skin tests or serologic assays to confirm previous infection with *B dermatitidis*.[6–8] As a result, our understanding of the geographic distribution, disease burden, and demographics of blastomycosis is based on case reporting. Ecologic studies of the organism have been limited by difficulty isolating the organism from soil[9–13] and the relatively short-lived conditions that support its growth.[14]

The traditional geographic distribution of blastomycosis has been restricted to southeastern and south central states that border the Mississippi and Ohio Rivers, the upper midwestern states, Canadian provinces near the great lakes, and a small area of New York and Canada adjacent to the St. Lawrence river (**Fig. 1**).[15,16] In more recent years, sporadic case reporting has identified the disease in Colorado, Texas, Kansas, and Nebraska.[17,18] Although these relatively isolated cases suggest that the geographic boundaries of

Division of Infectious Diseases, University of Alabama at Birmingham, THT 229, 1530 3rd Avenue South, Birmingham, AL 35294 0006, USA
* Corresponding author.
E-mail address: dr.mckinnell@yahoo.com (J.A. McKinnell).

Clin Chest Med 30 (2009) 227–239
doi:10.1016/j.ccm.2009.02.003

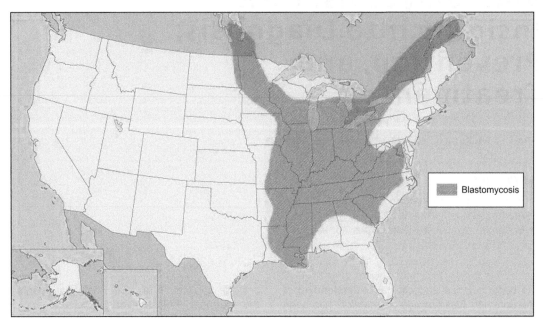

Fig. 1. The geographic distribution of *Blastomyces dermatitidis* in the continental Unites States. (*From* Watts B, Argekar P, Saint S, et al. Building a diagnosis from the ground up – a 49-year-old man came to the clinic with a 1-week history of suprapubic pain and fever. N Engl J Med 2007;356:1456–62; with permission. Copyright © 2007, Massachusetts Medical Society.)

blastomycosis are not rigid, the greatest burden of disease clearly lies within the traditional regions.

Attempts to estimate the burden of disease in the United States have met with some success. Within endemic regions, annual incidence estimates ranging from 0.3 to 1.8 cases per 100,000 have been reported by numerous studies.[13,19–22] More recently, a nationwide survey of hospitalizations showed that in certain regions as many as 7.4 hospital admissions per 1 million people are due to blastomycosis.[23] Given that these estimates are based on clinically confirmed cases of active disease, they underestimate the true burden of disease. In particular, it has been impossible to estimate the percentage of asymptomatic infections that go unreported.

The best-characterized epidemics of blastomycosis have occurred in Wisconsin and Ontario.[13,24,25] In contrast to previous reports, these studies do not support an independent association of age, race, or gender with *B dermatitidis* infection. Indeed, findings from both outbreaks indicate transmission is a geographically heterogeneous process, suggesting that previous reports of a male sex predominance and racial difference may have been more related to differences in exposure rather than intrinsic gender or racial differences. Studies in Wisconsin from 1986 to 1995 showed that incidence across 10 northern counties of the state ranged from 5.1 to

41.9 cases per 100,000 people.[26] Further analysis of this geographic heterogeneity uncovered subregions of hyperendemicity in the Eagle River area of Wisconsin and Kenora in northern Ontario (**Figs. 2 and 3**).[24,27]

On a microecologic scale, transmission of disease has long been linked to bodies of water.[27–32] The isolation of *B dermatitidis* from soil samples during an epidemic has allowed application of microecologic modeling to predict the presence of the fungus.[13,14,33] Modern methods of ecologic niche modeling allow for consolidation of multiple variables to more closely define characteristics associated with growth of the fungus.[34] This new technology has the potential to elucidate previously suspected microgeographic, seasonal, and climate conditions conducive to *B dermatitidis* primary infection.[25]

Further advancements in microecology have been made with geographic information systems (GIS). Similar to ecologic niche modeling, GIS systems capture, analyze and present multiple data variables, but using accurate global positioning systems have the ability to link these multiple variables to a specific location. Application of GIS technology has more specifically defined the types of watersheds that are at higher risk for blastomycosis. With close case-control methods, Baumgartner was able to describe an association with sandy rivers at less than 500 m

A

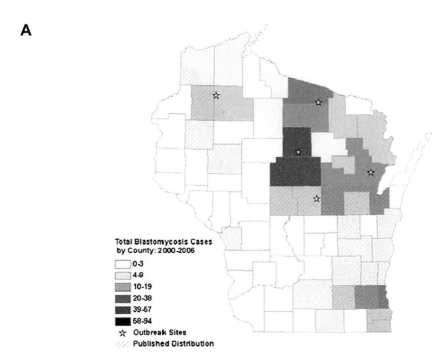

Total Blastomycosis Cases
by County: 2000-2006
- 0-3
- 4-9
- 10-19
- 20-38
- 39-57
- 58-94
☆ Outbreak Sites
/// Published Distribution

B

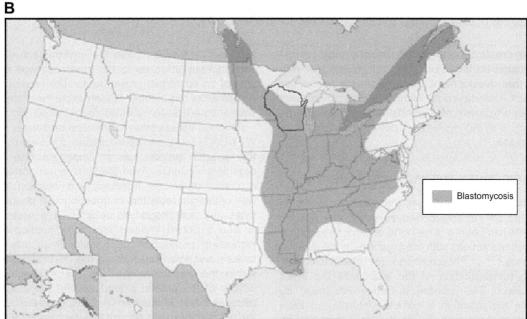

Blastomycosis

Fig. 2. Geographic distribution of *Blastomyces dermatitidis* in Wisconsin, 2000 to 2006. Clear variation exists between individual counties within the state despite close geographic proximity. (Fig. 2a: *From* Reed KD, Meece JK, Archer JR, et al. Ecologic niche modeling of Blastomyces dermatitidis in Wisconsin. PLoS ONE 2008;3(4):e2034. Fig. 2b: *From* Watts B, Argekar P, Saint S, et al. Building a diagnosis from the ground up – a 49-year-old man came to the clinic with a 1-week history of suprapubic pain and fever. N Engl J Med 2007;356:1456–62; with permission. Copyright © 2007, Massachusetts Medical Society.)

elevation. The authors connected these observations to differences in soil nutrients and drought conditions. They made similar observations about maximum lake depth and proposed an association with lake water mixing.[35] In a related study, associations with watersheds in urban areas were present.[36] These newer technologies combined with continued epidemiologic studies

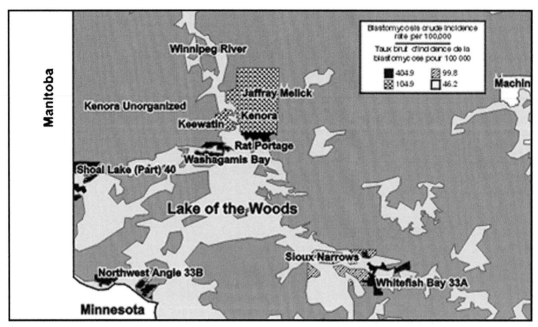

Fig. 3. Microgeographic distribution of *Blastomyces dermatitidis* in Kenora, Canada. Variation in burden of disease is evident on a local level, with clear areas of hyper endemic distribution. (*From* Dwight PJ, Naus M, Sarsfield P, et al. An outbreak of human blastomycosis: the epidemiology of blastomycosis in the Kenora catchment region of Ontario, Canada. Can Commun Dis Rep 2005;26(10):82–91.)

may create opportunities to further explore blastomycosis transmission. It is conceivable that with further development these information management systems could monitor for conditions that support growth of *B dermatitidis* and provide an early warning system for potential outbreaks of disease.

PATHOGENESIS AND VACCINE DEVELOPMENT

Since early observations that systemic infection with *B dermatitidis* follows an inhalation exposure, there has been a large body of work focusing on host interactions with the organism in the alveolar space.[5,15,37,38] Macrophages are critical to inhibiting transformation of the mold into the yeast phase.[39] The process is further influenced by lung surfactant in a complex interplay of local factors of immunity.[40] Unfortunately, investigation of *B dermatitidis* inhalation has not yet led to therapeutic or vaccine candidates. In contrast, recent research of the systemic host immune response has been promising.

T lymphocytes are the chief mediators of immunity to *B dermatitidis*.[41] Specifically, the TH-1 response is primarily responsible for effective immunologic control of infection.[42] The main antigen target for the human immune response has been identified as the WI-1 protein.[43,44] Study of the WI-1 antigen has shown that the protein is secreted by the yeast into the environment and subsequently attaches to the yeast cell wall by way of an epidermal growth factor–like receptor. As a result of this binding phenomenon, the protein was renamed blastomyces adhesion 1 (BAD1).[45–47]

Although the spectrum of immune responses to WI-1/BAD1 has yet to be elucidated, it is clear that this specific protein has an important role in organism virulence. WI-1/BAD1 is an important promoter of cellular adhesion and invasion by way of integrin receptors on mononuclear phagocytes and non-phagocytic cells.[47,48] The protein is also a potent immune modulator leading to increased production of transforming growth factor β and down-regulation of the TH-1 response within the alveolar space.[49,50] The modulatory effects of the protein extend beyond the lungs, because BAD1 blunts the TH-1 response outside the pulmonary space and impairs the complement cascade in peripheral blood.[51]

Investigation of the purified BAD1 protein as a potential target for vaccines or therapeutics has met with little success. Unfortunately, even in the presence of IL-12 as an adjuvant, this candidate vaccine did not lead to significant protective immunity.[52] In a related study looking at humoral responses, monoclonal antibodies to the protein were able to interfere with binding of the yeast to cells, but provided no protection to primary infection in vivo.[53]

An experimental strain of *B dermatitidis* lacking the BAD1 gene has resulted in a hypovirulent strain that might be a candidate for a live attenuated vaccine.[54]

Attempts to vaccinate mice with this attenuated yeast have shown promising results. In a healthy mouse model, the live attenuated vaccine showed significantly improved survival following experimental pulmonary infection.[55] In contrast to other T cell–mediated vaccines that have been developed for other bacterial and viral diseases, the attenuated *B dermatitidis* candidate affords durable immunity, more than 8 weeks after vaccination.[56–59] In experimental mice with interferon-γ and tumor necrosis factor-α cytokine deficiencies, immunity can still be attained after vaccination.[60] Although further exploration of the requisites for induction and maintenance of immunity are ongoing,[61–63] the plasticity of the vaccine suggests that it may have a role in patients who have an underlying immunodeficiency.[56] Early research into *B dermatitidis* pathogenesis has led to the possibility of a live attenuated vaccine for blastomycosis that can generate durable T cell–mediated immunity. An effective vaccine for blastomycosis would have significant implications for disease prevention and protection of at-risk populations.

CLINICAL MANIFESTATIONS AND NOVEL POPULATIONS

The range of clinical syndromes associated with blastomycosis infection is broad. Almost any organ system can be involved, with severity varying from mild to rapidly fatal. Most primary infections are asymptomatic or mild, usually go unrecognized, and resolve without treatment.[14,64,65] In contrast, acute respiratory distress syndrome (ARDS) due to *B dermatitidis* is a severe manifestation of disease, and is associated with a 50% to 89% mortality rate despite appropriate therapy.[66–69] There are many excellent reviews of the clinical presentation of blastomycosis[18,70–74]; this article provides a brief summary of common clinical syndromes and explores recent descriptions of the disease in novel populations.

The most common manifestation of blastomycosis infection is pulmonary involvement with either acute or chronic pneumonia. Patients who have acute pneumonia can present with mild flulike symptoms with nonproductive cough or more symptomatically with fever, productive cough, and pleuritic chest pain. Given the relatively nonspecific presentation, acute pneumonia due to *B dermatitidis* is rarely identified outside the

setting of epidemics and outbreak investigations and true incidence is unknown. Acute pulmonary blastomycosis typically resolves spontaneously without therapy.[15,31,75]

Chronic pneumonia is seen in 60% to 90% of patients who have proven *B dermatitidis* infection,[70] and is the most common clinical manifestation. Chronic pulmonary blastomycosis is characterized by low-grade fever, constitutional symptoms, and chronic cough with sputum production. Chest radiographs most commonly demonstrate nodular or lobar infiltrates, frequently with cavitations. Miliary disease, reticulonodular patterns, hilar adenopathy, and pleural effusion are reported but seen much less commonly.[76] In contrast to acute pneumonia, chronic pulmonary blastomycosis is an indolent process that tends to progress insidiously, although sudden clinical deterioration can occur.[74]

Cutaneous and subcutaneous involvement is the second most common manifestation of blastomycosis, and is seen in approximately 60% of patients. Although there are reports of disease due to direct inoculation, skin involvement is usually the result of secondary dissemination following inhalation exposure. Similar to pneumonia, skin and subcutaneous involvement have a multitude of clinical presentations. Cutaneous lesions are typically painless and most frequently on the head, neck, or extremities. Skin disease usually manifest as violaceous, ulcerative lesions or verrucous-type lesions that can be mistaken for squamous cell carcinoma or other chronic cutaneous infections. Patients may also present with subcutaneous nodules that often drain spontaneously and develop into chronic ulcerations with granulation and a necrotic border. Cutaneous disease is often a key component to diagnosis because tissue samples taken from the leading edge of the lesion yield a microscopic or culture diagnosis in 80% of cases.[74]

Other less common manifestations of extrapulmonary blastomycosis include osteoarticular disease, genitourinary involvement, and central nervous system involvement. Endocrine, cardiac, and ocular involvement are rarely reported.[15,64,71,77–80] With the exception of a few recent publications[81,82] that have added historical perspective on disease in the normal host, recent literature has focused on disease manifestation in the immunocompromised host.

Recognition and description of *B dermatitidis* infection in the expanding population of immunocompromised patients is a growing clinical problem and a current focus of interest. Reports from a retrospective study in Alabama have shown that between 1956 and 1977 only 2 of 75 patients (3%) who had blastomycosis were immunocompromised compared with 26 of 110 (24%) during the years 1978 to 1991. It is difficult to ascertain if this dramatic increase is due to a growing population of patients who have significant immune dysfunction or a markedly increased susceptibility to infection in the immunocompromised host. Unfortunately, published experience with blastomycosis in patients who have immunosuppression is relatively small. Nevertheless, a careful examination of available published reports suggests important differences in manifestations of disease and outcomes compared with the normal host.

Among patients who have undergone solid organ transplantation, published reports have primarily been limited to individual case reports or small case series.[83–90] The largest collection of solid organ transplant cases has come from the University of Wisconsin.[68] The experience of a major tertiary center within an endemic region suggests that blastomycosis is a rare complication following transplantation, affecting less than 1% of transplant patients.[68] Although rare in this population, the disease causes ARDS or miliary disease in 15% of transplant patients.[68,83] Because of the propensity for development of severe disease, most experts suggest that patients who have transplant-associated B dermatitidis infection be treated aggressively with a lipid formulation of amphotericin B initially.

Blastomycosis is known to occur in stem cell transplantation and in patients receiving chemotherapy, but there are few descriptions in these populations.[83,91,92] Current observations indicate that approximately 40% of these patients suffer rapidly fatal disseminated disease associated with ARDS and miliary infiltrates on chest radiographs. Infection in patients who have stem cell transplant and hematologic malignancies seem to have the most severe disease, associated with the poorest outcomes.

B dermatitidis infection among patients who have HIV is another novel population of interest. The disease has been most commonly described among those who have advanced HIV disease (CD4 < 200 cells/mL). It is believed that endogenous reactivation of disease may play an important role in up to 25% of AIDS-related cases.[18,93] Similar to other immunocompromised people, disease manifestations tend to be severe. Patients who have AIDS demonstrate central nervous system (CNS) involvement in 40% of cases. ARDS and miliary disease are seen almost in 20% of patients. Disease-related mortality approaches 40% in this population, with most deaths occurring within 3 weeks.[93]

Pregnant women are at risk for complicated infection with blastomycosis, likely because of pregnancy-related immune modulation.[94–99] When recognized and treated early, outcomes among these patients are similar to normal hosts who have blastomycosis. Although rare, intrauterine transmission has been described and does not seem to be associated with significant disease in the mother.[94,96,97]

Available published observations of blastomycosis in immunocompromised hosts indicate that disease is usually significantly more severe and is associated with a higher mortality. Extensive reviews of disease in the normal host have been previously published, and there exists an opportunity to systematically study blastomycosis in this growing population of patients. As our understanding of this disease in the immunocompromised host improves, clinicians will have more contextual data to inform their decisions on care and management of patients.

DIAGNOSIS

Delays in diagnosis have been a principle dilemma in the clinical care of patients who have blastomycosis. Given the chronic nature of the disease, nonspecific clinical presentation, and limited current diagnostic technology, approximately half of patients have symptoms for more than 1 month before a diagnosis is established.[80] Much of this delay is due to low clinical suspicion. In one study, the diagnosis was only suspected in 20% of patients at initial presentation.[73] In another study of patients who eventually died of blastomycosis, approximately two thirds were unsuspected at time of death or diagnosis was only made after the patient became gravely ill.[69] Improving the awareness of clinicians to the possibility of B dermatitidis infection is a key step to resolving the problem of delayed diagnosis.

Another significant factor in delay is that the diagnosis rests heavily on culture and histopathologic methods. As recently as 2002, a review of testing practices showed the diagnostic yield of culture to be remarkably high, 86% from sputum and 92% from bronchoscopic specimens. In the same review, however, the authors also found that clinicians only attempted rapid wet prep staining on 24% of sputum samples and 55% of bronchoscopic specimens.[100] A diagnostic strategy that relies on culture methods inevitably leads to significant delays because the organism may take several weeks to be isolated in culture. Cytologic and pathologic examinations in highly experienced centers have been shown to be specific, but the reproducibility of these results in less experienced centers is of concern. Fixed specimens can be sent for outside review or molecular methods of diagnosis.[101,102]

In addition to culture and histopathology, a crucial advancement in *B dermatitidis* diagnostics has been the development of rapid serologic assays. Historically, the clinical usefulness of serologic testing has been limited by lack of sensitivity and specificity. Purification of antigen and modern testing assays has resulted in promising, although not yet commercially viable, assays. Traditional serologic tests that depend on complement fixation (CF) or immunodiffusion (ID) techniques have yielded poor results.[100] The application of radioimmunoassay and ELISA has led to substantial improvements. For example, using the same antigen, comparison of CF with ID and ELISA demonstrated sensitivities of 9%, 28%, and 77%.[33] The dramatic improvements seen with these newer technologies have been reproduced in additional studies.[103–105]

Identification of novel antibody and antigen targets has created significant opportunities for new tests for *B dermatitidis*. The original antibody targets for serologic testing were based on unpurified filtrate specimens.[106,107] Targeting the more specific A-antigen yields sensitivity as high as 83%.[103,108] Unfortunately, the A-antigen serologic test is cross-reactive with *Histoplasma capsulatum*, limiting its clinical usefulness.[109] There was a brief attempt to commercialize the test (Premier Blastomyces Enzyme Immunoassay, Meridian Bioscience, Inc.), but it is currently not available.

The most recent attempt at developing a rapid and specific serologic test is based on the WI-1/BAD1 protein.[44] The BAD1 protein differs only slightly from the A-antigen, in that the BAD1 protein has no carbohydrate. The difference in molecular structure is important; carbohydrate seems to be the component of A-antigen that is cross-reactive to other endemic mycoses. Serologic tests using the WI-1/BAD1 assay do not cross-react with samples from patients who have histoplasmosis.[109] Attempts to use WI-1 antigen in a radioimmunoassay from patients in Wisconsin demonstrated 83% sensitivity and 95% specificity.[110] To our knowledge this rapid and specific serologic test is not yet commercially available, nor has the WI-1 antigen been evaluated with an ELISA-based assay.

Although serologic testing remains in the realm of research studies, techniques designed to look for antigen, as opposed to human antibodies, have lead to a commercially available, rapid diagnostic tool for blastomycosis. The routinely available assay (Miravista Diagnostics, Indianapolis, Indiana) can be used to detect *B dermatitidis* antigen in serum or urine samples. Both sandwich ELISA[111] and competitive binding inhibition ELISA[112] have been used to detect *B dermatitidis* antigen. Both are limited by significant cross-reactivity with *H capsulatum*, but current experience suggests that the antigen assays are extremely sensitive (93%), comparing favorably against serologic testing.[113] Furthermore, serial antigen assays may be a method to monitor disease progression.[114,115] As the role of antigen assays in clinical care is explored, attempts to separate *Histoplasma* antigen from *Blastomyces* antigen[116] and later-generation, more sensitive assays will help expand use into the clinical arena.[117] Regardless of the modality of choice, antigen assay or serologic testing, the field of rapid diagnostics for blastomycosis seems to be on the cusp of developing a specific, rapid assay with limited cross-reactivity to histoplasmosis.

TREATMENT

Recently released clinical practice guidelines support an approach of initial therapy with a lipid formulation of amphotericin B followed by consolidative therapy with itraconazole for patients who have moderately severe to severe forms of blastomycosis.[118,119] Data supporting amphotericin B use are strong; the medication has been shown effective in critically ill patients[120,121] and those who have CNS involvement.[122] Cure rates up to 97% have been reported in uncomplicated disease.[80,121,123] There are no comparative clinical trial efficacy data available, but animal data[124] and clinical experience[86,125–128] suggest that lipid formulations of amphotericin B are safer and as effective as amphotericin B deoxycholate; thus, these are preferred agents for treatment of severe blastomycosis.

Itraconazole has emerged as the preferred oral therapy for blastomycosis. Ketoconazole was plagued with significant adverse events and relatively high relapse rates (10%–14%).[80,118,129,130] Studies of fluconazole have been disappointing. Doses of 200 to 400 mg/d only led to cures in 65% of people.[131] Efficacy of fluconazole seems to be dose related, with efficacy approximately 87% at a fluconazole dose of 400 to 800 mg/d; these data compared favorably to itraconazole (90%–95%),[132] but the lower efficacy rates at standard doses of fluconazole has led most clinicians away from its use in the routine clinical setting. Because significantly higher doses (as much as 2 g/d) have been used in other fungal infections,[133] there may still be a role for fluconazole, although this has not been investigated. By comparison, itraconazole is reasonably been well tolerated and effective. A prospective trial using 200 mg of itraconazole per day showed cure rates of 90%, with rates approaching 95% in those who were compliant.[121,134] Higher doses of itraconazole (400 mg per day) did not significantly improve efficacy.[121,134]

Itraconazole has significant pharmacokinetic limitations. The oral capsule formulation depends on an acidic gastric environment for absorption.[135,136] Pharmacokinetic studies of the capsule form of itraconazole show inter- and intrasubject variability of drug absorption and metabolism.[137,138] Although oral itraconazole solution has improved absorption,[136,139,140] steady-state pharmacokinetics of itraconazole are not achieved for up to 2 weeks.[118] To adjust for irregular absorption of the drug, therapeutic monitoring of serum itraconazole concentration has been suggested.[118] A similar strategy has been used in histoplasmosis,[141,142] but adequate serum levels for successful treatment of blastomycosis and dose adjustment protocols for itraconazole have not been established.

To date, based on clinical data, there are few clear advantages of newer azoles over itraconazole for the treatment of blastomycosis. Voriconazole and posaconazole have shown impressive activity in animal models and in vitro testing.[143–147] Voriconazole has been used successfully for the treatment of blastomycosis.[68,127,148,149] It seems to be particularly promising in the management of CNS infections, and may be the oral drug of choice for this uncommon complication, but there are only limited reports of efficacy (see later discussion). There is little experience with posaconazole in the treatment of blastomycosis.

Blastomycosis involving the CNS is seen in less than 5% of healthy patients,[150] but as many as 40% of patients who have AIDS.[83,93] Guidelines support the use of a lipid formulation of amphotericin B compared with conventional amphotericin B based on a better safety profile[151] and limited published clinical experience.[127,128] Following initial therapy with amphotericin B, the choice of an oral agent for further therapy is unclear. Itraconazole has poor CNS penetration[152] and although fluconazole crosses the blood–brain barrier effectively, clinical failures have been described.[131,132,153,154] Voriconazole achieves good penetration into the CNS[147] and there have been several reports of successful therapy when used to treat CNS blastomycosis.[127,148,149] Voriconazole is well absorbed, but is associated with unpredictable serum levels, important drug–drug interactions, and significant adverse effects.[155–157]

In addition to drug selection, emerging developments in the management of the critically ill patient who has ARDS deserves mention. ARDS due to blastomycosis is associated with a 50% to 89% mortality rate.[66–69] Severe pulmonary disease may be more common in immunocompromised patients[67,83,93] and may represent a topic of growing concern for transplant and other immunosuppressed patients. Clinical experience suggests that a lipid formulation of amphotericin B should be used as initial therapy,[67,68] but given continued dismal results, many authors suggest a role for adjunctive steroids[158] and additional attention to endocrinologic manifestations, specifically adrenal insufficiency.[78,159] Further reports from medical centers in endemic areas will prove instrumental in clarifying the appropriate management of this severe clinical syndrome.

SUMMARY

Despite years of research and numerous sentinel discoveries, blastomycosis continues to present a challenge to the clinician and to the scientific community. Hobbled by the lack of rapid diagnostic testing, the clinician and epidemiologist are largely unable to rapidly identify the disease; this limits our understanding of the burden of disease, hampers our ability to identify people at risk, and leads to delayed treatment that may affect clinical care. Fortunately, innovations across several fields of study may lead to significant breakthroughs in the clinical care of blastomycosis. Description of *B dermatitidis* epidemiology and ecology is being revolutionized by modern information systems. Application of these information systems could lead to predictive models capable of providing more specific information regarding the risk for acquiring disease as it relates to geographic location and climate conditions. Similarly, recent pathophysiology research has led to improved diagnostic technology that has the potential to shorten time to diagnosis and initiation of appropriate therapy. With early reports that the newer azole antifungals may have a role in blastomycosis therapy, clinicians may be on the cusp of a new model of care. It is conceivable that blastomycosis could become a vaccine-preventable disease with an early warning system for potential outbreaks and clinical care may see options for rapid diagnostics and novel therapeutics.

REFERENCES

1. Gilchrist TC. Protozoan dermatitis. J Cutan Genitourin Dis 1894;12:496–9.
2. Gilchrist TC, Stokes WR. The presenece of an Oidium in the tissues of a case of pseudolupus vulgaris. Bull Johns Hopkins Hosp 1896;7:129–33.

3. Gilchrist TC, Stokes WR. A case of pseudolupus caused by blastomyces. J Exp Med 1898;3:53–78.
4. Martin DS, Smith DT. Blastomycosis. Am Rev Tuberc 1939;39:275–304, 488–515.
5. Schwarz J, Baum GL. Blastomycosis. Am J Clin Pathol 1951;21:999–1029.
6. Christie A, Peterson JC. Pulmonary calcifications in negative reactors to tuberculin. Am J Public Health 1945;35:1131–47.
7. Parsons RJ, Zaronfontis CJD. Histoplasmosis in man: report of 7 cases and a review of 71 cases. Arch Intern Med 1945;75:1–23.
8. Valdivia L, Nix D, Wright M, et al. Coccidioidomycosis as a common cause of community-acquired pneumonia. Emerg Infect Dis 2006;12:958–62.
9. Denton JF, Disalvo AF. Isolation of Blastomyces dermatitidis from natural sites at Augusta, Georgia. Am J Trop Med Hyg 1964;13:716–22.
10. Baumgardner DJ, Paretsky DP. The in vitro isolation of Blastomyces dermatitidis from a woodpile in north central Wisconsin, USA. Med Mycol 1999; 37:163–8.
11. Bakerspigel A, Kane J, Schaus D. Isolation of Blastomyces dermatitidis from an earthen floor in southwestern Ontario, Canada. J Clin Microbiol 1986;24: 890–1.
12. Sarosi GA, Serstock DS. Isolation of Blastomyces dermatitidis from pigeon manure. Am Rev Respir Dis 1976;114:1179–83.
13. Klein BS, Vergeront JM, DiSalvo AF, et al. Two outbreaks of blastomycosis along rivers in Wisconsin. Isolation of Blastomyces dermatitidis from riverbank soil and evidence of its transmission along waterways. Am Rev Respir Dis 1987;136:1333–8.
14. Klein BS, Vergeront JM, Weeks RJ, et al. Isolation of Blastomyces dermatitidis in soil associated with a large outbreak of blastomycosis in Wisconsin. N Engl J Med 1986;314:529–34.
15. Sarosi GA, Davies SF. Blastomycosis. Am Rev Respir Dis 1979;120:911–38.
16. Klein BS, Vergeront JM, Davis JP. Epidemiologic aspects of blastomycosis, the enigmatic systemic mycosis. Semin Respir Infect 1986;1:29–39.
17. De Groote MA, Bjerke R, Smith H, et al. Expanding epidemiology of blastomycosis: clinical features and investigation of 2 cases in Colorado. Clin Infect Dis 2000;30:582–4.
18. Pappas PG, Dismukes WE. Blastomycosis: Gilchrist's disease revisited. Curr Clin Top Infect Dis 2002;22:61–77.
19. Dworkin MS, Duckro AN, Proia L, et al. The epidemiology of blastomycosis in Illinois and factors associated with death. Clin Infect Dis 2005;41:e107–11.
20. Furcolow ML, Chick EW, Busey JF, et al. Prevalence and incidence studies of human and canine blastomycosis. 1. Cases in the United States, 1885-1968. Am Rev Respir Dis 1970;102:60–7.

21. Furcolow ML, Busey JF, Menges RW, et al. Prevalence and incidence studies of human and canine blastomycosis. II. Yearly incidence studies in three selected states, 1960–1967. Am J Epidemiol 1970; 92:121–31.
22. Cano MV, Ponce-de-Leon GF, Tippen S, et al. Blastomycosis in Missouri: epidemiology and risk factors for endemic disease. Epidemiol Infect 2003;131:907–14.
23. Chu JH, Feudtner C, Heydon K, et al. Hospitalizations for endemic mycoses: a population-based national study. Clin Infect Dis 2006;42:822–5.
24. Baumgardner DJ, Brockman K. Epidemiology of human blastomycosis in Vilas County, Wisconsin. II: 1991–1996. WMJ 1998;97:44–7.
25. Morris SK, Brophy J, Richardson SE, et al. Blastomycosis in Ontario, 1994–2003. Emerg Infect Dis 2006;12:274–9.
26. The Centers for Disease Control and Prevention. Blastomycosis–Wisconsin, 1986–1995. MMWR Morb Mortal Wkly Rep 1996;45:601–3.
27. Dwight PJ, Naus M, Sarsfield P, et al. An outbreak of human blastomycosis: the epidemiology of blastomycosis in the Kenora catchment region of Ontario, Canada. Can Commun Dis Rep 2000;26: 82–91.
28. Bradsher RW. Water and blastomycosis: don't blame beaver. Am Rev Respir Dis 1987;136: 1324–6.
29. Catherinot E, Rivaud E, Epardeau B, et al. A holiday in Canada. Lancet 2002;360:1564.
30. Parmar MS. Paradise – not without its plagues: overwhelming Blastomycosis pneumonia after visit to lakeside cottages in Northeastern Ontario. BMC Infect Dis 2005;5:30.
31. Vaaler AK, Bradsher RW, Davies SF. Evidence of subclinical blastomycosis in forestry workers in northern Minnesota and northern Wisconsin. Am J Med 1990;89:470–6.
32. Cockerill FR 3rd, Roberts GD, Rosenblatt JE, et al. Epidemic of pulmonary blastomycosis (Namekagon fever) in Wisconsin canoeists. Chest 1984;86: 688–92.
33. Klein BS, Vergeront JM, Kaufman L, et al. Serological tests for blastomycosis: assessments during a large point-source outbreak in Wisconsin. J Infect Dis 1987;155:262–8.
34. Reed KD, Meece JK, Archer JR, et al. Ecologic niche modeling of Blastomyces dermatitidis in Wisconsin. PLoS ONE 2008;3:e2034.
35. Baumgardner DJ, Steber D, Glazier R, et al. Geographic information system analysis of blastomycosis in northern Wisconsin, USA: waterways and soil. Med Mycol 2005;43:117–25.
36. Baumgardner DJ, Knavel EM, Steber D, et al. Geographic distribution of human blastomycosis cases in Milwaukee, Wisconsin, USA: association

with urban watersheds. Mycopathologia 2006;161: 275–82.

37. O'Neill RP, Penman RW. Clinical aspects of blastomycosis. Thorax 1970;25:708–15.

38. Wilson JW, Cawley EP, Weidman FD, et al. Primary cutaneous North American blastomycosis. AMA Arch Derm 1955;71:39–45.

39. Sugar AM, Picard M. Macrophage- and oxidant-mediated inhibition of the ability of live Blastomyces dermatitidis conidia to transform to the pathogenic yeast phase: implications for the pathogenesis of dimorphic fungal infections. J Infect Dis 1991;163:371–5.

40. Lekkala M, LeVine AM, Linke MJ, et al. Effect of lung surfactant collectins on bronchoalveolar macrophage interaction with Blastomyces dermatitidis: inhibition of tumor necrosis factor alpha production by surfactant protein D. Infect Immun 2006;74:4549–56.

41. Chang WL, Audet RG, Aizenstein BD, et al. T-cell epitopes and human leukocyte antigen restriction elements of an immunodominant antigen of Blastomyces dermatitidis. Infect Immun 2000;68:502–10.

42. Deepe GS Jr, Wuthrich M, Klein BS. Progress in vaccination for histoplasmosis and blastomycosis: coping with cellular immunity. Med Mycol 2005;43:381–9.

43. Klein BS, Sondel PM, Jones JM. WI-1, a novel 120-kilodalton surface protein on Blastomyces dermatitidis yeast cells, is a target antigen of cell-mediated immunity in human blastomycosis. Infect Immun 1992;60:4291–300.

44. Klein BS, Jones JM. Isolation, purification, and radiolabeling of a novel 120-kD surface protein on Blastomyces dermatitidis yeasts to detect antibody in infected patients. J Clin Invest 1990;85:152–61.

45. Brandhorst T, Wuthrich M, Finkel-Jimenez B, et al. A C-terminal EGF-like domain governs BAD1 localization to the yeast surface and fungal adherence to phagocytes, but is dispensable in immune modulation and pathogenicity of Blastomyces dermatitidis. Mol Microbiol 2003;48:53–65.

46. Brandhorst T, Klein B. Cell wall biogenesis of Blastomyces dermatitidis. Evidence for a novel mechanism of cell surface localization of a virulence-associated adhesin via extracellular release and reassociation with cell wall chitin. J Biol Chem 2000;275:7925–34.

47. Hogan LH, Josvai S, Klein BS. Genomic cloning, characterization, and functional analysis of the major surface adhesin WI-1 on Blastomyces dermatitidis yeasts. J Biol Chem 1995;270:30725–32.

48. Wiedemann A, Linder S, Grassl G, et al. Yersinia enterocolitica invasin triggers phagocytosis via beta1 integrins, CDC42Hs and WASp in macrophages. Cell Microbiol 2001;3:693–702.

49. Finkel-Jimenez B, Wuthrich M, Brandhorst T, et al. The WI-1 adhesin blocks phagocyte TNF-alpha production, imparting pathogenicity on Blastomyces dermatitidis. J Immunol 2001;166:2665–73.

50. Finkel-Jimenez B, Wuthrich M, Klein BS. BAD1, an essential virulence factor of Blastomyces dermatitidis, suppresses host TNF-alpha production through TGF-beta-dependent and -independent mechanisms. J Immunol 2002;168:5746–55.

51. Wuthrich M, Finkel-Jimenez B, Brandhorst TT, et al. Analysis of non-adhesive pathogenic mechanisms of BAD1 on Blastomyces dermatitidis. Med Mycol 2006;44:41–9.

52. Wuthrich M, Chang WL, Klein BS. Immunogenicity and protective efficacy of the WI-1 adhesin of Blastomyces dermatitidis. Infect Immun 1998;66:5443–9.

53. Wuthrich M, Klein BS. Investigation of anti-WI-1 adhesin antibody-mediated protection in experimental pulmonary blastomycosis. J Infect Dis 2000;181:1720–8.

54. Brandhorst TT, Wuthrich M, Warner T, et al. Targeted gene disruption reveals an adhesin indispensable for pathogenicity of Blastomyces dermatitidis. J Exp Med 1999;189:1207–16.

55. Wuthrich M, Filutowicz HI, Klein BS. Mutation of the WI-1 gene yields an attenuated blastomyces dermatitidis strain that induces host resistance. J Clin Invest 2000;106:1381–9.

56. Cutler JE, Deepe GS Jr, Klein BS. Advances in combating fungal diseases: vaccines on the threshold. Nat Rev Microbiol 2007;5:13–28.

57. Shedlock DJ, Shen H. Requirement for CD4 T cell help in generating functional CD8 T cell memory. Science 2003;300:337–9.

58. Shen H, Whitmire JK, Fan X, et al. A specific role for B cells in the generation of CD8 T cell memory by recombinant Listeria monocytogenes. J Immunol 2003;170:1443–51.

59. Sun JC, Bevan MJ. Defective CD8 T cell memory following acute infection without CD4 T cell help. Science 2003;300:339–42.

60. Wuthrich M, Filutowicz HI, Warner T, et al. Requisite elements in vaccine immunity to Blastomyces dermatitidis: plasticity uncovers vaccine potential in immune-deficient hosts. J Immunol 2002;169:6969–76.

61. Wuthrich M, Warner T, Klein BS. CD28 is required for optimal induction, but not maintenance, of vaccine-induced immunity to Blastomyces dermatitidis. Infect Immun 2005;73:7436–41.

62. Wuthrich M, Warner T, Klein BS. IL-12 is required for induction but not maintenance of protective, memory responses to Blastomyces dermatitidis: implications for vaccine development in immune-deficient hosts. J Immunol 2005;175:5288–97.

63. Wuthrich M, Fisette PL, Filutowicz HI, et al. Differential requirements of T cell subsets for CD40 costimulation in immunity to Blastomyces dermatitidis. J Immunol 2006;176:5538–47.

64. Recht LD, Philips JR, Eckman MR, et al. Self-limited blastomycosis: a report of thirteen cases. Am Rev Respir Dis 1979;120:1109–12.

65. Tosh FE, Hammerman KJ, Weeks RJ, et al. A common source epidemic of North American blastomycosis. Am Rev Respir Dis 1974;109: 525–9.

66. Lemos LB, Baliga M, Guo M. Acute respiratory distress syndrome and blastomycosis: presentation of nine cases and review of the literature. Ann Diagn Pathol 2001;5:1–9.

67. Meyer KC, McManus EJ, Maki DG. Overwhelming pulmonary blastomycosis associated with the adult respiratory distress syndrome. N Engl J Med 1993; 329:1231–6.

68. Gauthier GM, Safdar N, Klein BS, et al. Blastomycosis in solid organ transplant recipients. Transpl Infect Dis 2007;9:310–7.

69. Vasquez JE, Mehta JB, Agrawal R, et al. Blastomycosis in northeast Tennessee. Chest 1998;114: 436–43.

70. Abernathy RS. Clinical manifestations of pulmonary blastomycosis. Ann Intern Med 1959;51:707–27.

71. Bradsher RW. Clinical features of blastomycosis. Semin Respir Infect 1997;12:229–34.

72. Bradsher RW, Chapman SW, Pappas PG. Blastomycosis. Infect Dis Clin North Am 2003;17:21–40, vii.

73. Lemos LB, Baliga M, Guo M. Blastomycosis: The great pretender can also be an opportunist. Initial clinical diagnosis and underlying diseases in 123 patients. Ann Diagn Pathol 2002;6:194–203.

74. Kwon-Chung KJ, Bennett JE. Medical mycology. Philadelphia: Lea & Febiger; 1992.

75. Sarosi GA, Davies SF, Phillips JR. Self-limited blastomycosis: a report of 39 cases. Semin Respir Infect 1986;1:40–4.

76. Brown LR, Swensen SJ, Van Scoy RE, et al. Roentgenologic features of pulmonary blastomycosis. Mayo Clin Proc 1991;66:29–38.

77. Halvorsen RA, Duncan JD, Merten DF, et al. Pulmonary blastomycosis: radiologic manifestations. Radiology 1984;150:1–5.

78. Witorsch P, Utz JP. North American blastomycosis: a study of 40 patients. Medicine (Baltimore) 1968; 47:169–200.

79. Moore RM, Green NE. Blastomycosis of bone. A report of six cases. J Bone Joint Surg Am 1982;64:1097–101.

80. Chapman SW, Lin AC, Hendricks KA, et al. Endemic blastomycosis in Mississippi: epidemiological and clinical studies. Semin Respir Infect 1997;12:219–28.

81. Pariseau B, Lucarelli MJ, Appen RE. A concise history of ophthalmic blastomycosis. Ophthalmology 2007;114:e27–32.

82. Gottlieb JR, Eismont FJ. Nonoperative treatment of vertebral blastomycosis osteomyelitis associated with paraspinal abscess and cord compression. A case report. J Bone Joint Surg Am 2006;88:854–6.

83. Pappas PG, Threlkeld MG, Bedsole GD, et al. Blastomycosis in immunocompromised patients. Medicine (Baltimore) 1993;72:311–25.

84. Butka BJ, Bennett SR, Johnson AC. Disseminated inoculation blastomycosis in a renal transplant recipient. Am Rev Respir Dis 1984;130:1180–3.

85. Hii JH, Legault L, DeVeber G, et al. Successful treatment of systemic blastomycosis with high-dose ketoconazole in a renal transplant recipient. Am J Kidney Dis 1990;15:595–7.

86. Linden P, Williams P, Chan KM. Efficacy and safety of amphotericin B lipid complex injection (ABLC) in solid-organ transplant recipients with invasive fungal infections. Clin Transplant 2000;14:329–39.

87. Pechan WB, Novick AC, Lalli A, et al. Pulomary nodules in a renal transplant recipient. J Urol 1980;124:111–4.

88. Serody JS, Mill MR, Detterbeck FC, et al. Blastomycosis in transplant recipients: report of a case and review. Clin Infect Dis 1993;16:54–8.

89. Walker K, Skelton H, Smith K. Cutaneous lesions showing giant yeast forms of Blastomyces dermatitidis. J Cutan Pathol 2002;29:616–8.

90. Winkler S, Stanek G, Hubsch P, et al. Pneumonia due to blastomyces dermatitidis in a European renal transplant recipient. Nephrol Dial Transplant 1996;11:1376–9.

91. Isotalo PA, Ford JC, Veinot JP. Miliary blastomycosis developing in an immunocompromised host with chronic lymphocytic leukaemia. Pathology 2002;34:293–5.

92. Kauffman CA. Endemic mycoses in patients with hematologic malignancies. Semin Respir Infect 2002;17:106–12.

93. Pappas PG, Pottage JC, Powderly WG, et al. Blastomycosis in patients with the acquired immunodeficiency syndrome. Ann Intern Med 1992;116:847–53.

94. Lemos LB, Soofi M, Amir E. Blastomycosis and pregnancy. Ann Diagn Pathol 2002;6:211–5.

95. Ismail MA, Lerner SA. Disseminated blastomycosis in a pregnant woman: review of amphotericin B usage during pregnancy. Am Rev Respir Dis 1982;126:350–3.

96. Tuthill SW. Disseminated blastomycosis with intra-uterine transmission. South Med J 1985;78:1526–7.

97. Maxson S, Miller SF, Tryka AF, et al. Perinatal blastomycosis: a review. Pediatr Infect Dis J 1992;11:760–3.

98. MacDonald D, Alguire PC. Adult respiratory distress syndrome due to blastomycosis during pregnancy. Chest 1990;98:1527–8.

99. Young L, Schutze GE. Perinatal blastomycosis: the rest of the story. Pediatr Infect Dis J 1995;14:83.

100. Martynowicz MA, Prakash UB. Pulmonary blastomycosis: an appraisal of diagnostic techniques. Chest 2002;121:768–73.

101. Kappe R, Okeke CN, Fauser C, et al. Molecular probes for the detection of pathogenic fungi in the presence of human tissue. J Med Microbiol 1998;47:811–20.

102. Bialek R, Gonzalez GM, Begerow D, et al. Coccidioidomycosis and blastomycosis: advances in molecular diagnosis. FEMS Immunol Med Microbiol 2005;45:355–60.

103. Bradsher RW, Pappas PG. Detection of specific antibodies in human blastomycosis by enzyme immunoassay. South Med J 1995;88:1256–9.

104. Lambert RS, George RB. Evaluation of enzyme immunoassay as a rapid screening test for histoplasmosis and blastomycosis. Am Rev Respir Dis 1987;136:316–9.

105. Lo CY, Notenboom RH. A new enzyme immunoassay specific for blastomycosis. Am Rev Respir Dis 1990;141:84–8.

106. Kaufman L, McLaughlin DW, Clark MJ, et al. Specific immunodiffusion test for blastomycosis. Appl Microbiol 1973;26:244–7.

107. Martin DS. Serologic studies on North American blastomycosis; studies with soluble antigens from untreated and sonic-treated yeast-phase cells of Blastomyces dermatitidis. J Immunol 1953;71:192–201.

108. Green JH, Harrell WK, Johnson JE, et al. Preparation of reference antisera for laboratory diagnosis of blastomycosis. J Clin Microbiol 1979;10:1–7.

109. Klein BS, Jones JM. Purification and characterization of the major antigen WI-1 from Blastomyces dermatitidis yeasts and immunological comparison with A antigen. Infect Immun 1994;62:3890–900.

110. Soufleris AJ, Klein BS, Courtney BT, et al. Utility of anti-WI-1 serological testing in the diagnosis of blastomycosis in Wisconsin residents. Clin Infect Dis 1994;19:87–92.

111. Durkin M, Witt J, Lemonte A, et al. Antigen assay with the potential to aid in diagnosis of blastomycosis. J Clin Microbiol 2004;42:4873–5.

112. Shurley JF, Legendre AM, Scalarone GM. Blastomyces dermatitidis antigen detection in urine specimens from dogs with blastomycosis using a competitive binding inhibition ELISA. Mycopathologia 2005;160:137–42.

113. Spector D, Legendre AM, Wheat J, et al. Antigen and antibody testing for the diagnosis of blastomycosis in dogs. J Vet Intern Med 2008;22:839–43.

114. Tarr M, Marcinak J, Mongkolrattanothai K, et al. Blastomyces antigen detection for monitoring progression of blastomycosis in a pregnant adolescent. Infect Dis Obstet Gynecol 2007; [article 89059].

115. Mongkolrattanothai K, Peev M, Wheat LJ, et al. Urine antigen detection of blastomycosis in pediatric patients. Pediatr Infect Dis J 2006;25:1076–8.

116. Shurley JF, Scalarone GM. Isoelectric focusing and ELISA evaluation of a Blastomyces dermatitidis human isolate. Mycopathologia 2007;164:73–6.

117. Hage CA, Davis TE, Egan L, et al. Diagnosis of pulmonary histoplasmosis and blastomycosis by detection of antigen in bronchoalveolar lavage fluid using an improved second-generation enzyme-linked immunoassay. Respir Med 2007;101:43–7.

118. Chapman SW, Dismukes WE, Proia LA, et al. Clinical practice guidelines for the management of blastomycosis: 2008 update by the Infectious Diseases Society of America. Clin Infect Dis 2008;46:1801–12.

119. Bradsher RW Jr. Pulmonary blastomycosis. Semin Respir Crit Care Med 2008;29:174–81.

120. Parker JD, Doto IL, Tosh FE. A decade of experience with blastomycosis and its treatment with amphotericin B. A National Communicable Disease Center Cooperative Mycoses Study. Am Rev Respir Dis 1969;99:895–902.

121. Bradsher RW. Histoplasmosis and blastomycosis. Clin Infect Dis 1996;22(Suppl 2):S102–11.

122. Friedman JA, Wijdicks EF, Fulgham JR, et al. Meningoencephalitis due to Blastomyces dermatitidis: case report and literature review. Mayo Clin Proc 2000;75:403–8.

123. Abernathy RS. Amphotericin therapy of North American blastomycosis. Antimicrobial Agents Chemother (Bethesda) 1966;6:208–11.

124. Clemons KV, Stevens DA. Comparative efficacies of amphotericin B lipid complex and amphotericin B deoxycholate suspension against murine blastomycosis. Antimicrobial Agents Chemother 1991; 35:2144–6.

125. Cook PP. Amphotericin B lipid complex for the treatment of recurrent blastomycosis of the brain in a patient previously treated with itraconazole. South Med J 2001;94:548–9.

126. Perfect JR. Treatment of non-Aspergillus moulds in immunocompromised patients, with amphotericin B lipid complex. Clin Infect Dis 2005;40(Suppl 6): S401–8.

127. Panicker J, Walsh T, Kamani N. Recurrent central nervous system blastomycosis in an immunocompetent child treated successfully with sequential liposomal amphotericin B and voriconazole. Pediatr Infect Dis J 2006;25:377–9.

128. Chowfin A, Tight R, Mitchell S. Recurrent blastomycosis of the central nervous system: case report and review. Clin Infect Dis 2000;30:969–71.

129. Treatment of blastomycosis and histoplasmosis with ketoconazole. Results of a prospective randomized clinical trial. National Institute of Allergy and Infectious Diseases Mycoses Study Group. Ann Intern Med 1985;103:861–72.

130. Bradsher RW, Rice DC, Abernathy RS. Ketoconazole therapy for endemic blastomycosis. Ann Intern Med 1985;103:872–9.

131. Pappas PG, Bradsher RW, Chapman SW, et al. Treatment of blastomycosis with fluconazole: a pilot

study. The National Institute of Allergy and Infectious Diseases Mycoses Study Group. Clin Infect Dis 1995;20:267–71.

132. Pappas PG, Bradsher RW, Kauffman CA, et al. Treatment of blastomycosis with higher doses of fluconazole. The National Institute of Allergy and Infectious Diseases Mycoses Study Group. Clin Infect Dis 1997;25:200–5.

133. Galgiani JN, Ampel NM, Blair JE, et al. Coccidioidomycosis. Clin Infect Dis 2005;41:1217–23.

134. Dismukes WE, Bradsher RW Jr, Cloud GC, et al. Itraconazole therapy for blastomycosis and histoplasmosis. NIAID Mycoses Study Group. Am J Med 1992;93:489–97.

135. Barone JA, Koh JG, Bierman RH, et al. Food interaction and steady-state pharmacokinetics of itraconazole capsules in healthy male volunteers. Antimicrobial Agents Chemother 1993;37:778–84.

136. Cartledge JD, Midgely J, Gazzard BG. Itraconazole solution: higher serum drug concentrations and better clinical response rates than the capsule formulation in acquired immunodeficiency syndrome patients with candidosis. J Clin Pathol 1997;50:477–80.

137. Hardin TC, Graybill JR, Fetchick R, et al. Pharmacokinetics of itraconazole following oral administration to normal volunteers. Antimicrobial Agents Chemother 1988;32:1310–3.

138. Poirier JM, Berlioz F, Isnard F, et al. Marked intra- and inter-patient variability of itraconazole steady state plasma concentrations. Therapie 1996;51:163–7.

139. Stevens DA. Itraconazole in cyclodextrin solution. Pharmacotherapy 1999;19:603–11.

140. Barone JA, Moskovitz BL, Guarnieri J, et al. Enhanced bioavailability of itraconazole in hydroxypropyl-beta-cyclodextrin solution versus capsules in healthy volunteers. Antimicrobial Agents Chemother 1998;42:1862–5.

141. Huet E, Hadji C, Hulin A, et al. Therapeutic monitoring is necessary for the association itraconazole and efavirenz in a patient with AIDS and disseminated histoplasmosis. AIDS 2008;22:1885–6.

142. Koo HL, Hamill RJ, Andrade RA. Drug-drug interaction between itraconazole and efavirenz in a patient with AIDS and disseminated histoplasmosis. Clin Infect Dis 2007;45:e77–9.

143. Li RK, Ciblak MA, Nordoff N, et al. In vitro activities of voriconazole, itraconazole, and amphotericin B against Blastomyces dermatitidis, Coccidioides immitis, and Histoplasma capsulatum. Antimicrobial Agents Chemother 2000;44:1734–6.

144. Espinel-Ingroff A. Comparison of In vitro activities of the new triazole SCH56592 and the echinocandins MK-0991 (L-743,872) and LY303366 against opportunistic filamentous and dimorphic fungi and yeasts. J Clin Microbiol 1998;36:2950–6.

145. Sugar AM, Liu XP. In vitro and in vivo activities of SCH 56592 against Blastomyces dermatitidis. Antimicrobial Agents Chemother 1996;40:1314–6.

146. Sugar AM, Liu XP. Efficacy of voriconazole in treatment of murine pulmonary blastomycosis. Antimicrobial Agents Chemother 2001;45:601–4.

147. Lutsar I, Roffey S, Troke P. Voriconazole concentrations in the cerebrospinal fluid and brain tissue of guinea pigs and immunocompromised patients. Clin Infect Dis 2003;37:728–32.

148. Bakleh M, Aksamit AJ, Tleyjeh IM, et al. Successful treatment of cerebral blastomycosis with voriconazole. Clin Infect Dis 2005;40:e69–71.

149. Borgia SM, Fuller JD, Sarabia A, et al. Cerebral blastomycosis: a case series incorporating voriconazole in the treatment regimen. Med Mycol 2006;44:659–64.

150. Lemos LB, Guo M, Baliga M. Blastomycosis: organ involvement and etiologic diagnosis. A review of 123 patients from Mississippi. Ann Diagn Pathol 2000;4:391–406.

151. Groll AH, Giri N, Petraitis V, et al. Comparative efficacy and distribution of lipid formulations of amphotericin B in experimental Candida albicans infection of the central nervous system. J Infect Dis 2000;182:274–82.

152. Harley WB, Lomis M, Haas DW. Marked polymorphonuclear pleocytosis due to blastomycotic meningitis: case report and review. Clin Infect Dis 1994;18:816–8.

153. Pearson GJ, Chin TW, Fong IW. Case report: treatment of blastomycosis with fluconazole. Am J Med Sci 1992;303:313–5.

154. Taillan B, Ferrari E, Cosnefroy JY, et al. Favourable outcome of blastomycosis of the brain stem with fluconazole and flucytosine treatment. Ann Med 1992;24:71–2.

155. Johnson LB, Kauffman CA. Voriconazole: a new triazole antifungal agent. Clin Infect Dis 2003;36:630–7.

156. Smith J, Safdar N, Knasinski V, et al. Voriconazole therapeutic drug monitoring. Antimicrobial Agents Chemother 2006;50:1570–2.

157. Denning DW, Ribaud P, Milpied N, et al. Efficacy and safety of voriconazole in the treatment of acute invasive aspergillosis. Clin Infect Dis 2002;34:563–71.

158. Lahm T, Neese S, Thornburg AT, et al. Corticosteroids for blastomycosis-induced ARDS: a report of two patients and review of the literature. Chest 2008;133:1478–80.

159. Abernathy RS, Melby JC. Addison's disease in North American blastomycosis. N Engl J Med 1962;266:552–4.

Coccidioidomycosis: A Review of Recent Advances

Neil M. Ampel, MD

KEYWORDS

• Coccidioidomycosis • Coccidioides • Fungi

Coccidioidomycosis is one of three dimorphic endemic mycoses recognized in North America. Over the past decade, the disease has been resurgent, particularly in the southwest United States.[1] With this increase in incidence have come new observations and insights and reexamination of past issues. This article explores some of these areas by focusing principally on recent publications that are of importance.

DISCOVERY AND EARLY HISTORY

Odds[2] and Hirschmann[3] have recently augmented our understanding of the early history of coccidioidomycosis and have added to the excellent histories of Smith[4] and Deresinki.[5] The disease was first described in 1892 by Alejandro Posadas, an Argentinean medical student. The patient, Domingo Escurra, was a soldier serving in northern Argentina who presented with several years of progressive cutaneous lesions of the face, arm, and trunk. Posadas examined the material from Escurra's lesions and saw organisms resembling protozoa. In 1894, Thorne and Rixford[6,7] presented the clinical histories of two similar cases in California involving Azorean emigrants. Subsequently, Rixford and Gilchrist[8] exhaustively reviewed these cases, including their pathology.

For the next 20 years coccidioidomycosis was considered to be a disfiguring, frequently fatal illness. Observations suggested that in many instances, however, coccidioidomycosis followed a more benign course. Most striking was the case of Harold Chope, a medical student at Stanford University, who accidentally inhaled a culture of Coccidioides in 1929. After initial pulmonary symptoms and the development of erythema nodosum, he subsequently completely recovered.[3,9] Following this, Dixon began exploring a symptom complex known as "Valley Fever," consisting of cough, pleuritic chest pain, fever, and rash, frequently seen in the San Joaquin Valley of California. He found that it was common to isolate Coccidioides from the sputum of such patients, that the patients frequently manifested strong reactions to coccidioidal skin tests, and the patients usually completely recovered. In collaboration with Giffords, cases of Valley Fever were carefully detailed.[10] Coccidioidomycosis was now seen as a relatively benign pulmonary infection.

The early history of coccidioidomycosis ends with Charles E. Smith. With his coworkers, he was able to describe the panoply of manifestations that occurs with coccidioidal infection, from benign pulmonary illness to disease disseminated beyond the thoracic cavity. In addition, Smith and his colleagues[11] developed important diagnostic tools, such as the coccidioidin skin test and serologic tests, that remain useful to this day. In one landmark study Smith and his colleagues performed a prospective study at four army air fields in the San Joaquin Valley. Using a questionnaire and repeated testing with the skin test reagent coccidioidin, he was able to demonstrate that 60% of new cases of coccidioidal infection were completely asymptomatic. Moreover, he showed that people who lose or never demonstrate skin test reactivity are more likely to develop disseminated disease outside of the thoracic cavity. He also found that disseminated disease was more likely among black army corpsman and that they

College of Medicine, University of Arizona, Medical Service (1-111), SAVAHCS, 3601 South Sixth Avenue, Tucson, AZ 85723, USA
E-mail address: nampel@email.arizona.edu

Clin Chest Med 30 (2009) 241–251
doi:10.1016/j.ccm.2009.02.004
0272-5231/09/$ – see front matter. Published by Elsevier Inc.

were less likely to manifest coccidioidin reactivity. Finally, he and his colleagues showed that meningitis was the one form of disseminated coccidioidomycosis that could occur in the face of a persistently positive coccidioidin skin test.

THE ORGANISM

In 1896, Rixford and Gilchrist[8] named the organism that they identified Coccidioides immitis and considered it protozoan in nature. Ophüls[12] was subsequently able to prove that the organism was a fungus and showed that it was dimorphic. Although structures consistent with classification of Coccidioides as an ascomycetous fungus had been observed, further taxonomy was stymied for many years because of a lack of evidence of sexual reproduction. Molecular methods that became available in the 1990s, however, allowed for improved analysis of the evolutionary relationship between Coccidioides and other fungi. For example, Bowman and colleagues[13] analyzed 18S ribosomal DNA sequences among C immitis and found it was closely related to two pathogenic ascomycetes, Histoplasma capsulatum and Blastomyces dermatitidis. Pan and colleagues,[14] using a combination of biochemical, immunologic, and genetic analyses, were able to demonstrate a close relationship between C immitis and Uncinocarpus reseii, a nonpathogenic species of Malbranchea.

Although there is still no direct observation of sexual reproduction by Coccidioides, there has been accumulating evidence for genetic recombination. Burt and colleagues[15] examined 30 clinical isolates of Coccidioides using population and phylogenetic analysis and found that biparental sex is a regular part of the life cycle of Coccidioides. Koufopanou and coworkers[16] observed two reproductively isolated groups by examining five different genes of Coccidioides. More recently, Mandel and colleagues[17] have shown that Coccidioides contains mating-type loci similar to those found in other sexually reproducing ascomycetes. Moreover, they were able to identify these loci in 3 of 11 geographic isolates. It had been assumed that only asexual spores were produced in the environment, but these data challenge that assumption.

During the last decade, M.C. Fisher and colleagues[18] have further defined the phylogeny of Coccidioides. Using patient isolates of Coccidioides from a 1993 to 1994 epidemic of coccidioidomycosis in Kern County, California, they examined two classes of genetic markers: single nucleotide polymorphisms (SNPs) and short tandem repeats (STRs). The data demonstrated that there was extensive genetic diversity in the fungal isolates, precluding the concept that the epidemic was due to the emergence of a pathogenic clone of Coccidioides. In another study, examining nine microsatellite loci of 161 clinical and two environmental isolates, they were able to demonstrate geographic partitioning of the organism in North America, with clustering in the San Joaquin Valley of California, in Arizona, and in Texas. Among South American isolates, there was limited geographic diversity, which seemed to have evolved from a single clade in Texas some 9000 to 140,000 years ago. They postulated that this evolution was consistent with dispersal through a mammalian host and suggested that Coccidioides could have arrived in South America coincident with man.[19] The work culminated with the recognition that the fungus genetically consisted of two species. The name C immitis was retained for a species that seems to be geographically limited to the San Joaquin Valley. The new species, C posadasii, was named for Posadas, who described the first case. This species inhabits all other coccidioidal endemic regions.[20] Although this genetic speciation has been confirmed,[21] there are concerns regarding speciation on other levels. For example, little or no morphologic difference exists between them and there are no apparent clinical or immunologic differences when infection occurs by the two different Coccidioides species.

ECOLOGY AND CLIMATE

Although Coccidioides has been frequently cultured from clinical material, it was not isolated from the environment until 1932 when it was found in soil from beneath a bunk house in Delano, California, where cases of coccidioidomycosis had occurred.[22] Subsequent efforts to consistently isolate Coccidioides from the environment have been less than fruitful, particularly in recent years. For example, Greene and colleagues[23] were only able to isolate the organism four times in 720 specimens using molecular techniques; this has made it difficult to ascertain the soil attributes that sustain Coccidioides.

F.S. Fisher and colleagues have examined sites where Coccidioides has consistently been isolated or where human infection has been known to have repeatedly occurred. Their interest started with an outbreak of coccidioidomycosis in 2001 in Dinosaur National Monument in northeastern Utah, an area well outside the known endemic region for coccidioidomycosis. In that instance, 10 individuals developed coccidioidomycosis after working in an Amerindian archaeologic site named Swelter Shelter, a south-facing indentation in a sandstone cliff with a rock overhang. Notably, workers excavating Swelter Shelter in 1964 to 1965 may have also developed coccidioidomycosis.[24] Using this site and three others, various soil conditions were examined at depths between 2 and 20 cm. At these sites, median temperatures ranged from 11.7°C to 27.9°C. Soils tended to be fine and silty have less than 10% clay. Vegetation type did not predict whether coccidioidomycosis was associated with a particular site.[25] These data suggest that Coccidioides resides in specific geoclimatic foci and may persist there for prolonged periods.

Coccidioidomycosis has been frequently linked to climatic factors but until recently there have been few systemic explorations of meteorologic factors associated with the development of infection. Using reports of symptomatic cases of coccidioidomycosis in Pima County, Arizona from 1948 through 1998 in combination with monthly climate data for southeastern Arizona, Kolivras and Comrie[26] were able to develop a predictive model. This model gained validation when it was independently applied to Maricopa County, Arizona using data from 1998 to 2001.[27] Factors such as the Palmer drought severity index, wind velocity, temperature and cumulative rainfall 7 months prior were significantly associated with an increased risk for coccidioidomycosis in subsequent months or even years. Although still imperfect, particularly because the model relies on reports of symptomatic cases rather than soil isolates of Coccidioides, such multifactorial models suggest that climate plays an important role in the risk for developing coccidioidomycosis within endemic regions.

EPIDEMIOLOGY

Arizona currently accounts for 60% of all cases of symptomatic coccidioidomycosis reported in the United States. In 2006 there were more than 5000 cases reported to the state and only slightly less than this in 2007.[28] The incidence of reported cases in Arizona was first noticed to increase in the early 1990s,[29] increasing from 7 cases per 100,000 in 1990 to nearly 15 per 100,000 in 1995. Cases were concentrated in four counties, Maricopa, Pima, Pinal, and Mohave, which contained 80% of the state's population. Men and older individuals, particularly those older than 60 years, were more likely to be reported. To examine this more closely, Leake and colleagues[30] performed a case-control study, comparing people 60 years or older with a diagnosis of coccidioidomycosis between 1990 and 1996, to two control groups, one identified by random digit dialing and another that contained subjects who had been serologically tested for coccidioidomycosis and were found to be negative. Those who had symptomatic coccidioidomycosis had resided in the state an average of 6.5 years, significantly less than the 19.5 and 11.0 years for the two control groups. In addition, the cases were more likely to have various comorbidities, including congestive heart failure, chronic lung disease, cancer, and use of corticosteroid drugs, than the controls.

The incidence of reported symptomatic coccidioidomycosis has continued to increase into the current decade,[31] with an estimated incidence of 75 per 100,000 in 2007.[28] The geography of the disease remains the same as a decade ago, with most cases reported from Maricopa, Pinal, and Pima counties, which are located in the south-central part of the state. Moreover, men and older individuals continue to account for a disproportionate number of cases. Enhanced surveillance performed in 2007 by the Arizona State Department of Health has demonstrated the profound effect that the disease has had on the state and on the individuals. For example, hospital admissions due to coccidioidomycosis in 2007 were associated with costs of $86 million. People diagnosed with coccidioidomycosis in Arizona missed an average of 1 month of work.

Although the state of Arizona made coccidioidomycosis a laboratory reportable disease in 1997, this only partially explains the continued increase. Current theories include a continued influx into the state of older, nonimmune individuals who have comorbidities, who are more likely to develop symptomatic illness; a heightened awareness of the disease, leading to an increase in testing and reporting; changes in climate conducive to the growth of the fungus; and soil disruption in native desert areas leading to greater airborne propagation of the organism.[28]

The impact of coccidioidomycosis in Arizona is not limited to humans. There are reports of nonhuman primates being highly susceptible.[32] Moreover, domestic animals are also at risk; dogs and cats develop symptomatic disease. Shubitz and colleagues[33] recently performed a serosurvey of dogs in Pima and Maricopa counties. Among 104 dogs that were followed for 1 year, 28 (27%) developed coccidioidal antibodies. In the same study, a cross-sectional analysis revealed that 32 of 381 (8%) dogs had positive antibody tests.

California, particularly the southern portion of the San Joaquin Valley, is the other major region of coccidioidal endemicity in the United States. To determine the impact of coccidioidomycosis on California, Flaherman and coworkers[34] examined inpatient hospital discharge data from 1997 through 2002. They found 7457 hospital admissions were associated with coccidioidomycosis and that 3707 (50%) of these were principally for coccidioidomycosis. The annual hospitalization rate was 3.7 per 100,000 residents and the annual mortality rate was 2.1 per million residents. Kern, Los Angeles, and San Diego counties had the highest number of hospitalizations.

Like Arizona, California has experienced increases in the number of cases over the past few decades. A striking increase in the number of cases in Ventura County occurred after the Northridge earthquake in January, 1994. Satellite images clearly demonstrated dust clouds associated with landslides that occurred in the aftermath of the temblor.[35] Pappagianis[36] described a spike in the incidence of cases reported from Kern County in the southern San Joaquin Valley in the early 1990s associated with prolonged drought interspersed by intense rains. A subsequent case-control study performed there from 1995 through 1996[37] revealed an incidence of 86 cases per 100,000, similar to that currently seen in Arizona. Crum and colleagues[38] examined the incidence of coccidioidomycosis among military trainees at Fort Irwin, a known coccidioidal endemic area located in the Mojave Desert. Over 5 weeks, 1 definite and 2 possible cases of coccidioidomycosis were identified, for an estimated annual incidence of 6% to 32%. The most recent and perhaps most striking outbreak in California has been reported at the Pleasant Valley State Prison, located on the western side of the San Joaquin Valley not far from where Smith conducted his prospective studies on coccidioidomycosis among army air corpsmen in the early 1940s. During 2003, 127 new cases of coccidioidomycosis were observed at the prison. It is presumed that the extraordinary increase was associated with housing prisoners originally from regions not endemic for coccidioidomycosis combined with construction causing soil disturbance.[39] The epidemic has continued, as recently reported by the New York Times.[40]

IMMUNOLOGY

Studies early in the twentieth century demonstrated that the expression of delayed-type hypersensitivity is important in predicting control of coccidioidal infection in humans.[41] These and subsequent studies have led to the conclusion that the cellular immune response is the critical element in controlling coccidioidomycosis. Recent studies in humans have shed some light on the mechanisms of that process.

One area of interest is the role of antigen presentation on immune response in coccidioidomycosis. As Smith and colleagues[11] demonstrated, patients who have disseminated disease do not consistently express delayed-type hypersensitivity to injected coccidioidin. We and others have observed similar findings using in vitro measures of cellular immune response.[42–44] To examine this further, John Richards, Douglas Lake, and I[45] generated human monocyte-derived dendritic cells from subjects who had various forms of coccidioidomycosis. We were able to show that lymphocytes from individuals who had disseminated coccidioidomycosis could respond to a coccidioidal antigen complex when it was presented with mature dendritic cells. Moreover, the lymphocytes from these donors were functionally normal, suggesting that the defect in host immunity was in antigen presentation. In follow-up work, Dionne and colleagues[46] demonstrated that mature dendritic cells can phagocytose and process whole coccidioidal spherules, eventually presenting antigen on their surface in association with HLA-DR. This process could be blocked by mannan, suggesting that mannose receptors play a role in the initial phagocytosis.

The in situ immunologic response to coccidioidal infection has not been frequently observed in humans. Modlin and colleagues[47] used immunohistochemical techniques to perform a limited study on skin biopsies from patients who had coccidioidomycosis that had disseminated to this site. More recently, Li and coworkers[48] explored the in situ events in surgically excised human pulmonary coccidioidal granulomata. A striking observation was the finding of perigranulomatous clusters of lymphoid tissue consisting predominantly of CD20+ cells surrounded by smaller numbers of CD4+ and CD8+ lymphocytes. These B-cell clusters were associated with relatively increased numbers of cells producing the down-regulating cytokine IL-10 compared with cells producing IFN-γ. Since this report, others have observed B-cell clusters in other pulmonary inflammatory conditions. For example, Tsai and coworkers[49] found them in an experimental murine model of pulmonary tuberculosis. These clusters were not observed early but were prominent 1 month after infection. Similar clusters were observed in biopsies from patients who had idiopathic pulmonary fibrosis.[50]

Over the last 2 decades, there has been a great deal of interest in developing a vaccine for coccidioidomycosis, and Cole and colleagues[51] have argued that such a vaccine is feasible. A murine model has been developed involving either intraperitoneal or intranasal injection of Coccidioides.

Susceptibility varies among different inbred mouse strains, with BALB/c being most susceptible, followed by C57BL/6, and then DBA/2.[51] Outbred Swiss-Webster mice are very resistant to the development of illness after coccidioidal infection. Cole and coworkers[51] have demonstrated that inoculation of BALB/c mice with live but avirulent C posadasii, produced through deletion of a single chitin synthase gene (Δchs5), can subsequently completely protect these mice from a subsequent lethal intranasal challenge with the wild-type strain. Enthusiasm for this approach has been dampened, however, because of concerns about toxicity and compositional variability when using live organisms as immunogens.

There have been several recent studies of recombinant protein antigens as vaccine candidates using the murine model of coccidioidomycosis. Shubitz and colleagues[52] have explored the protective efficacy of two recombinant coccidioidal antigens. Initially, they subcutaneously injected BALB/c mice with rAg2/PRA, a proline-rich 194–amino acid protein derived from coccidioidal spherules and expressed by Escherichia coli, in combination with the adjuvant monophosphoryl lipid A. One month later, the mice were challenged intranasally with Coccidioides. Although there were significant reductions in mortality compared with unvaccinated mice, protection was lost at high inocula. Results were slightly better when rAg2/PRA was given intranasally or when C57BL/6 mice, a more resistant strain, were used. In comparison, subcutaneous vaccination with whole, killed spherules resulted in complete survival at all but the highest inocula. Since then, this group has shown that inoculation with a chimeric antigen expressed in the yeast vector Saccharomyces cerevisiae that contains the first 106 amino acids of Ag2/PRA (Ag2/PRA$_{1-106}$) and another peptide, Coccidioides-specific antigen (CSA), was more protective than either recombinant peptide alone.[53]

Most recently, Shubitz and colleagues[54] have shown that the histologic pulmonary events of coccidioidal infection after vaccination of the susceptible C57BL/6 and DBA/2 mouse strains with the Ag2/PRA$_{1-106}$/CSA chimera is distinct from the native response of the resistant Swiss-Webster strain. Specifically, Swiss-Webster mice develop significantly less inflammation and demonstrate mature granulomata, including the perigranulomatous lymphoid aggregates noted by Li and colleagues[48] in humans.

In a similar manner, Tarcha and coworkers[55] have shown that a recombinant aspartyl protease expressed by E coli protected C57BL/6 from lethal challenge when combined with the synthetic oligodeoxynucleotide adjuvant CpG. Tarcha and colleagues[56] subsequently demonstrated that combining three E coli–expressed recombinant peptides, including aspartyl protease, was more protective than any single antigen.

Although these results are encouraging, several concerns regarding the murine model of coccidioidomycosis must be noted. First, as demonstrated by Shubitz and colleagues,[54] different inbred mouse strains display different susceptibilities to challenge and different responses to immunization. This finding suggests that the recombinant antigens currently tested may not be useful in humans, in whom there is wide genetic diversity. Second, the murine model, in which death occurs within days after intranasal challenge with even low inocula of Coccidioides, differs dramatically from the human disease, in which most cases result in asymptomatic illness and the development of long-lived immunity. Cole and his laboratory have recently attempted to address this problem, however. They found that although subcutaneous inoculation of rAg2/PRA combined with CpG protected C57BL/6 mice against lethal intranasal challenge of Coccidioides for the first 50 days, mice subsequently became ill and died over the next 40 days. They subsequently were able to detect and express a homolog of Ag2/PRA called PRP2. When rAg2/PRA and rPRP2 were combined as a vaccine with CpG as the adjuvant, there was a significantly lower tissue fungal burden 90 days post infection and significantly greater protection from death after 120 days.[57]

DIAGNOSIS

Diagnosis of coccidioidomycosis depends on direct histologic identification of the fungus in tissue or respiratory secretions, culture, or serology. Although serology is probably the method relied on most frequently, the sensitivity and specificity of the various assays are in question. Although the tube-precipitin (TP) and complement-fixation (CF) assays originally developed by Smith are time honored, few laboratories perform these today. Like these tests, immunodiffusion (IDTP and IDCF) assays seem to have few if any false-positive results.

A commercial enzyme immunoassay (EIA) that detects IgM and IgG antibodies is available but neither its sensitivity nor its specificity is known. Particular concern has focused on the specificity of an isolated IgM. Blair and Currier[58] recently reviewed the records of 405 patients in whom EIA demonstrated either IgM, IgG, or both. Among

706 tests, 37 (5%) tests in 28 patients revealed an isolated IgM. In 7 of these patients, the diagnosis of coccidioidomycosis was confirmed by either culture or histology. In 21 others, an immunodiffusion serologic assay was positive and the clinical and radiographic presentations were compatible with coccidioidomycosis. Coccidioidomycosis thus seemed likely in all cases.

There is a pressing need for assays that are based on the direct detection of the organism that are rapid, sensitive, and specific. In that regard, a commercial enzyme immunoassay for the detection of *Histoplasma antigenuria* has existed for many years. Kuberski and colleagues[59] noted that this test was positive in 11 of 19 (58%) patients who had established coccidioidomycosis. As a follow-up, Durkin and colleagues[60] reported their results for an enzyme immunoassay specifically for coccidioidal antigenuria. Using rabbit antibody raised against galactomannan isolated from *C immitis* and *C posadasii*, they studied 24 patients who had a diagnosis of coccidioidomycosis. The *Coccidioides* enzyme immunoassay detected urinary antigen in 17 (71%). Although these results are promising, it must be realized that 19 (79%) of these patients were immunocompromised, principally because of HIV infection and solid organ transplantation, and that 7 died of their disease. The sensitivity of the *Coccidioides antigenuria* assay in less-compromised patients who had milder forms of coccidioidomycosis is not currently known.

Although no commercial genomic test currently exists for coccidioidomycosis, there are several studies demonstrating the usefulness of polymerase chain reaction (PCR) in establishing the diagnosis. Initially, Bialek and colleagues[61] developed a safe DNA extraction procedure for *Coccidioides*, necessary because of the extreme hazard presented by this organism when grown in the laboratory. Next they produced nested PCR and real-time PCR assays using Ag2/PRA as the target. Ag2/PRA was chosen because, although it exists only in single copy in the genome, it is highly conserved and unique to *Coccidioides*. They were able to detect *Coccidioides* in three biopsy specimens in which coccidioidal spherules were seen and ascertained a sensitivity of 1 to 10 organisms per sample. No amplification occurred when other fungi were tested. In a study from Brazil, de Aguiar Cordeiro and coworkers[62] used a slight modification of Bialek's method on a poor-quality sputum specimen in which a coccidioidal spherule was seen and clearly detected the appropriate 342–base pair product by PCR. This method was also recently used to confirm a diagnosis of coccidioidal pericarditis.[63]

COCCIDIOIDOMYCOSIS IN SPECIAL HOSTS

Patients who have suppressed cellular immunity are at increased risk for developing symptomatic coccidioidomycosis. One group of particular interest is those who have HIV infection. In the late 1980s, we conducted a prospective observational study of coccidioidomycosis among HIV-infected people living in Tucson, Arizona. We found that 13 patients, 24% of the cohort, developed coccidioidomycosis by 41 months of follow-up.[64] Death attributable to coccidioidomycosis occurred in 5 (38%). Less than a decade later and after the introduction of potent antiretroviral therapy, Woods and colleagues[65] offered epidemiologic evidence of a decline in symptomatic coccidioidomycosis among people in Arizona infected with HIV. We recently found that the prevalence of coccidioidomycosis in the same HIV clinic cited previously[64] was only 11% over a 5-year period. Infection was primarily focal pulmonary, frequently asymptomatic, and no deaths were attributable to it.[66] Based on this, it seems that the frequency of symptomatic and severe coccidioidomycosis during HIV infection has declined with the advent of potent antiretroviral therapy.

Biologic inhibitors of inflammation are being increasingly used to treat rheumatic and other conditions but are potent immunosuppressives. In particular, inhibitors of tumor necrosis factor-α (TNF-α) have been associated with an increased risk for tuberculosis and histoplasmosis.[67] In a study conducted among five rheumatology practices within the coccidioidal endemic region, Bergstrom and coworkers[68] identified 13 patients who developed active disease while on these drugs. Twelve of these cases were associated with the anti–TNF-α monoclonal antibody infliximab. Nine of the cases were focal pulmonary disease and resolved with antifungal therapy but the other 4 were disseminated and 2 of these patients died. The relative risk for developing coccidioidomycosis while on infliximab was calculated to be fivefold that of other treatments. This study suggests that patients need to be followed closely for the development of coccidioidomycosis on infliximab. Although there are no data, empiric antifungal therapy before starting this agent should be considered if there is any evidence of active coccidioidomycosis, such as a positive coccidioidal serology.

Blair has extensively studied the risk for coccidioidomycosis among patients in an orthoptic solid organ transplantation program located in the endemic region. In one study,[69] charts of 820 transplantation recipients were reviewed.

Forty-seven (5.7%) had evidence of coccidioido-mycosis. Of the 3 patients who had active infection at the time of transplantation, 2 received antifungal therapy and did well. The third was not diagnosed until after transplantation and developed dissemi-nated disease. The other 44 patients were offered antifungal prophylaxis before transplantation. Seven did not complete the course, however. Among them, 1 developed worsening pulmonary symptoms associated with a coccidioidal cavity. Based on this and other experience, Blair points out that a history of prior coccidioidomycosis does not contraindicate transplantation. Identifica-tion and treatment with antifungal agents of such patients seems prudent.[70]

A recent concern is infection with *Coccidioides* derived from the transplanted organ. In one report, two solid organ transplant recipients developed disseminated coccidioidomycosis and died after receiving organs from a donor with a history of disseminated cutaneous coccidioidomycosis that was not known at the time of donation. A third organ recipient was treated for 3 months with itra-conazole and did well.[71] It is clear, however, that organ donation from people who have coccidioidal infection does not always result in active infection. For example, Blair and Mulligan found that 12 possible organ donors among 568 (2.1%) living in the coccidioidal endemic area had a positive serology for *Coccidioides*. Three of these 12 donated a kidney and one became a liver donor. None of the recipients developed active coccidioidomycosis.[72]

CLINICAL PRESENTATION

Within the endemic area, a concern exists that primary pulmonary coccidioidomycosis is being confused with community-acquired pneumonia of a bacterial cause. This confusion is problematic because patients may be prescribed antibacterials inappropriately or may have a subsequent compli-cation, such as fatigue.[73] Moreover, unnecessary laboratory testing may be done because the diag-nosis is not established. Valdivia and colleagues specifically examined this question by enrolling patients who had a lower respiratory tract syndrome of less than 1 month's duration from three primary care sites in Tucson, Arizona. Among 55 patients, 16 (27%) had at least one positive coccidioidal serologic test during the time of diagnosis. Antibacterials were prescribed in 46 (84%) and all patients were improved by 6 months after enrollment. Despite this study's limitations, including small size and the positive serologic test not definitively establish that the current syndrome was due to coccidioidomycosis,

the results suggest that primary pulmonary coccidioidomycosis is underdiagnosed in the endemic area.

Although several epidemiologic studies have clearly demonstrated that symptomatic coccidioi-domycosis is more likely to occur among the elderly,[28,29] the reason for this is unclear. Blair and coworkers[74] recently performed a retrospec-tive review of 396 patients reported to the Arizona State Health Department from 1999 to 2003 with coccidioidomycosis to ascertain if there were differences in clinical illness and outcome based on age. Among these patients, 186 were younger than 60 years of age and 210 were aged 60 years or older. No clear differences were seen based on age in this study. There was a potential bias, however, in that younger patients who were referred for care were more likely to have dissem-inated disease and to require hospitalization. More studies are needed in this area.

THERAPY

Azole antifungals have become the standard therapy in many cases of coccidioidomycosis.[75] There are clear differences in the efficacy between different azoles for treatment of different fungal diseases, however. For example, fluconazole is superior to itraconazole for the treatment of cryp-tococcosis, whereas itraconazole is superior to fluconazole for the treatment of histoplasmosis and blastomycosis. In a landmark study, Galgiani and colleagues[76] performed a randomized, double-blind, placebo-controlled trial comparing fluconazole, 400 mg daily, to itraconazole, 200 mg twice daily as a capsule, for the treatment of coccidioidomycosis among 198 patients who had chronic pulmonary, soft tissue, or skeletal disseminated coccidioidomycosis. After 8 months, 50% of patients treated with fluconazole and 63% of those who had received itraconazole had responded, a nonsignificant difference. By 12 months, a follow-up time outside the original protocol, these differences in response persisted and just achieved statistical significance in favor of itraconazole. Moreover, itraconazole was clearly superior to fluconazole for the treatment of skeletal coccidioidomycosis. Although it is known that the capsule formulation of itraconazole can have variable absorption, serum levels of itra-conazole did not predict response.

Newer triazole antifungals have become avail-able over the last few years that could be useful for the treatment of coccidioidomycosis. Unfortu-nately, they have not been as rigorously studied as earlier therapies. Posaconazole is structurally similar to itraconazole. Gonzalez and colleagues[77] showed that it has approximately the same activity against *Coccidioides* as itraconazole in vitro, but demonstrated sterilization of lungs and spleens in more than 70% of animals in an in vivo murine model, a result not achieved with itraconazole. Three clinical trials of posaconazole have been published.[78–80] They are small, non-randomized, and contain overlapping subjects. They suggest that posaconazole can be useful in patients who have failed previous azole therapy for coccidioidomycosis. Voriconazole is another new triazole and is structurally related to fluconazole. Only case reports of treatment of coccidioidomycosis have been reported and all, not surprisingly, suggest efficacy.[81–83]

Amphotericin B, as the deoxycholate formulation, was first used for the treatment of coccidioidomycosis in the 1950s.[84] Since then, new lipid-dispersal formulations with reduced renal toxicity have become available. There have been no clinical trials comparing these new formulations to deoxycholate amphotericin B. *Coccidioides* strains seem to be more susceptible to these lipid preparations than to deoxycholate amphotericin B, however.[85] Moreover, Clemons and colleagues[86] have examined the role of intravenous liposomal amphotericin B in a murine model of coccidioidal meningitis, in which deoxycholate amphotericin B is ineffective, and found evidence of efficacy. Clinical studies are clearly needed.

There have been two reports of clinical efficacy of the echinocandin antifungal caspofungin in cases of coccidioidomycosis[87,88] and caspofungin therapy was associated with prolonged survival compared with controls in a murine model.[89] Without clinical studies, however, the use of echinocandin antifungals for the treatment of coccidioidomycosis should be approached with caution.

Nikkomycin Z is a competitive inhibitor of chitin synthase. Hector and coworkers[90] demonstrated complete protection after intranasal inoculation of *Coccidioides* in a murine model of coccidioidomycosis at a dose of 20 mg/kg given orally twice daily. Moreover, at a dose of 50 mg/kg daily, only one colony of *Coccidioides* was identified in the lungs of treated animals, far superior to what was achieved with fluconazole and another experimental azole. This finding has led to interest in this drug for human disease[91] and a study is ongoing.

A continuing controversy is whether symptomatic patients who have primary pulmonary coccidioidomycosis should be treated with antifungal agents. Potential benefits of therapy might include more rapid resolution of illness or the prevention of subsequent complications, such as extrathoracic dissemination. Even with azole antifungals, however, there are potential complications and increased monetary costs. The current guidelines from the Infectious Diseases Society of America suggest some latitude in this regard.[75] The optimal approach to this question would be to perform a randomized clinical trial, but this has been logistically difficult to achieve. Since 1998, we have followed a prospective, observational cohort of patients who have a diagnosis of coccidioidomycosis at the Southern Arizona Veterans Affairs Health Care System in Tucson, Arizona. Among this group, we examined the outcome of 105 subjects who had primary pulmonary coccidioidomycosis.[92] Among these, 54 were prescribed antifungals and 51 were not. Patients prescribed therapy had a higher clinical severity score than those not prescribed therapy, but there were no other clinical differences. In follow-up, all of the patients not prescribed therapy did well without recurrence of disease. In addition, there was no difference in the rate of clinical improvement between those treated and those not. Among those prescribed therapy, all those who remained on therapy had no recurrences. Eight patients in whom therapy was subsequently discontinued developed recurrences of coccidioidomycosis, however. In 3 cases, extrathoracic dissemination had occurred despite prolonged initial antifungal therapy. These results suggest that many patients who have primary pneumonia will not benefit from antifungal therapy and that, for those who are treated, close follow-up is required when that treatment is discontinued.

REFERENCES

1. CDC. Notifiable diseases/deaths in selected cities weekly information. MMWR Morb Mortal Wkly Rep 2006;55(50):1365.

2. Odds FC. Coccidioidomycosis: flying conidia and severed heads. Mycologist 2003;17(1):37–40.

3. Hirschmann JV. The early history of coccidioidomycosis: 1892–1945. Clin Infect Dis 2007;44(9):1202–7.

4. Smith CE, editor. Reminiscences of the flying chlamydospore and its allies. The second symposium on coccidioidomycosis. Phoenix (AZ): University of Arizona Press; 1967. p. xiii–xxii.

5. Deresinski SC. History of coccidioidomycosis: "dust to dust." In: Stevens DA, editor. Coccidioidomycosis a text. New York: Plenum Medical Book Company; 1980. p. 1–20.

6. Thorne WS. A case of protozoic skin disease. Occidental Medical Times 1894;8(12):703–4.

7. Rixford E. A case of protozoic dermatitis. Occidental Medical Times 1894;8(12):704–7.

8. Rixford E, Gilchrist TC. Two cases of protozoon (coccidioidal) infection of the skin and other organs. Johns Hopkins Hosp Rep 1896;1:209–68.

9. Dickson EC. Primary coccidioidomycosis. The initial acute infection which results in coccidioidal granuloma. Ann Rev Tuberc 1938;38:722–9.
10. Dickson EC, Gifford MA. *Coccidioides* infection (coccidioidomycosis). II. The primary type of infection. Arch Intern Med 1938;62:853–71.
11. Smith CE, Beard RR, Whiting EG, et al. Varieties of coccidioidal infection. Am J Public Health 1946;36:1394–402.
12. Ophüls W. Further observations on a pathogenic mould formerly described as a protozoan (*Coccidioides immitis*; *Coccidioides pyogenes*). J Exp Med 1905;6:443–85.
13. Bowman B, Taylor JW, White TJ. Molecular evolution of the fungi: human pathogens. Mol Biol Evol 1992;9(5):893–904.
14. Pan S, Sigler L, Cole G. Evidence for a phylogenetic connection between *Coccidioides immitis* and *Uncinocarpus reesii* (Onygenaceae). Microbiology 1994;140(6):1481–94.
15. Burt A, Carter DA, Koenig GL, et al. Molecular markers reveal cryptic sex in the human pathogen *Coccidioides immitis*. Proc Natl Acad Sci U S A 1996;93:770–3.
16. Koufopanou V, Burt A, Szaro T, et al. Gene genealogies, cryptic species, and molecular evolution in the human pathogen *Coccidioides immitis* and relatives (Ascomycota, Onygenales). Mol Biol Evol 2001;18(7):1246–58.
17. Mandel MA, Barker BM, Kroken S, et al. Genomic and population analyses of the mating type loci in *Coccidioides* species reveal evidence for sexual reproduction and gene acquisition. Eukaryot Cell 2007;6(7):1189–99.
18. Fisher M, Koenig G, White T, et al. Pathogenic clones versus environmentally driven population increase: analysis of an epidemic of the human fungal pathogen *Coccidioides immitis*. J Clin Microbiol 2000;38(2):807–13.
19. Fisher M, Koenig G, White T, et al. Biogeographic range expansion into South America by *Coccidioides immitis* mirrors New World patterns of human migration. Proc Natl Acad Sci U S A 2001;98:4558–62.
20. Fisher M, Koenig G, White T, et al. Molecular and phenotypic description of *Coccidioides posadasii* sp. nov., previously recognized as the non-California population of *Coccidioides immitis*. Mycol Soc America 2002;73–84.
21. Barker BM, Jewell KA, Kroken S, et al. The population biology of *Coccidioides*: epidemiologic implications for disease outbreaks. Ann N Y Acad Sci 2007;1111:147–63.
22. Stewart RA, Meyer KF. Isolation of *Coccidioides immitis* (Stiles) from the soil. Proc Soc Exp Biol Med 1932;29:937–8.
23. Greene DR, Koenig G, Fisher MC, et al. Soil isolation and molecular identification of *Coccidioides immitis*. Mycologia 2000;92(3):406–10.
24. Petersen LR, Marshall SL, Barton-Dickson C, et al. Coccidioidomycosis among workers at an archeological site, northeastern Utah. Emerg Infect Dis 2004;10(4):637–42.
25. Fisher FS, Bultman MW, Jonhson SM, et al. *Coccidioides* niches and habitat parameters in the southwestern United States. A matter of scale. Ann N Y Acad Sci 2007;1111:47–72.
26. Kolivras KN, Comrie AC. Modeling valley fever (coccidioidomycosis) incidence on the basis of climate conditions. Int J Biometeorol 2003;47(2):87–101.
27. Park BJ, Sigel K, Vaz V, et al. An epidemic of coccidioidomycosis in Arizona associated with climatic changes, 1998–2001. J Infect Dis 2005;191(11):1981–7.
28. Valley fever annual report 2007. Arizona Department of Health Services; 2008.
29. Ampel NM, Mosley DG, England B, et al. Coccidioidomycosis in Arizona: increase in incidence from 1990 to 1995. Clin Infect Dis 1998;27(6):1528–30.
30. Leake JA, Mosley DG, England B, et al. Risk factors for acute symptomatic coccidioidomycosis among elderly persons in Arizona, 1996–1997. J Infect Dis 2000;181(4):1435–40.
31. Sunenshine RH, Anderson S, Erhart L, et al. Public health surveillance for coccidioidomycosis in Arizona. Ann N Y Acad Sci 2007;1111:96–102.
32. Beaman L, Holmberg C, Henrickson R, et al. The incidence of coccidioidomycosis among nonhuman primates housed outdoors at the California Primate Research Center. J Med Primatol 1980;9(4):254–61.
33. Shubitz LF, Butkiewicz CD, Dial SM, et al. Incidence of *Coccidioides* infection among dogs residing in a region in which the organism is endemic. J Am Vet Med Assoc 2005;226(11):1846–50.
34. Flaherman VJ, Hector R, Rutherford GW. Estimating severe coccidioidomycosis in California. Emerg Infect Dis 2007;13(7):1087–90.
35. Schneider E, Hajjeh RA, Spiegel RA, et al. A coccidioidomycosis outbreak following the Northridge, Calif, earthquake. JAMA 1997;277(11):904–8.
36. Pappagianis D. Marked increase in cases of coccidioidomycosis in California: 1991, 1992, and 1993. Clin Infect Dis 1994;19(Suppl 1):S14–8.
37. Rosenstein NE, Emery KW, Werner SB, et al. Risk factors for severe pulmonary and disseminated coccidioidomycosis: Kern County, California, 1995–1996. Clin Infect Dis 2001;32(5):708–15.
38. Crum NF, Potter M, Pappagianis D. Seroincidence of Coccidioidomycosis during military desert training exercises. J Clin Microbiol 2004;42(10):4552–5.
39. Pappagianis D. Coccidioidomycosis in California state correctional institutions. Ann N Y Acad Sci 2007;1111:103–11.
40. McKinley J. Infection hits a California prison hard. The New York Times. 2007.

41. Ampel NM. Measurement of cellular immunity in human coccidioidomycosis. Mycopathologia 2003; 156(4):247–62.

42. Ampel NM, Kramer LA, Li L, et al. In vitro whole-blood analysis of cellular immunity in patients with active coccidioidomycosis by using the antigen preparation T27K. Clin Diagn Lab Immunol 2002; 9(5):1039–43.

43. Catanzaro A, Spitler LE, Moser KM. Cellular immune response in coccidioidomycosis. Cell Immunol 1975;15(2):360–71.

44. Cox RA, Brummer E, Lecara G. In vitro lymphocyte responses of coccidioidin skin test-positive and -negative persons to coccidioidin, spherulin, and a Coccidioides cell wall antigen. Infect Immun 1977;15(3):751–5.

45. Richards JO, Ampel NM, Lake DF. Reversal of coccidioidal anergy in vitro by dendritic cells from patients with disseminated coccidioidomycosis. J Immunol 2002;169(4):2020–5.

46. Dionne SO, Podany AB, Ruiz YW, et al. Spherules derived from Coccidioides posadasii promote human dendritic cell maturation and activation. Infect Immun 2006;74(4):2415–22.

47. Modlin RL, Segal GP, Hofman FM, et al. In situ localization of T lymphocytes in disseminated coccidioidomycosis. J Infect Dis 1985;151(2):314–9.

48. Li L, Dial SM, Schmelz M, et al. Cellular immune suppressor activity resides in lymphocyte cell clusters adjacent to granulomata in human coccidioidomycosis. Infect Immun 2005;73(7):3923–8.

49. Tsai MC, Chakravarty S, Zhu G, et al. Characterization of the Tuberculous granuloma in murine and human lungs: cellular composition and relative tissue oxygen tension. Cell Microbiol 2006;8(2):218–32.

50. Marchal-Somme J, Uzunhan Y, Marchand-Adam S, et al. Cutting edge: nonproliferating mature immune cells form a novel type of organized lymphoid structure in idiopathic pulmonary fibrosis. J Immunol 2006;176(10):5735–9.

51. Cole GT, Xue JM, Okeke CN, et al. A vaccine against coccidioidomycosis is justified and attainable. Med Mycol 2004;42(3):189–216.

52. Shubitz L, Peng T, Perrill R, et al. Protection of mice against Coccidioides immitis intranasal infection by vaccination with recombinant antigen 2/PRA. Infect Immun 2002;70(6):3287–9.

53. Shubitz LF, Yu JJ, Hung CY, et al. Improved protection of mice against lethal respiratory infection with Coccidioides posadasii using two recombinant antigens expressed as a single protein. Vaccine 2006; 24(31–32):5904–11.

54. Shubitz LF, Dial SM, Perrill R, et al. Vaccine-induced cellular immune responses differ from innate responses in susceptible and resistant strains of mice infected with Coccidioides posadasii. Infect Immun 2008;76:5553–64.

55. Tarcha EJ, Basrur V, Hung CY, et al. A recombinant aspartyl protease of Coccidioides posadasii induces protection against pulmonary coccidioidomycosis in mice. Infect Immun 2006;74(1):516–27.

56. Tarcha EJ, Basrur V, Hung CY, et al. Multivalent recombinant protein vaccine against coccidioidomycosis. Infect Immun 2006;74(10):5802–13.

57. Herr RA, Hung CY, Cole GT. Evaluation of two homologous proline-rich proteins of Coccidioides posadasii as candidate vaccines against coccidioidomycosis. Infect Immun 2007;75(12):5777–87.

58. Blair JE, Currier JT. Significance of isolated positive IgM serologic results by enzyme immunoassay for coccidioidomycosis. Mycopathologia 2008;166(2): 77–82.

59. Kuberski T, Myers R, Wheat LJ, et al. Diagnosis of coccidioidomycosis by antigen detection using cross-reaction with a Histoplasma antigen. Clin Infect Dis 2007;44(5):e50–4.

60. Durkin M, Connolly P, Kuberski T, et al. Diagnosis of coccidioidomycosis with use of the Coccidioides antigen enzyme immunoassay. Clin Infect Dis 2008;47(8):e69–73.

61. Bialek R, Kern J, Herrmann T, et al. PCR assays for identification of Coccidioides posadasii based on the nucleotide sequence of the antigen 2/proline-rich antigen. J Clin Microbiol 2004;42(2):778–83.

62. de Aguiar Cordeiro R, Nogueira Brilhante RS, Gadelha Rocha MF, et al. Rapid diagnosis of coccidioidomycosis by nested PCR assay of sputum. Clin Microbiol Infect 2007;13(4):449–51.

63. Brilhante RS, Cordeiro RA, Rocha MF, et al. Coccidioidal pericarditis: a rapid presumptive diagnosis by an in-house antigen confirmed by mycological and molecular methods. J Med Microbiol 2008; 57(Pt 10):1288–92.

64. Ampel NM, Dols CL, Galgiani JN. Coccidioidomycosis during human immunodeficiency virus infection: results of a prospective study in a coccidioidal endemic area. Am J Med 1993;94(3): 235–40.

65. Woods CW, McRill C, Plikaytis BD, et al. Coccidioidomycosis in human immunodeficiency virus-infected persons in Arizona, 1994–1997: incidence, risk factors, and prevention. J Infect Dis 2000; 181(4):1428–34.

66. Masannat FY, Ampel NM. Coccidioidomycosis in patients with HIV infection in the age of potent antiretroviral therapy: a cohort analysis. Annual Meetings of the 48th ICAAC/46th IDSA Meeting; Washington, DC, 2008.

67. Winthrop KL, Yamashita S, Beekmann SE, et al. Mycobacterial and other serious infections in patients receiving anti-tumor necrosis factor and other newly approved biologic therapies: case finding through the Emerging Infections Network. Clin Infect Dis 2008;46(11):1738–40.

68. Bergstrom L, Yocum DE, Ampel NM, et al. Increased risk of coccidioidomycosis in patients treated with tumor necrosis factor alpha antagonists. Arthritis Rheum 2004;50(6):1959–66.

69. Blair JE, Kusne S, Carey EJ, et al. The prevention of recrudescent coccidioidomycosis after solid organ transplantation. Transplantation 2007;83(9): 1182–7.

70. Blair JE. Approach to the solid organ transplant patient with latent infection and disease caused by *Coccidioides* species. Curr Opin Infect Dis 2008;21(4):415–20.

71. Wright PW, Pappagianis D, Wilson M, et al. Donor-related coccidioidomycosis in organ transplant recipients. Clin Infect Dis 2003;37(9):1265–9.

72. Blair JE, Mulligan DC. Coccidioidomycosis in healthy persons evaluated for liver or kidney donation. Transpl Infect Dis 2007;9(1):78–82.

73. Muir Bowers J, Mourani JP, Ampel NM. Fatigue in coccidioidomycosis. Quantification and correlation with clinical, immunological, and nutritional factors. Med Mycol 2006;44(7):585–90.

74. Blair JE, Mayer AP, Currier J, et al. Coccidioidomycosis in elderly persons. Clin Infect Dis 2008;47:1513–8.

75. Galgiani JN, Ampel NM, Blair JE, et al. Coccidioidomycosis. Clin Infect Dis 2005;41(9):1217–23.

76. Galgiani JN, Catanzaro A, Cloud GA, et al. Comparison of oral fluconazole and itraconazole for progressive, nonmeningeal coccidioidomycosis. A randomized, double-blind trial. Mycoses Study Group. Ann Intern Med 2000;133(9):676–86.

77. Gonzalez GM, Tijerina R, Najvar LK, et al. In vitro and in vivo activities of posaconazole against *Coccidioides immitis*. Antimicrobial Agents Chemother 2002;46(5):1352–6.

78. Anstead GM, Corcoran G, Lewis J, et al. Refractory coccidioidomycosis treated with posaconazole. Clin Infect Dis 2005;40(12):1770–6.

79. Catanzaro A, Cloud GA, Stevens DA, et al. Safety, tolerance, and efficacy of posaconazole therapy in patients with nonmeningeal disseminated or chronic pulmonary coccidioidomycosis. Clin Infect Dis 2007; 45(5):562–8.

80. Stevens DA, Rendon A, Gaona-Flores V, et al. Posaconazole therapy for chronic refractory coccidioidomycosis. Chest 2007;132(3):952–8.

81. Cortez KJ, Walsh TJ, Bennett JE. Successful treatment of coccidioidal meningitis with voriconazole. Clin Infect Dis 2003;36(12):1619–22.

82. Prabhu RM, Bonnell M, Currier BL, et al. Successful treatment of disseminated nonmeningeal coccidioidomycosis with voriconazole. Clin Infect Dis 2004; 39(7):e74–7.

83. Proia LA, Tenorio AR. Successful use of voriconazole for treatment of *Coccidioides meningitis*. Antimicrobial Agents Chemother 2004;48(6):2341.

84. Fiese MJ. Treatment of disseminated coccidioidomycosis with amphotericin B: report of a case. Calif Med 1957;86:119–20.

85. Gonzalez GM, Tijerina R, Sutton DA, et al. In vitro activities of free and lipid formulations of amphotericin B and nystatin against clinical isolates of *Coccidioides immitis* at various saprobic stages. Antimicrobial Agents Chemother 2002;46(5):1583–5.

86. Clemons KV, Sobel RA, Williams PL, et al. Efficacy of intravenous liposomal amphotericin B (AmBisome) against coccidioidal meningitis in rabbits. Antimicrobial Agents Chemother 2002;46(8):2420–6.

87. Antony S. Use of the echinocandins (caspofungin) in the treatment of disseminated coccidioidomycosis in a renal transplant recipient. Clin Infect Dis 2004; 39(6):879–80.

88. Hsue G, Napier JT, Prince RA, et al. Treatment of meningeal coccidioidomycosis with caspofungin. J Antimicrob Chemother 2004;54(1):292–4.

89. Gonzalez GM, Gonzalez G, Najvar LK, et al. Therapeutic efficacy of caspofungin alone and in combination with amphotericin B deoxycholate for coccidioidomycosis in a mouse model. J Antimicrob Chemother 2007;60(6):1341–6.

90. Hector RF, Zimmer BL, Pappagianis D. Evaluation of nikkomycins X and Z in murine models of coccidioidomycosis, histoplasmosis, and blastomycosis. Antimicrobial Agents Chemother 1990;34(4):587–93.

91. Galgiani JN. Coccidioidomycosis: changing perceptions and creating opportunities for its control. Ann N Y Acad Sci 2007;1111:1–18.

92. Ampel NM, Giblin A, Mourani JP, et al. Factors and outcomes associated with the decision to treat primary pulmonary coccidioidomycosis. Clin Infect Dis 2009;48:172–8.

Cryptococcosis: An Emerging Respiratory Mycosis

Shaunna M. Huston, RN, BSc[a], Christopher H. Mody, MD[b,c],*

KEYWORDS

- Cryptococcus neoformans • Cryptococcus gattii
- HIV • Epidemiology • Management

It has been more than a century since *Cryptococcus* was first described in 1894,[1] but only in the last 30 years have investigators begun to understand this complex and devastating organism. Moreover, despite current treatment, patients continue to die of cryptococcosis.[2,3] *Cryptococcus neoformans* has gained increasing importance with the advent of HIV infections and the increased use of solid-organ transplantation and immunosuppressive therapies.[4] More recently, the Vancouver outbreak of *Cryptococcus gattii* has brought attention to the pathogen because of the frequency with which it causes infections in otherwise healthy, immunocompetent individuals.[5,6] The potential for mortality, the prevalence of acute and chronic debilitation, and the ability of *Cryptococcus* to infect immunocompetent as well as immunocompromised individuals makes the study of this organism important. Current regimens have improved outcomes, highlighting the importance of appropriate management. Despite these advances, however, cryptococcosis remains an important cause of morbidity and mortality. Because it sometimes is difficult to establish a diagnosis, it is important to have a high index of clinical suspicion and appropriate testing. Moreover, despite a high standard of medical care, patients die from infections with highly virulent *Cryptococcus* strains, as recently reported on Vancouver Island,[7,8]

underscoring the importance of understanding the epidemiology of the organism. It is hoped that future studies will improve the understanding of the pathogenesis and host response and facilitate management of cryptococcosis through the advent of more efficient diagnostics, the development of more effective, available, and less toxic anti-fungal agents, and the introduction of prophylactic regimens.

CRYPTOCOCCUS—EMERGING AND RECLASSIFIED

Genetic studies have defined two main human pathogenic species of *Cryptococcus*: *Cryptococcus neoformans* and *Cryptococcus gattii*. In humans, infections by other cryptococcal species such as *Cryptococcus laurentii* are rare.[9] The current literature suggests that the infective particle of *Cryptococcus* is acquired from the environment rather than by transmission from person to person, suggesting that the ecologic niche is important.[10–12] The environmental reservoir for *C. neoformans* is primarily pigeon guano. *C. gattii* is found predominantly in tropical and subtropical trees, in most cases eucalyptus trees.[10–12] As a result of its environmental reservoir, infections caused by *C. neoformans* occur worldwide. By contrast, *C. gattii* has a more limited distribution, classically to northern Australia and Papua New

[a] Department of Medical Science, University of Calgary, 3330 Hospital Drive NW, Calgary, Alberta, Canada T2N 4N1
[b] Department of Microbiology and Infectious Diseases, University of Calgary, 3330 Hospital Drive NW, Calgary, Alberta, Canada T2N 4N1
[c] Department of Internal Medicine, University of Calgary, 3330 Hospital Drive NW, Calgary, Alberta, Canada T2N 4N1
* Corresponding author. Room 4AA14, Health Research Innovation Centre, University of Calgary, Calgary, Alberta, Canada T2N 4N1.
E-mail address: cmody@ucalgary.ca (C.H. Mody).

Clin Chest Med 30 (2009) 253–264
doi:10.1016/j.ccm.2009.02.006

Guinea and more recently Vancouver Island and the surrounding area. Interestingly, although eucalyptus trees are found on Vancouver Island, C. gattii is found in association with other species of trees, especially Red alder and Douglas fir.[13,14] In addition, the incidence of C. gattii infection on Vancouver Island is second only to that in Northern Australia, and the mortality on Vancouver Island is the highest worldwide.[7,15,16] It is tempting to speculate that the phenotypic changes that allow C. gattii to occupy non-eucalyptus environmental niches on Vancouver Island also may confer hypervirulence (ie, the ability to elude host defense and increased mortality). Perhaps future knowledge of Cryptococcus ecologic niches may improve the understanding of mechanisms of host evasion.

C. neoformans and C. gattii are within the phylum Basidiomycota and are fungal pathogens that produce progeny through asexual and sexual means. Asexual reproduction occurs through simple budding and by haploid fruiting.[17] Simple budding is the reproductive mechanism that occurs within the human host.[17] Sexual reproduction has the advantage of increasing genetic diversity and therefore has the potential to promote hypervirulence and antifungal resistance. It generally occurs through crossing of an α-mating type with an a-mating type, resulting in the production of filaments and basidiospores. The α-mating type of Cryptococcus are found in higher numbers worldwide, are more virulent, and show increased central nervous system (CNS) infectivity.[18–20] Same-sex α–α-mating is thought to have occurred with the hypervirulent C. gattii on Vancouver Island,[21] which is associated with CNS involvement and death.[7,8] Cryptococcus yeast or the small (2 μm) basidiospores are inhaled and cause the initial pulmonary Cryptococcus infection.[22,23] Unfortunately, in many individuals, Cryptococcus also disseminates by an unknown mechanism throughout the body.[24–27] Of particular importance, it crosses the blood–brain barrier, resulting in meningitis and meningoencephalitis, which are associated with a much higher mortality.[4,5,28]

There also is evidence of Cryptococcus latency. Individuals develop infections from strains that can be identified by their environmental origin months or even years after the exposure. For example, immigrants from Africa have presented with infections caused by African strains of C. neoformans years after immigrating to other parts of the world.[29] C. gattii infection has occurred many months after exposure on Vancouver Island.[29–31] Moreover, isolates extracted from the same patient over time are identical by polymerase-chain reaction identification, suggesting relapse rather than a new environmental exposure.[22,32]

Therefore, a heightened awareness for cryptococcosis is appropriate, because in areas with a low prevalence of cryptococcosis patients may present with disease resulting from exposure that occurred months or years earlier.

HOST IMMUNE RESPONSE DURING CRYPTOCOCCOSIS

Opportunistic pathogens exploit a break in the host line of defense, whereas non-opportunistic pathogens induce a critical defect in the immune system or bypass normal mechanisms of defense to infect their hosts. C. neoformans preferentially infects immunocompromised individuals.[33–39] Indeed, CD4 and CD8 cells are required for effective elimination of Cryptococcus in murine models, and loss of T-cell function (as occurs with HIV infection) confers susceptibility in humans.[40–43] This finding suggests that C. neoformans possesses a sufficient complement of virulence factors to bypass the initial innate immune host defense. The polysaccharide capsule is the most potent C. neoformans virulence factor.[44] The capsule binds to complement molecules efficiently; however, despite the importance of complement in phagocytic cell recognition of other pathogens, phagocytic cells show variable ability to bind complement-opsonized C. neoformans.[45–47] Cryptococcus also evades the innate immune system through the production of antioxidants such as melanin, superoxide dismutase, thioredoxin reductase, and mannitol that neutralize specific innate host effector molecules.[48–51] Other virulence factors include phospholipase, which functions through destabilization of host cell membranes, urease, which alters pH, and proteinases, which degrade host proteins.[52–55] Other aspects of virulence are the α-mating type and the ability of Cryptococcus to survive at body temperature (37°C).[19] In the future, boosting the innate immune system by targeting one or more of these virulence factors during cryptococcosis may result in improved outcomes. By contrast, as discussed later, C. gattii infects immunocompetent individuals more frequently than immunosuppressed hosts, suggesting that it possesses additional mechanisms that induce a state of immunosuppression in the host.[15]

EPIDEMIOLOGY
Cryptococcosis and HIV Infection

Cryptococcus infections were less common before the advent of HIV infections.[35,38,39] HIV-infected patients are at high risk of cryptococcosis, at least in part because of the reduction in CD4 T-cell function.[40–43] In France, 86% of individuals presenting with cryptococcosis between 1985 and 1993 were HIV positive.[38] Cryptococcosis infection still seems to be most prevalent in HIV-positive individuals in sub-Saharan Africa and Thailand.[4,56] The incidence of cryptococcosis infection has decreased modestly where improved anti-HIV therapies are available, but it remains a frequent and devastating problem.[35,57]

Cryptococcosis and Non-HIV Immunosuppressed Individuals

Although persons infected with HIV constitute the largest population of severely immunocompromised individuals in the world today, increasing numbers of Cryptococcus infections are associated with underlying lung disease, liver disease, renal disease, increased use of immunosuppressive drugs (eg, corticosteroids, cyclosporine, azathioprine, cytotoxic chemotherapy, tacrolimus, and biologic agents), solid-organ transplantation, autoimmune disease, and malignancies.[24,38,58] Interestingly, patients receiving cyclosporine treatment after solid-organ transplantation have an increased incidence of cryptococcosis even though cyclosporine is a potent antifungal agent.[59,60] One retrospective study demonstrated that the incidence of cryptococcosis was increasing in the 1970s, before the HIV epidemic. This increase was thought to be related to expanding numbers of transplant recipients or the use of cancer therapies.[35,61] It also is evident, at least in industrialized countries, that the number of these individuals has continued to increase. For example, azathioprine is a common immunosuppressive treatment for autoimmune disease,[37,62,63] and the use of azathioprine has led to immunosuppression and susceptibility to cryptococcosis.[36,63] Transplant recipients also may receive immunosuppressive drugs, such as rabbit anti-thymocyte globulin (ATG) and alemtuzumab (anti-CD52), that lead to increased susceptibility to cryptococcosis.[33,34] Treatments for cancer patients have improved during the past few decades, but many of these regimens suppress the host immune system, rendering the individuals susceptible to cryptococcosis.[64] Studies are under way to determine the most effective immunosuppressive regimens that do not render the individual susceptible to infections such as cryptococcosis and methods to restore protection in these immunosuppressed patients.[65]

Cryptococcosis in Immunocompetent Individuals

C. neoformans and C. gattii recently were classified as two different species based on genetic studies. It also is evident that the risk factors for these pathogens are different.[9] In one retrospective study in Vancouver, from 1997 to 2002, C. gattii was 4.8 times more common in immunocompetent hosts than in immunosuppressed hosts, and the reverse was true for C. neoformans.[7] A retrospective study conducted in Australia suggested that C. gattii causes more severe disease and has a worse clinical outcome than C. neoformans because of increased cerebral involvement.[66] These studies suggest that the virulence mechanisms used by C. gattii are different from or possibly are more profound than those used by C. neoformans. Because C. gattii infections are less frequent than C. neoformans infections (95% of cryptococcosis cases are caused by C. neoformans var grubii), however, and because the two species have been classified separately only recently, there is little information on the specific host-immune responses to C. gattii.[67,68] On the other hand, the recent C. gattii outbreak on Vancouver Island, which has resulted in the highest reported cryptococcosis-related mortality, has directed attention toward C. gattii.[4–6,8,69,70]

CLINICAL FEATURES OF CRYPTOCOCCOSIS

Clinical findings associated with cryptococcosis generally are caused by pulmonary and neurologic abnormalities, although Cryptococcus has the capacity to disseminate to most organs of the body, including the skin, joints, prostate, and eye.[24–27] In addition, underlying immunodeficiencies, including HIV infection, malignancies, chronic hepatic failure, chronic renal failure, chronic lung disease, rheumatologic disease, solid-organ transplantation (liver, heart, kidney and lung), bone marrow transplantation, and glucocorticoid therapy may attenuate the signs and symptoms observed during cryptococcosis.[24,58] Therefore, the clinical suspicion for cryptococcosis in immunodeficient patients should be high.

The clinical presentation may depend on the underlying risk factors. For example, in patients who had underlying chronic liver disease, only 11% had pulmonary involvement, 24% had involvement of a different organ, and 66% had CNS involvement. By contrast, in patients who had chronic lung disease, 78% had pulmonary involvement, 5% had involvement of a different organ, and only 16% had CNS disease.[24] Clearly the underlying risk factors influence the manifestations of disease.

Central Nervous System Cryptococcosis

Meningitis and meningoencephalitis are commonly the result of dissemination of Cryptococcus from the lungs. Studies suggest that HIV co-infection is associated with enhanced CNS infection, whereas symptomatic pulmonary disease is more evident in patients who do not have HIV.[15,71] In a South African population with a high seroprevalence for HIV, 97% of patients who had cryptococcosis had CNS involvement.[4] Similar results were observed in Australia and New Zealand in patients who had HIV: 128 of 139 HIV-positive patients who had cryptococcosis had CNS involvement. In contrast, only 16% to 21% of HIV-negative patients presented with *Cryptococcus* CNS involvement.[71,72] These data suggest that the specific immune changes associated with HIV may alter the host barriers to the CNS, allowing *Cryptococcus* to disseminate preferentially to this site. Interestingly *C. gattii* does not follow this trend: enhanced *C. gattii* CNS involvement is observed in HIV-negative patients.[30,66] Intensive research in the area of CNS dissemination of *Cryptococcus* is under way to determine and potentially to manipulate the mechanisms involved.[73,74]

Neurologic signs and symptoms of meningitis including neck stiffness, headache, fever, and altered mental status should raise suspicion of cryptococcosis.[75–77] Diagnosis of cryptococcosis with CNS involvement is based on positive *Cryptococcus* antigen titer, culture, or visualizing the organism by India ink staining of cerebral spinal fluid (CSF) (**Fig. 1**).[75] *Cryptococcus* polysaccharide capsular antigen can be detected in most fluids and tissues of the body by a latex agglutination test or ELISA and is helpful to confirm involvement.[78,79] Sensitivity of the latex test is reported to be 93% to 100% with a specificity of 93% to 98% and up to 7% false-positive results. Factors that cause false-positive tests include methods used for testing (increased incubation time with human serum), the presence of hydroxyethyl starches, disinfectants, or soaps, positive rheumatoid factor, or the presence of *Stomatococcus mucilaginosus*, *Trichosporon beigelii*, or *Klebsiella pneumoniae* (**Box 1**).[80–86] False-negative results are attributed mainly to a prozone effect or to a low fungal burden (see **Box 1**).[87–89] ELISA shows comparable sensitivity and specificity (99% and 97%, respectively).[90] When these methods are used to detect *Cryptococcus* antigen, an increase in antigen titer during initial therapy may not indicate an increase in viable fungal load, because these antibodies also detect dead organisms and *Cryptococcus* fragments. The quantitative colony-forming unit assay is a measure of *Cryptococcus* viability and therefore is important for diagnosis and for continued assessment of the infection. *Cryptococcus* preferentially grows on media at 30°C to 35°C. Canavanine-glycine-bromthymol blue

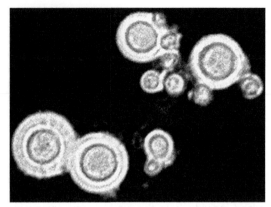

Fig. 1. India ink preparation of *C. neoformans* depicting unique capsule morphology.

medium is a selective medium used to differentiate *C. gattii* from *C. neoformans*.[91] India ink staining also is used to identify the capsule, which is unique to *Cryptococcus*; but it does not distinguish between viable and nonviable cells (see **Fig. 1**).

Recently, it has become evident that in some cases the level of inflammatory response does not reflect the burden of pathogens. This discrepancy is especially apparent in the immune reconstitution inflammatory syndrome (IRIS). IRIS occurs following the initiation of anti-retroviral therapy and when doses of immunosuppressive drugs are reduced in patients who have received a solid-organ transplant.[92–95] Indeed, it also may occur in normal patients.[96] In the presence of *Cryptococcus* infection, these individuals show an enhanced inflammatory response that is out of proportion to the burden of viable organisms.[92,94] The overt clinical signs and symptoms

---

Box 1
Factors causing false-negative or false-positive results when using the latex agglutination test for identification of *Cryptococcus* antigen[80–89]

False-negative results

Prozone effect

Low fungal burden

False-positive results

Positive rheumatoid factor

Increased incubation time with human serum

Presence of hydroxyethyl starches

Disinfectants or soaps

Stomatococcus mucilaginosus

Trichosporon beigelii

Klebsiella pneumoniae

make it quite difficult to distinguish IRIS from worsening infection, and appropriate management can be extremely challenging.

Pulmonary Cryptococcosis

Although inhalation is the mechanism of entry, studies have found that as few as 2% of HIV-positive patients present with pulmonary symptoms. In HIV-negative patients, however, 35% to 77% of those infected with *Cryptococcus* have at least some pulmonary involvement.[30,71,72,97,98] Signs and symptoms of pulmonary involvement include cough (often dry), chest tightness, sputum, and fever, although a few cases in each series were asymptomatic.[72,77,99,100] Pleural effusions, nodules, dense consolidation, ground-glass opacities, reticular or reticulonodular densities, and adenopathy have been observed in both HIV-negative and HIV-positive patients.[101–104] Severe cases of respiratory cryptococcosis in HIV-negative patients resulted in acute respiratory failure.[101,102] Cryptococcosis should be considered in the differential diagnosis of pulmonary nodules, masses, or interstitial pneumonitis identified by chest radiograph or CT scan (**Figs. 2** and **3**).[72,99,100] Diagnosis of pulmonary cryptococcosis is based on positive bronchial alveolar lavage, *Cryptococcus* antigen titer, positive cultures, or India ink staining.

TREATMENT OF CRYPTOCOCCOSIS

Currently, recommendations for treatment of the two species, *C. gattii* and *C. neoformans*, are quite similar, although these recommendations may change in the future. These recommendations are categorized by the host immune status (HIV positive or HIV negative) and organ involvement (respiratory cryptococcosis with or without CNS involvement) and include the use of antifungal agents (azoles, polyene, and nucleoside analogues), CSF drainage, and, occasionally, surgical resection.[77]

Amphotericin B

The mainstay of treatment for severe infections is amphotericin B deoxycholate. Amphotericin B is a polyene agent that has an affinity for fungal sterols and upon binding results in destabilization of the fungal cell membrane and death.[105] Unfortunately, the use of amphotericin B can be limited by side effects.[106] Thus, slow intravenous administration along with frequent monitoring of electrolytes, liver function, renal function, complete blood cell counts, and prothrombin time is recommended. It has been shown that flucytosine, when given along with amphotericin B, resulted in fewer

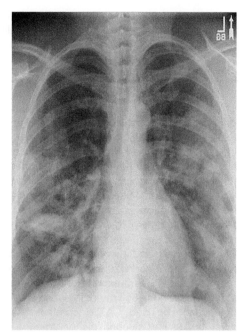

Fig. 2. Frontal projection of a chest roentgenograph from a patient who has *C. gattii* infection. Patchy and nodular parenchymal areas of opacification can be seen throughout both lung fields with a mid- and lower-zone predominance.

relapses and failures than amphotericin B alone, even when the duration of therapy was shorter.[107] Additionally, recent studies show that lipid preparations of amphotericin B (liposomal amphotericin B or amphotericin B lipid complex) decrease nephrotoxicity and other side effects and may be used at higher doses.[108] Although lipid preparations of amphotericin B frequently are used by expert

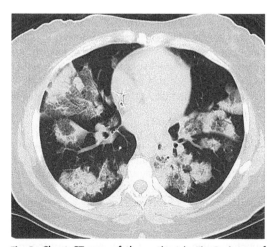

Fig. 3. Chest CT scan of the patient in **Fig. 2**. Areas of dense consolidation and an area of ground-glass opacification are present.

consultants, the superiority of these agents has not been demonstrated in high-quality studies.[105,108]

Azoles

Oral antifungal agents are effective against *Cryptococcus* infections. Interestingly, although amphotericin B is effective in eliminating *Cryptococcus*, it is less efficient in penetrating the blood–brain barrier than azoles such as fluconazole. Therefore azoles have some advantages in meningitis and meningoencephalitis.[105,108] In addition, azole compounds have less toxicity than amphotericin B. Azole compounds target the conversion of lanosterol to ergosterol, resulting in destabilization of the fungal membrane.[105] Azoles that have been studied in cryptococcosis include fluconazole and itraconazole.[109,110] Fluconazole penetrates the CNS, and expert consultants have used high doses (400–800 mg daily) when amphotericin B cannot be used.[77] ATS recommendations suggest the use of fluconazole or itraconazole in mild cryptococcosis and fluconazole after the initial 2 weeks of amphotericin B for treatment of disseminated disease or CNS involvement.[105] Effective treatment of cryptococcosis takes weeks to months, depending on the degree of immunosuppression and severity of the illness, and requires regular reassessment for relapse. Although there is a paucity of studies supporting the use of combined drug therapies, the ATS guidelines indicate that they might be employed.

Nucleoside Analogues

Nucleoside analogues such as flucytosine have been used in treatment of cryptococcosis since the early 1970s.[111] Flucytosine interrupts nucleotide synthesis associated with replication and was used extensively in the pre-HIV era. Unfortunately, the use of this drug alone resulted in *Cryptococcus* resistance.[112] Flucytosine does improve outcomes when used in combination with amphotericin B for individuals who have more extensive disseminated disease, although toxicity can limit its use.[105,107,113]

Immunocompetent Patients

In immunocompetent patients the severity of cryptococcosis varies widely. ATS guidelines indicate that serum antigen titers should be obtained in all immunocompetent patients who have cryptococcosis. If titers are positive or there is any suspicion of CNS involvement, patients should have a lumbar puncture with CSF cultures and cryptococcal antigen titers because of the high mortality associated with CNS involvement.[101] If the patient is asymptomatic and has no evidence of parenchymal disease (colonization only), negative serum antigen titers, and no immunosuppression, treatment may be withheld.[72] Patients who have parenchymal disease, positive serum antigen titers, or immunosuppression should undergo treatment even if there is no evidence of meningitis, because it is not possible to predict in which patients *Cryptococcus* might disseminate to the CNS. Consequently, even asymptomatic patients who fulfill these criteria should be considered for treatment (fluconazole, 200–400 mg/day for up to 6 months followed by 6 months of follow-up monitoring). If fluconazole cannot be used, itraconazole is an alternative,[114] although its penetration to the CNS is inferior to that of fluconazole. The presence of CNS or disseminated *Cryptococcus* should prompt consideration of an initial 2 weeks of amphotericin B, 0.7 to 1 mg/kg/day, with or without flucytosine, 100 mg/kg/day (in four divided doses), followed by fluconazole, 400 mg/day, for 10 weeks. An alternative regimen is amphotericin B, 0.7 to 1 mg/kg/day, with or without flucytosine, 100 mg/kg/day (in four divided doses), for 6 to 10 weeks. An interim assessment at 2 to 3 weeks often is used to ensure clinical response to therapy. On completion of the recommended regimen, follow-up assessment is required, including signs, symptoms, antigen titers, and cultures, because therapy may be extended if cure is not established.[105]

Immunocompromised Patients

Both HIV-positive and HIV-negative immunocompromised infected patients should receive antifungal treatments, even if they are asymptomatic. All immunocompromised patients who have cryptococcosis should have serum antigen titers obtained and a lumbar puncture performed with CSF cultures and cryptococcal antigen titers to determine CNS involvement.[101] In the case of asymptomatic or pulmonary involvement with or without positive serum antigen and in the absence of disseminated or CNS involvement, immunocompromised patients presenting with positive cryptococcal cultures should receive fluconazole, 200 to 400 mg/day, for 6 to 12 months with follow-up prophylaxis. CNS disease and evidence of dissemination to other sites is associated with higher mortality than pulmonary cryptococcosis alone; therefore more aggressive treatments are required, including 2 weeks of amphotericin B, 0.7 to 1 mg/kg/day, with or without flucytosine, 100 mg/kg/day (in four divided doses), followed by fluconazole, 400 mg/day, for 8 weeks (alternatively, amphotericin B, 0.7–1 mg/kg/day, with or without flucytosine, 100 mg/kg/day [in four divided doses] for 6–10 weeks).[115,116] Lipid formulations of amphotericin B, 3 to 6 mg/kg/day for 6 to 10 weeks, can be used as an alternative if the patient is at high risk for nephrotoxicity or has severe cryptococcosis.[105,108] In addition, following the initial course of therapy, immunocompromised patients usually are supplied with prophylactic therapy (fluconazole, 200 mg/day) and signs, symptoms, antigen titers, and cultures are assessed to determine if continued treatment is required.[105]

HIV is a special case in the immunosuppressed population. The ATS guidelines suggest that patients who have HIV and who have CD4 counts lower than 100/μL in the absence of positive cryptococcal cultures or antigen titers should receive prophylactic treatment with fluconazole, 200 mg/day. In addition, upon initiation of antifungal therapy in patients who have HIV, antiretroviral therapy should be delayed for 8 to 10 weeks because of the association of the combination of these treatments with IRIS.[92,93,95] Upon completion of therapy, antifungal prophylaxis should be continued until the CD4 count is higher than 100/μL, HIV RNA levels have become and remained undetectable for 3 months, and the patient has been stable for 1 to 2 years.[105,117,118] It also should be noted that, in rare cases, CNS involvement, including paradoxic intracranial cryptococcoma and intramedullary abscesses, has occurred during restoration of the immune system related to antiretroviral therapy.[119,120]

Additional Management for Immunocompetent or Immunosuppressed Patients

The ATS guidelines recommend intermittent CSF drainage for individuals who have meningitis and high CSF pressures (> 250 mm) after CT or MRI to rule out a cerebral mass effect.[77,105,116] Alternative methods to decrease CSF pressure include ventriculoperitoneal shunts, temporary ventriculostomy, and mannitol therapy. Acetazolamide and other diuretics therapies are to be avoided.[75,116,121–124] Surgical resection of *Cryptococcus* in refractory cases has been associated with improved outcome, but this practice is not common.[125,126] Other antifungal agents, including voriconazole and posaconazole, show promise in the treatment of cryptococcosis; however, no randomized clinical trials have been done that confirm their efficacy.[127] Echinocandins inhibit 1,3-β-d-glucan synthases[105] and therefore have poor activity against cryptococcal glucan synthases.[128] Echinocandins are not effective against cryptococcosis and therefore should not be

used.[129–131] If the patient exhibits signs and symptoms of IRIS, corticosteroids may be of use; however, corticosteroids also can contribute to worsening of the infection.[132]

Prevention of Cryptococcosis

Prevention of *Cryptococcus* infections would be an ideal goal. Avoiding the organism has not been found practical or effective, however, even in discrete geographic outbreaks[133] In the future, approaches might be available to enhance host immune responses. Levitz and colleagues[134] are studying a *Cryptococcus* mannosylated protein vaccine with the goal of increasing the T-helper cell 1–specific host immune response to *C. neoformans.* In murine models the efficiency of this vaccine is greatly enhanced in association with the TLR9 ligand CpG.[134] It is hoped that the prevention of cryptococcosis through vaccines or boosting immunity will prevent or eliminate the disease.

SUMMARY

Cryptococcus infects humans throughout the world and without treatment results in high mortality.[8] It is encouraging that recent advances in treatments have improved outcomes, but morbidity and mortality continue to be associated with *Cryptococcus* infection. Perhaps in the future improved understanding of this organism will lead to improved therapies that will eliminate *C. neoformans* and *C. gattii.*

REFERENCES

1. Safelice F. Contributo alla morfologia e biologia dei blastomiceti che si sviluppano nei succhi di alcuni frutti. Ann Ig 1894;4:463–95.
2. French N, Gray K, Watera C, et al. Cryptococcal infection in a cohort of HIV-1-infected Ugandan adults. AIDS 2002;16(7):1031–8.
3. Lara-Peredo O, Cuevas LE, French N, et al. Cryptococcal infection in an HIV-positive Ugandan population. J Infect 2000;41(2):195.
4. McCarthy KM, Morgan J, Wannemuehler KA, et al. Population-based surveillance for cryptococcosis in an antiretroviral-naive South African province with a high HIV seroprevalence. AIDS 2006;20(17):2199–206.
5. Mitchell TG, Perfect JR. Cryptococcosis in the era of AIDS—100 years after the discovery of Cryptococcus neoformans. Clin Microbiol Rev 1995;8(4):515–48.
6. Kidd SE, Hagen F, Tscharke RL, et al. A rare genotype of Cryptococcus gattii caused the cryptococcosis outbreak on Vancouver Island

(British Columbia, Canada). Proc Natl Acad Sci U S A 2004;101(49):17258–63.

7. Hoang LM, Maguire JA, Doyle P, et al. Cryptococcus neoformans infections at Vancouver Hospital and Health Sciences Centre (1997–2002): epidemiology, microbiology and histopathology. J Med Microbiol 2004;53(Pt 9):935–40.

8. Bartlett KH, Kidd SE, Kronstad JW. The Emergence of Cryptococcus gattii in British Columbia and the Pacific Northwest. Curr Infect Dis Rep 2008;10(1):58–65.

9. Kwon-Chung K, Boekhout T, Fell J, et al. Proposal to conserve the name Cryptococcus gattii against C. bondurianus and C. bacillisporus (Basidiomycota, Hymenomyceter, Tremellomycetidae). Taxon 2002;51(4):804–6.

10. Gugnani HC, Mitchell TG, Litvintseva AP, et al Isolation of Cryptococcus gattii and Cryptococcus neoformans var. grubii from the flowers and bark of Eucalyptus trees in India. Med Mycol 2005;43(6):565–9.

11. Escandon P, Quintero E, Granados D, et al. [Isolation of Cryptococcus gattii serotype B from detritus of Eucalyptus trees in Colombia]. Biomedica 2005;25(3):390–7 [in Spanish].

12. Pfeiffer T, Ellis D. Environmental isolation of Cryptococcus neoformans gattii from California. J Infect Dis 1991;163(4):929–30.

13. Kidd SE, Chow Y, Mak S, et al. Characterization of environmental sources of the human and animal pathogen Cryptococcus gattii in British Columbia, Canada, and the Pacific Northwest of the United States. Appl Environ Microbiol 2007;73(5):1433–43.

14. Kidd SE, Bach PJ, Hingston AO, et al. Cryptococcus gattii dispersal mechanisms, British Columbia, Canada. Emerg Infect Dis 2007;13(1):51–7.

15. Chen S, Sorrell T, Nimmo G, et al. Epidemiology and host- and variety-dependent characteristics of infection due to Cryptococcus neoformans in Australia and New Zealand. Australasian Cryptococcal Study Group. Clin Infect Dis 2000;31(2):499–508.

16. Sorrell TC. Cryptococcus neoformans variety gattii. Med Mycol 2001;39(2):155–68.

17. Wickes BL, Mayorga ME, Edman U, et al. Dimorphism and haploid fruiting in Cryptococcus neoformans: association with the alpha-mating type. Proc Natl Acad Sci U S A 1996;93(14):7327–31.

18. Kwon-Chung KJ, Bennett JE. Distribution of alpha and alpha mating types of Cryptococcus neoformans among natural and clinical isolates. Am J Epidemiol 1978;108(4):337–40.

19. Kwon-Chung KJ, Edman JC, Wickes BL. Genetic association of mating types and virulence in Cryptococcus neoformans. Infect Immun 1992;60(2):602–5.

20. Nielsen K, Cox GM, Litvintseva AP, et al. Cryptococcus neoformans {alpha} strains preferentially disseminate to the central nervous system during coinfection. Infect Immun 2005;73(8):4922–33.

21. Fraser JA, Giles SS, Wenink EC, et al. Same-sex mating and the origin of the Vancouver Island Cryptococcus gattii outbreak. Nature 2005;437(7063):1360–4.

22. Sorrell TC, Chen SC, Ruma P, et al. Concordance of clinical and environmental isolates of Cryptococcus neoformans var. gattii by random amplification of polymorphic DNA analysis and PCR fingerprinting. J Clin Microbiol 1996;34(5):1253–60.

23. Yamamoto Y, Kohno S, Koga H, et al. Random amplified polymorphic DNA analysis of clinically and environmentally isolated Cryptococcus neoformans in Nagasaki. J Clin Microbiol 1995;33(12):3328–32.

24. Pappas PG, Perfect JR, Cloud GA, et al. Cryptococcosis in human immunodeficiency virus-negative patients in the era of effective azole therapy. Clin Infect Dis 2001;33(5):690–9.

25. Wilson ML, Sewell LD, Mowad CM. Primary cutaneous cryptococcosis during therapy with methotrexate and adalimumab. J Drugs Dermatol 2008;7(1):53–4.

26. Caballes RL, Caballes RA Jr. Primary cryptococcal prostatitis in an apparently uncompromised host. Prostate 1999;39(2):119–22.

27. Sheu SJ, Chen YC, Kuo NW, et al. Endogenous cryptococcal endophthalmitis. Ophthalmology 1998;105(2):377–81.

28. Bicanic T, Harrison TS. Cryptococcal meningitis. Br Med Bull 2004;72:99–118.

29. Garcia-Hermoso D, Janbon G, Dromer F. Epidemiological evidence for dormant Cryptococcus neoformans infection. J Clin Microbiol 1999;37(10):3204–9.

30. Levy R, Pitout J, Long P, et al. Late presentation of Cryptococcus gattii meningitis in a traveller to Vancouver Island: a case report. Can J Infect Dis Med Microbiol 2007;18(3):197–9.

31. MacDougall L, Fyfe M. Emergence of Cryptococcus gattii in a novel environment provides clues to its incubation period. J Clin Microbiol 2006;44(5):1851–2.

32. Meyer W, Marszewska K, Amirmostofian M, et al. Molecular typing of global isolates of Cryptococcus neoformans var. neoformans by polymerase chain reaction fingerprinting and randomly amplified polymorphic DNA—a pilot study to standardize techniques on which to base a detailed epidemiological survey. Electrophoresis 1999;20(8):1790–9.

33. Silveira FP, Husain S, Kwak EJ, et al. Cryptococcosis in liver and kidney transplant recipients receiving anti-thymocyte globulin or alemtuzumab. Transpl Infect Dis 2007;9(1):22–7.

34. Wu G, Vilchez RA, Eidelman B, et al. Cryptococcal meningitis: an analysis among 5,521 consecutive organ transplant recipients. Transpl Infect Dis 2002;4(4):183–8.

35. Chayakulkeeree M, Perfect JR. Cryptococcosis. Infect Dis Clin North Am 2006;20(3):507–44, v–vi.

36. Kozic H, Riggs K, Ringpfeil F, et al. Disseminated *Cryptococcus neoformans* after treatment with infliximab for rheumatoid arthritis. J Am Acad Dermatol 2008;58(5 Suppl 1):S95–6.

37. Stangel M, Muller M, Marx P. Adverse events during treatment with high-dose intravenous immunoglobulins for neurological disorders. Eur Neurol 1998;40(3):173–4.

38. Dromer F, Mathoulin S, Dupont B, et al. Epidemiology of cryptococcosis in France: a 9-year survey (1985–1993). French Cryptococcosis Study Group. Clin Infect Dis 1996;23(1):82–90.

39. Mirza SA, Phelan M, Rimland D, et al. The changing epidemiology of cryptococcosis: an update from population-based active surveillance in 2 large metropolitan areas, 1992–2000. Clin Infect Dis 2003;36(6):789–94.

40. Crowe SM, Carlin JB, Stewart KI, et al. Predictive value of CD4 lymphocyte numbers for the development of opportunistic infections and malignancies in HIV-infected persons. J Acquir Immune Defic Syndr 1991;4(8):770–6.

41. Mody CH, Chen GH, Jackson C, et al. Depletion of murine CD8+ T cells in vivo decreases pulmonary clearance of a moderately virulent strain of *Cryptococcus neoformans*. J Lab Clin Med 1993;121(6): 765–73.

42. Mody CH, Lipscomb MF, Street NE, et al. Depletion of CD4+ (L3T4+) lymphocytes in vivo impairs murine host defense to *Cryptococcus neoformans*. J Immunol 1990;144(4):1472–7.

43. Mody CH, Paine R 3rd, Jackson C, et al. CD8 cells play a critical role in delayed type hypersensitivity to intact *Cryptococcus neoformans*. J Immunol 1994;152(8):3970–9.

44. Dykstra MA, Friedman L, Murphy JW. Capsule size of *Cryptococcus neoformans*: control and relationship to virulence. Infect Immun 1977;16(1):129–35.

45. Kozel TR, Gotschlich EC. The capsule of *Cryptococcus neoformans* passively inhibits phagocytosis of the yeast by macrophages. J Immunol 1982;129(4):1675–80.

46. Kelly RM, Chen J, Yauch LE, et al. Opsonic requirements for dendritic cell-mediated responses to *Cryptococcus neoformans*. Infect Immun 2005; 73(1):592–8.

47. Kozel TR, Wilson MA, Murphy JW. Early events in initiation of alternative complement pathway activation by the capsule of *Cryptococcus neoformans*. Infect Immun 1991;59(9):3101–10.

48. Kwon-Chung KJ, Rhodes JC. Encapsulation and melanin formation as indicators of virulence in *Cryptococcus neoformans*. Infect Immun 1986; 51(1):218–23.

49. Jacobson ES, Jenkins ND, Todd JM. Relationship between superoxide dismutase and melanin in a pathogenic fungus. Infect Immun 1994;62(9):4085–6.

50. Wong B, Perfect JR, Beggs S, et al. Production of the hexitol D-mannitol by *Cryptococcus neoformans* in vitro and in rabbits with experimental meningitis. Infect Immun 1990;58(6):1664–70.

51. Missall TA, Lodge JK. Thioredoxin reductase is essential for viability in the fungal pathogen *Cryptococcus neoformans*. Eukaryot Cell 2005;4(2):487–9.

52. Chen LC, Blank ES, Casadevall A. Extracellular proteinase activity of *Cryptococcus neoformans*. Clin Diagn Lab Immunol 1996;3(5):570–4.

53. Cox GM, Mukherjee J, Cole GT, et al. Urease as a virulence factor in experimental cryptococcosis. Infect Immun 2000;68(2):443–8.

54. Chen SC, Wright LC, Santangelo RT, et al. Identification of extracellular phospholipase B, lysophospholipase, and acyltransferase produced by *Cryptococcus neoformans*. Infect Immun 1997;65(2):405–11.

55. Ghannoum MA. Potential role of phospholipases in virulence and fungal pathogenesis. Clin Microbiol Rev 2000;13(1):122–43, table of contents.

56. Kuroki M, Phichaichumpon C, Yasuoka A, et al. Environmental isolation of *Cryptococcus neoformans* from an endemic region of HIV-associated cryptococcosis in Thailand. Yeast 2004;21(10): 809–12.

57. van Elden LJ, Walenkamp AM, Lipovsky MM, et al. Declining number of patients with cryptococcosis in the Netherlands in the era of highly active antiretroviral therapy. AIDS 2000;14(17):2787–8.

58. Baddley JW, Perfect JR, Oster RA, et al. Pulmonary cryptococcosis in patients without HIV infection: factors associated with disseminated disease. Eur J Clin Microbiol Infect Dis 2008;27(10):937–43.

59. Mody CH, Toews GB, Lipscomb MF. Cyclosporin A inhibits the growth of Cryptococcus neoformans in a murine model. Infect Immun 1988;56(1):7–12.

60. Mody CH, Toews GB, Lipscomb MF. Treatment of murine cryptococcosis with cyclosporin-A in normal and athymic mice. Am Rev Respir Dis 1989;139(1):8–13.

61. Anekthananon T, Ratanasuwan W, Techasathit W, et al. HIV infection/acquired immunodeficiency syndrome at Siriraj Hospital, 2002: time for secondary prevention. J Med Assoc Thai 2004; 87(2):173–9.

62. Carroll RR, Noyes WD, Kitchens CS. High-dose intravenous immunoglobulin therapy in patients with immune thrombocytopenic purpura. JAMA 1983;249(13):1748–50.

63. Sethi NK, Torgovnick J, Sethi PK. Cryptococcal meningitis after Imuran (azathioprine) therapy for autoimmune hepatitis. Eur J Gastroenterol Hepatol 2007;19(10):913–4.

64. Safdieh JE, Mead PA, Sepkowitz KA, et al. Bacterial and fungal meningitis in patients with cancer. Neurology 2008;70(12):943–7.

65. Husain S, Wagener MM, Singh N. *Cryptococcus neoformans* infection in organ transplant recipients: variables influencing clinical characteristics and outcome. Emerg Infect Dis 2001;7(3):375–81.

66. Mitchell DH, Sorrell TC, Allworth AM, et al. Cryptococcal disease of the CNS in immunocompetent hosts: influence of cryptococcal variety on clinical manifestations and outcome. Clin Infect Dis 1995; 20(3):611–6.

67. Bennett JE, Kwon-Chung KJ, Howard DH. Epidemiologic differences among serotypes of *Cryptococcus neoformans*. Am J Epidemiol 1977;105(6): 582–6.

68. Kwon-Chung KJ, Bennett JE. Epidemiologic differences between the two varieties of *Cryptococcus neoformans*. Am J Epidemiol 1984;120(1):123–30.

69. Kidd SE, Guo H, Bartlett KH, et al. Comparative gene genealogies indicate that two clonal lineages of *Cryptococcus gattii* in British Columbia resemble strains from other geographical areas. Eukaryot Cell 2005;4(10):1629–38.

70. MacDougall L, Kidd SE, Galanis E, et al. Spread of *Cryptococcus gattii* in British Columbia, Canada, and detection in the Pacific Northwest, USA. Emerg Infect Dis 2007;13(1):42–50.

71. Jongwutiwes U, Sungkanuparph S, Kiertiburanakul S. Comparison of clinical features and survival between cryptococcosis in human immunodeficiency virus (HIV)-positive and HIV-negative patients. Jpn J Infect Dis 2008;61(2):111–5.

72. Nadrous HF, Antonios VS, Terrell CL, et al. Pulmonary cryptococcosis in nonimmunocompromised patients. Chest 2003;124(6):2143–7.

73. Charlier C, Nielsen K, Daou S, et al. Evidence for a role of monocytes in dissemination and brain invasion by *Cryptococcus neoformans*. Infect Immun 2009;77(1):120–7.

74. Jong A, Wu CH, Shackleford GM, et al. Involvement of human CD44 during *Cryptococcus neoformans* infection of brain microvascular endothelial cells. Cell Microbiol 2008;10(6):1313–26.

75. Johnston SR, Corbett EL, Foster O, et al. Raised intracranial pressure and visual complications in AIDS patients with cryptococcal meningitis. J Infect 1992;24(2):185–9.

76. Antinori S, Galimberti L, Magni C, et al. Cryptococcus neoformans infection in a cohort of Italian AIDS patients: natural history, early prognostic parameters, and autopsy findings. Eur J Clin Microbiol Infect Dis 2001;20(10):711–7.

77. Saag MS, Graybill RJ, Larsen RA, et al. Practice guidelines for the management of cryptococcal disease. Infectious Diseases Society of America. Clin Infect Dis 2000;30(4):710–8.

78. Eckert TF, Kozel TR. Production and characterization of monoclonal antibodies specific for *Cryptococcus neoformans* capsular polysaccharide. Infect Immun 1987;55(8):1895–9.

79. Baughman RP, Rhodes JC, Dohn MN, et al. Detection of cryptococcal antigen in bronchoalveolar lavage fluid: a prospective study of diagnostic utility. Am Rev Respir Dis 1992;145(5):1226–9.

80. McFadden DC, Zaragoza O, Casadevall A. Immunoreactivity of cryptococcal antigen is not stable under prolonged incubations in human serum. J Clin Microbiol 2004;42(6):2786–8.

81. Millon L, Barale T, Julliot MC, et al. Interference by hydroxyethyl starch used for vascular filling in latex agglutination test for cryptococcal antigen. J Clin Microbiol 1995;33(7):1917–9.

82. Blevins LB, Fenn J, Segal H, et al. False-positive cryptococcal antigen latex agglutination caused by disinfectants and soaps. J Clin Microbiol 1995; 33(6):1674–5.

83. McManus EJ, Bozdech MJ, Jones JM. Role of the latex agglutination test for cryptococcal antigen in diagnosing disseminated infections with *Trichosporon beigelii*. J Infect Dis 1985; 151(6):1167–9.

84. Bennett JE, Bailey JW. Control for rheumatoid factor in the latex test for cryptococcosis. Am J Clin Pathol 1971;56(3):360–5.

85. MacKinnon S, Kane JG, Parker RH. False-positive cryptococcal antigen test and cervical prevertebral abscess. JAMA 1978;240(18):1982–3.

86. Tanner DC, Weinstein MP, Fedorciw B, et al. Comparison of commercial kits for detection of cryptococcal antigen. J Clin Microbiol 1994;32(7): 1680–4.

87. Gray LD, Roberts GD. Experience with the use of pronase to eliminate interference factors in the latex agglutination test for cryptococcal antigen. J Clin Microbiol 1988;26(11):2450–1.

88. Stoeckli TC, Burman WJ. Inactivated pronase as the cause of false-positive results of serum cryptococcal antigen tests. Clin Infect Dis 2001;32(5):836–7.

89. Stamm AM, Polt SS. False-negative cryptococcal antigen test. JAMA 1980;244(12):1359.

90. Gade W, Hinnefeld SW, Babcock LS, et al. Comparison of the PREMIER cryptococcal antigen enzyme immunoassay and the latex agglutination assay for detection of cryptococcal antigens. J Clin Microbiol 1991;29(8):1616–9.

91. Min KH, Kwon-Chung KJ. The biochemical basis for the distinction between the two *Cryptococcus neoformans* varieties with CGB medium. Zentralbl Bakteriol Mikrobiol Hyg [A] 1986;261(4): 471–80.

92. Shelburne SA 3rd, Darcourt J, White AC Jr, et al. The role of immune reconstitution inflammatory syndrome in AIDS-related *Cryptococcus*

neoformans disease in the era of highly active anti-retroviral therapy. Clin Infect Dis 2005;40(7): 1049–52.

93. Jenny-Avital ER, Abadi M. Immune reconstitution cryptococcosis after initiation of successful highly active antiretroviral therapy. Clin Infect Dis 2002; 35(12):e128–33.

94. Singh N, Lortholary O, Alexander BD, et al. An immune reconstitution syndrome-like illness associated with *Cryptococcus neoformans* infection in organ transplant recipients. Clin Infect Dis 2005; 40(12):1756–61.

95. King MD, Perlino CA, Cinnamon J, et al. Paradoxical recurrent meningitis following therapy of cryptococcal meningitis: an immune reconstitution syndrome after initiation of highly active antiretroviral therapy. Int J STD AIDS 2002;13(10):724–6.

96. Ecevit IZ, Clancy CJ, Schmalfuss IM, et al. The poor prognosis of central nervous system cryptococcosis among nonimmunosuppressed patients: a call for better disease recognition and evaluation of adjuncts to antifungal therapy. Clin Infect Dis 2006;42(10):1443–7.

97. Oliveira Fde M, Severo CB, Guazzelli LS, et al. Cryptococcus gattii fungemia: report of a case with lung and brain lesions mimicking radiological features of malignancy. Rev Inst Med Trop Sao Paulo 2007;49(4):263–5.

98. Sweeney DA, Caserta MT, Korones DN, et al. A ten-year-old boy with a pulmonary nodule secondary to *Cryptococcus neoformans*: case report and review of the literature. Pediatr Infect Dis J 2003;22(12):1089–93.

99. Yang CJ, Hwang JJ, Wang TH, et al. Clinical and radiographic presentations of pulmonary cryptococcosis in immunocompetent patients. Scand J Infect Dis 2006;38(9):788–93.

100. Nunez M, Peacock JE Jr, Chin R Jr. Pulmonary cryptococcosis in the immunocompetent host. Therapy with oral fluconazole: a report of four cases and a review of the literature. Chest 2000; 118(2):527–34.

101. Vilchez RA, Linden P, Lacomis J, et al. Acute respiratory failure associated with pulmonary cryptococcosis in non-aids patients. Chest 2001;119(6): 1865–9.

102. Aberg JA, Mundy LM, Powderly WG. Pulmonary cryptococcosis in patients without HIV infection. Chest 1999;115(3):734–40.

103. Cameron ML, Bartlett JA, Gallis HA, et al. Manifestations of pulmonary cryptococcosis in patients with acquired immunodeficiency syndrome. Rev Infect Dis 1991;13(1):64–7.

104. Zinck SE, Leung AN, Frost M, et al. Pulmonary cryptococcosis: CT and pathologic findings. J Comput Assist Tomogr 2002;26(3):330–4.

105. Limper AH, Knox KS, Sarosi GA, et al. American Thoracic society statement on treatment of fungal infections in adult pulmonary and critical care patients. Am J Respir Crit Care Med 2009, in review.

106. Olivero JJ, Lozano-Mendez J, Ghafary EM, et al. Mitigation of amphotericin B nephrotoxicity by mannitol. Br Med J 1975;1(5957):550–1.

107. Bennett JE, Dismukes WE, Duma RJ, et al. A comparison of amphotericin B alone and combined with flucytosine in the treatment of cryptococcal meningitis. N Engl J Med 1979;301(3):126–31.

108. Coukell AJ, Brogden RN. Liposomal amphotericin B. Therapeutic use in the management of fungal infections and visceral leishmaniasis. Drugs 1998;55(4): 585–612.

109. Stern JJ, Hartman BJ, Sharkey P, et al. Oral fluconazole therapy for patients with acquired immunodeficiency syndrome and cryptococcosis: experience with 22 patients. Am J Med 1988;85(4):477–80.

110. Viviani MA, Tortorano AM, Langer M, et al. Experience with itraconazole in cryptococcosis and aspergillosis. J Infect 1989;18(2):151–65.

111. Block ER, Bennett JE. Pharmacological studies with 5-fluorocytosine. Antimicrobial Agents Chemother 1972;1(6):476–82.

112. Utz JP, Tynes BS, Shadomy HJ, et al. 5-Fluorocytosine in human cryptococcosis. Antimicrob Agents Chemother (Bethesda) 1968;8:344–6.

113. Bicanic T, Wood R, Meintjes G, et al. High-dose amphotericin B with flucytosine for the treatment of cryptococcal meningitis in HIV-infected patients: a randomized trial. Clin Infect Dis 2008; 47(1):123–30.

114. Denning DW, Tucker RM, Hanson LH, et al. Itraconazole in opportunistic mycoses: cryptococcosis and aspergillosis. J Am Acad Dermatol 1990; 23(3 Pt 2):602–7.

115. van der Horst CM, Saag MS, Cloud GA, et al. Treatment of cryptococcal meningitis associated with the acquired immunodeficiency syndrome. National Institute of Allergy and Infectious Diseases Mycoses Study Group and AIDS Clinical Trials Group. N Engl J Med 1997;337(1):15–21.

116. Graybill JR, Sobel J, Saag M, et al. Diagnosis and management of increased intracranial pressure in patients with AIDS and cryptococcal meningitis. The NIAID Mycoses Study Group and AIDS Co-operative Treatment Groups. Clin Infect Dis 2000; 30(1):47–54.

117. Mussini C, Pezzotti P, Miro JM, et al. Discontinuation of maintenance therapy for cryptococcal meningitis in patients with AIDS treated with highly active antiretroviral therapy: an international observational study. Clin Infect Dis 2004; 38(4):565–71.

118. Vibhagool A, Sungkanuparph S, Mootsikapun P, et al. Discontinuation of secondary prophylaxis for cryptococcal meningitis in human immunodeficiency virus-infected patients treated with highly

active antiretroviral therapy: a prospective, multi-center, randomized study. Clin Infect Dis 2003; 36(10):1329–31.

119. Rambeloarisoa J, Batisse D, Thiebaut JB, et al. Intramedullary abscess resulting from disseminated cryptococcosis despite immune restoration in a patient with AIDS. J Infect 2002;44(3):185–8.

120. Breton G, Seilhean D, Cherin P, et al. Paradoxical intracranial cryptococcoma in a human immunodeficiency virus-infected man being treated with combination antiretroviral therapy. Am J Med 2002;113(2):155–7.

121. Fessler RD, Sobel J, Guyot L, et al. Management of elevated intracranial pressure in patients with Cryptococcal meningitis. J Acquir Immune Defic Syndr Hum Retrovirol 1998;17(2):137–42.

122. Liliang PC, Liang CL, Chang WN, et al. Shunt surgery for hydrocephalus complicating cryptococcal meningitis in human immunodeficiency virus-negative patients. Clin Infect Dis 2003;37(5):673–8.

123. Liliang PC, Liang CL, Chang WN, et al. Use of ventriculoperitoneal shunts to treat uncontrollable intracranial hypertension in patients who have cryptococcal meningitis without hydrocephalus. Clin Infect Dis 2002;34(12):E64–8.

124. Park MK, Hospenthal DR, Bennett JE. Treatment of hydrocephalus secondary to cryptococcal meningitis by use of shunting. Clin Infect Dis 1999;28(3):629–33.

125. Kishi K, Fujii T, Takaya H, et al. Pulmonary coccidioidomycosis found in healthy Japanese individuals. Respirology 2008;13(2):252–6.

126. Liu M, Jiang GN [Surgical treatment of pulmonary cryptococcosis]. Zhonghua Jie He He Hu Xi Za Zhi 2006;29(5):307–9 [in Chinese].

127. Kantarcioglu AS, Boekhout T, Yucel A, et al. Susceptibility testing of Cryptococcus diffluens against amphotericin B, flucytosine, fluconazole, itraconazole, voriconazole and posaconazole. Med Mycol 2008;25:1–8.

128. Feldmesser M, Kress Y, Mednick A, et al. The effect of the echinocandin analogue caspofungin on cell wall glucan synthesis by Cryptococcus neoformans. J Infect Dis 2000; 182(6):1791–5.

129. Cappelletty D, Eiselstein-McKitrick K. The echinocandins. Pharmacotherapy 2007;27(3):369–88.

130. Cornely OA. Aspergillus to Zygomycetes: causes, risk factors, prevention, and treatment of invasive fungal infections. Infection 2008;36(4): 296–313.

131. Cuenca-Estrella M, Gomez-Lopez A, Mellado E, et al. Head-to-head comparison of the activities of currently available antifungal agents against 3,378 Spanish clinical isolates of yeasts and filamentous fungi. Antimicrobial Agents Chemother 2006;50(3):917–21.

132. Seaton RA, Verma N, Naraqi S, et al. The effect of corticosteroids on visual loss in Cryptococcus neoformans var. gattii meningitis. Trans R Soc Trop Med Hyg 1997;91(1):50–2.

133. Chambers C, MacDougall L, Li M, et al. Tourism and specific risk areas for Cryptococcus gattii, Vancouver Island, Canada. Emerg Infect Dis 2008;14(11):1781–3.

134. Dan JM, Wang JP, Lee CK, et al. Cooperative stimulation of dendritic cells by Cryptococcus neoformans mannoproteins and CpG oligodeoxynucleotides. PLoS ONE 2008;3(4):e2046.

Pneumocystis Pneumonia: Current Concepts in Pathogenesis, Diagnosis, and Treatment

Bryan J. Krajicek, MD, Charles F. Thomas, Jr, MD,
Andrew H. Limper, MD*

KEYWORDS

- Pneumocystis pneumonia
- Opportunistic infection
- Acquired immunodeficiency syndrome (AIDS)
- Immune suppression • Inflammation

Pneumocystis jirovecii (formerly *P carinii*) is an ascomycetous fungus that causes opportunistic infection, particularly pneumonia, in patients who have impaired immunity. Pneumocystis pneumonia (PCP) continues to be a devastating AIDS-defining illness in patients who have HIV infection.[1] PCP also occurs in other non-HIV immunosuppressed patients, particularly those receiving immunosuppressive agents in the settings of malignancy, organ transplantation, and various rheumatologic and hematologic conditions. PCP in these patients frequently occurs as a result of adjusting the dosage of immunosuppressants.[2,3] The number of patients who are receiving chronic immunosuppressive medications or who have an impaired immune system placing them at risk for PCP is increasing.[4] The diagnosis of PCP continues to be challenging, despite advances in laboratory technology. Early treatment is beneficial, particularly in patients who have PCP who do not have HIV, whose prognosis is dismal once mechanical ventilation for respiratory failure is required.[5] The mortality rate of PCP in patients who have or do not have AIDS ranges from 10% to 60% depending on the population at risk, with immunocompromised cancer patients having the highest mortality.[4,6] This article summarizes recent advances resulting from studies of the cell biology and genetics of *Pneumocystis* and reviews current epidemiologic, diagnostic, and treatment modalities for PCP.

TAXONOMY OF *PNEUMOCYSTIS*

The taxonomy of *Pneumocystis* has changed considerably over the years. Carlos Chagas, who believed that he had discovered a new trypanosomal life form in his guinea pig model of trypanosome infection, first identified members of the current *Pneumocystis* fungal genus in 1909. Antonio Carinii later identified similar organisms in 1910, again believing that they also represented a new trypanosomal life form. In 1912, the Delanoës recognized that the organism represented a uniquely different species and named it *Pneumocystis carinii*, highlighting its unique tropism for the lung and giving credit to Carinii, rather than Chagas.[7]

Pneumocystis carinii was initially classified as a protozoan based on the histologic characteristics of its trophozoite and cyst life forms and its

Division of Pulmonary and Critical Care Medicine, Mayo Clinic, 200 First Street SW, Rochester, MN 55905, USA
* Corresponding author.
E-mail address: limper.andrew@mayo.edu (A.H. Limper).

Clin Chest Med 30 (2009) 265–278
doi:10.1016/j.ccm.2009.02.005
0272-5231/09/$ – see front matter © 2009 Elsevier Inc. All rights reserved.

treatment response with the anti-protozoan medication pentamidine, the first agent found effective against this newly discovered microbe. In 1988, *P carinii* was phylogenetically reclassified within the fungal kingdom after sequencing of the small ribosomal RNA subunit and the discovery that it possessed homology to ascomycetous fungi.[8] Since its initial discovery, a unique form of *Pneumocystis* has been identified in virtually every mammal investigated, including rats, mice, ferrets, swine, sheep, various primates, bats, and cetacean host species. Each form of *Pneumocystis* possesses unique genetic characteristics and strict host specificity. The explanation for such strict host specificity has not been determined and is largely unprecedented in the fungi. The form that infects humans has recently been renamed *Pneumocystis jirovecii*, after the pathologist Jirovec who first reported the organism in humans.[9]

PATHOGENESIS AND LIFE CYCLE OF *PNEUMOCYSTIS*

The transmission of *Pneumocystis* organisms between hosts is not fully understood. Early studies noted the identification of *Pneumocystis* nucleic acids in ambient air and pond water.[7] It remains uncertain, however, whether there is an ecologic niche or reservoir for *Pneumocystis* outside of the mammalian host. Currently, animal and human studies favor an airborne transmission model for PCP with person-to-person spread being the most likely mode of infection acquisition. Several recent observations have described the detection of small numbers of *Pneumocystis* organisms in individuals who have normal immunity or HIV but who do not have evidence of active infection or clinical disease.[10,11] On repeat sampling of such individuals, the organisms often is not detected again, suggesting that temporary asymptomatic carriage of *P jirovecii* does occur. In addition, an increasing number of reports have described the occurrence of asymptomatic pulmonary colonization by *P jirovecii* in otherwise immunocompetent hosts who have underlying lung disease, such as chronic obstructive lung disease or interstitial lung disease.[12–16]

The current inability to propagate *Pneumocystis* outside of the host lung has been a major obstacle to studying the life cycle and genetics of this opportunistic fungal pathogen.[1] *Pneumocystis* can proliferate transiently in low numbers in the presence of lung epithelial cells in tissue-culture medium. Sustained in vitro growth has not been achieved despite multiple attempts to simulate the environment of the alveoli. Pneumonia models in immune-suppressed animals remain the main source of organisms for laboratory studies, yet these approaches have numerous inherent difficulties. Although the study of *Pneumocystis* has been hindered by the inability to isolate the fungus in pure culture, the use of molecular techniques and genomic analysis has recently brought many insights into its complex pathogenesis and life cycle.[7]

According to current information, *Pneumocystis* exists almost exclusively within lung alveoli in the infected host. Attachment of *Pneumocystis* to the alveolar epithelium strongly promotes proliferation of the organism.[17] Studies in which organism attachment to alveoli was prevented by physical or chemical means resulted in inhibition of organism proliferation.[18] Although organism attachment to alveoli epithelial cells is essential for *Pneumocystis* infection and propagation, invasion of host cells is not common. Disseminated *Pneumocystis* infection has rarely been reported and occurs only in the setting of overwhelming infection or severe immunosuppression.[19]

There are at least two unique morphologic life cycle forms of *Pneumocystis*, the trophic form and the cyst form (**Fig. 1**). The trophic form measures 1 to 4 μm in diameter and the mature cyst is 8 to 10 μm in diameter. The trophic forms predominate over the cyst forms by approximately 10:1 during infection of the lung. During infection, most trophic forms are haploid and it has been hypothesized that trophic forms can conjugate and develop into cysts. Microscopic observation of life cycle forms has led to a proposed *Pneumocystis* life cycle model (**Fig. 2**). Three intermediate cyst stages (early, intermediate, and late precysts) containing complements of two, four, and eight nuclei have been visualized by electron microscopy.[20] The mature cyst contains eight intracystic nuclei. It has been suggested that trophic forms originate from the intracystic nuclei of the mature cyst as it ruptures and then undergo vegetative growth or conjugation to re-form the cyst forms. In addition to this form of sexual reproduction, it is hypothesized that trophic forms also may undergo haploid mitosis and binary fission as a form of asexual reproduction.[7]

The proposed *Pneumocystis* life cycle described above is based solely on the microscopic observation of life cycle forms. The inability to propagate *Pneumocystis* outside the host lung has prevented isolation of its life cycle forms in pure in vitro culture. Although this proposed model is compatible with the life cycle of other ascomycetous fungi, it seems clear that study of *Pneumocystis* will advance rapidly once the organism can be cultured outside of the mammalian host.

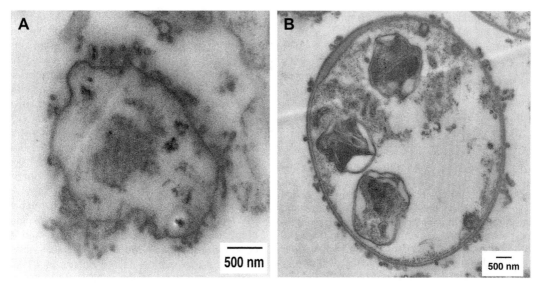

Fig. 1. Electron microscopic imaging of isolated *Pneumocystis* life cycle forms. (*A*) *Pneumocystis* trophic forms demonstrated by transmission electron microscopy. These simple forms are 1 to 4 μm in diameter and have a simple plasma membrane often with filopodial projections. (*B*) *Pneumocystis* cyst forms are larger (~8–10 μm in diameter) and are characterized by a rigid b-glucan–rich cyst wall. Cysts contain up to eight intracystic bodies, which will be released to generate new trophic forms.

IMPLICATIONS OF *PNEUMOCYSTIS* GENOMIC ANALYSIS

Use of *Pneumocystis* genome analysis has led to major advances in our understanding of *Pneumocystis* biology during the past decade. Key proteins involved in cell cycle control, cell wall assembly, signal transduction cascades, and metabolic pathways have been identified.[7] Each offers the potential for yielding novel drug targets in the treatment of PCP. Currently known molecules with defined functions in *Pneumocystis* metabolic pathways include dihydropteroate synthase (DHPS) and dihydrofolate reductase (DHFR), the molecular targets of the first-line medications sulfamethoxazole and trimethoprim. Although their clinical significance remains controversial, mutations in the DHFR enzyme and DHPS gene have been increasingly found in patients who have PCP.[21–24] Furthermore, mutations in the cytochrome *b* gene, identified in the mitochondria of *Pneumocystis*, have been shown to confer resistance to atovaquone, an important second-line therapy for PCP.[25] Recent studies suggest that addition of caspofungin, a medication targeting *Pneumocystis* glucan synthetase (GSC1) thereby inhibiting fungal cell wall beta-1,3-glucan synthesis, to conventional treatment with trimethoprim-sulfamethoxazole (TMP-SMX) may theoretically provide synergistic activity in severe PCP in patients who do not have HIV.[26] The identification of additional therapeutic targets is anticipated following the completion of the *Pneumocystis* genome project, which will be increasingly important given increasing concerns for emerging resistance to current pharmacologic agents.

EPIDEMIOLOGY OF *PNEUMOCYSTIS* PNEUMONIA

The number of patients who have an altered immune system or who are receiving chronic immunosuppressive medications and are thus at a risk for PCP is rapidly growing.[4] PCP remains the most prevalent opportunistic infection in patients who have AIDS, even in the era of highly active antiretroviral therapy (HAART).[27,28] Other individuals at risk for contracting PCP include patients who have hematologic or solid malignancies, individuals receiving immunosuppressive medications, transplant recipients, and those who have an altered immune system.[1,4] Patients who have cancer may present with PCP before receiving chemotherapy likely resulting from malignancy-related immune depression.[5] Although corticosteroids remain the most recognized immunosuppressive medication associated with *Pneumocystis* infection, PCP has been reported with many nonsteroid immune modulating medications. Several recent reports describe the development of PCP in patients who have autoimmune diseases or malignancy being treated with the monoclonal antibodies adalimumab, infliximab, etanercept, or rituximab.[29–34] The true incidence of PCP in

Proposed Life Cycle of *Pneumocystis*

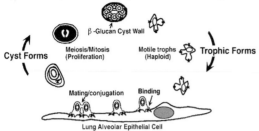

Fig. 2. Proposed life cycle of *Pneumocystis*. Motile *Pneumocystis* forms bind tightly to lung alveolar epithelial cells. Growing evidence supports a sexual conjugation-mating phase followed by meiosis and mitosis resulting in a mature cyst containing eight intracystic bodies. The cyst ruptures releasing the intracystic bodies as new trophic forms. The trophic forms are haploid and it is further proposed that they may also undergo asexual proliferation through haploid mitosis.

patients being treated with these novel biologic agents is unknown. Accordingly, care providers must be aware of PCP as a possible complication of their use and remain vigilant for this complication.

CLINICAL FEATURES OF *PNEUMOCYSTIS PNEUMONIA*

The diagnosis of PCP is challenging for primary care physicians, internists, infectious disease specialists, and pulmonary and critical care specialists alike. Physicians caring for immunocompromised patients should maintain a high index of suspicion for PCP. Although PCP is most frequently associated with AIDS, several groups of immunocompromised patients who do not have AIDS are also at risk of for developing PCP. The clinical features and symptoms of PCP differ in patients who have or do not have AIDS.

In patients infected with HIV, PCP is a common AIDS-defining illness, with patients developing the subacute onset of progressive dyspnea, a nonproductive cough or cough productive of clear sputum, malaise, and a low-grade fever. These symptoms may develop over several weeks. PCP occurs most frequently in patients who have HIV with a CD4+ count less than 200 cells per cubic millimeter. A more acute illness with symptoms including a cough productive of purulent sputum or rigors should suggest an alternate infectious diagnosis, such as bacterial pneumonia or tuberculosis. Compared with patients who do not have HIV, patients infected with HIV often present with a higher arterial oxygen tension and a lower alveolar–arterial oxygen gradient, and

a better clinical outcome.[35] This better outcome is not related to HAART.[36] The physical examination, including lung auscultation, is often unremarkable. A recent review of patients who had HIV with PCP revealed an overall hospital mortality of 11.6%, with mortality in patients requiring intensive care of 29.0%. Mechanical ventilation, development of pneumothoraces, or low serum albumin were independent predictors of increased mortality in these patients. Furthermore, the diagnosis of PCP in patients using HAART most likely represented failing HAART regimens or noncompliance with HAART regimens.[37]

Immunocompromised patients who do not have HIV typically present more acutely with fulminate respiratory failure associated with fever and dry cough and frequently require mechanical ventilation. Acute respiratory failure occurs in 43% of patients who do not have AIDS who develop PCP, and the overall mortality of PCP in patients who do not have AIDS may be as high as 40%.[3] Symptoms may correlate with the titration of immunosuppressants (particularly corticosteroids) or may be associated with an immunosuppressant dosage increase (such as cytotoxic agents). Evidence suggests that great than 90% of the PCP cases in patients who did not have AIDS occurred when the patients had received systemic corticosteroids within 1 month of the PCP diagnosis.[3] In that study, most patients who had PCP had received a corticosteroid dose equivalent to 16 mg or greater administered for at least 8 weeks.

The typical chest radiographic features of PCP in patients who are HIV-positive or HIV-negative are bilateral, symmetric, fine reticular interstitial infiltrates involving the perihilar areas, becoming more homogenous and diffuse as the severity of infection increases (**Fig. 3**). A wide variety of radiographic findings has been shown with PCP. Less common patterns include upper lobe involvement in patients receiving aerosolized pentamidine, solitary or multiple nodular opacities (which commonly cavitate), lobar infiltrates, pneumatoceles, and pneumothoraces. Although uncommon, lymphadenopathy and pleural effusion have also been reported.[38,39] A high-resolution CT scan is more sensitive than the chest radiograph and may demonstrate changes suggestive of PCP even when chest radiographic findings are normal.

DIAGNOSIS OF *PNEUMOCYSTIS PNEUMONIA*

The clinical diagnosis of PCP is complicated by the nonspecific signs and symptoms of PCP and because *Pneumocystis* is an intractable organism that currently cannot be isolated or sustained in

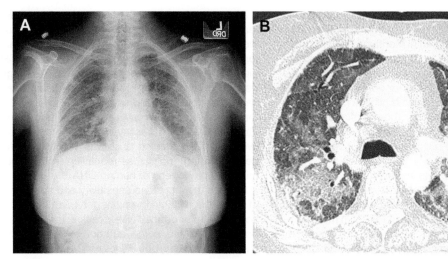

Fig. 3. Radiographic imaging of PCP. (*A*) A 66-year-old woman treated with corticosteroids chronically for polymyalgia rheumatica. The standard chest radiograph reveals perihilar alveolar and interstitial infiltrates. (*B*) CT scan on the same patient demonstrating perihilar ground glass and scattered linear infiltrates. Bronchoalveolar lavage confirmed *Pneumocystis* organisms.

culture. Routine diagnosis of this fungal pathogen has traditionally relied on microscopic visualization. For years, the gold standard has been microscopic examination of either Giemsa, methenamine silver, or direct immunofluorescence stains of bronchoalveolar lavage (BAL) fluid or induced sputum.[40,41] These methods depend on the quality of the sample, the organism burden, and the experience of the laboratory staff. Recently, molecular techniques, such as polymerase chain reaction (PCR), have been developed to assist in the clinical diagnosis of PCP.

Clinical Samples for Pneumocystis Identification

No combination of symptoms, signs, blood chemistries, or radiographic findings is diagnostic of PCP. As such, identification of *Pneumocystis* in a clinically relevant sample is necessary to make a diagnosis. Bronchoscopy with BAL is the preferred diagnostic procedure with reported sensitivities ranging from 89% to greater than 98%.[42] Some institutions rely on induced sputum (IS) or oropharyngeal (OPW) wash samples as the initial diagnostic procedure. Although a less invasive approach, these specimens have in general yielded lower sensitivities when analyzed with current microscopic or molecular technologies. A recent study confirmed the low diagnostic yield of induced sputum and recommended BAL sampling as the initial diagnostic test for PCP, particularly in patients who are HIV-negative.[43]

Microscopic Visualization with Conventional Stains

Pneumocystis trophic forms or cysts obtained from induced sputum, BAL fluid, or lung tissue can be visualized with the use of various tinctorial histochemical stains. Trophic forms can be detected using Papanicolaou, Gram-Weigert, or modified Wright Giemsa (Diff-Quik) stains. Cysts can be stained with Grocott-Gomori methenamine-silver (GMS), cresyl echt violet, toluidine blue O stain, or calcofluor white (CW) fungal stain. CW is quick and simple to use and has the added advantage of detecting other fungi present in the specimen. Several studies support the usefulness of CW stain for the routine laboratory detection of *Pneumocystis*.[44,45] The use of CW and other stains requires expertise on the part of the reader to differentiate *Pneumocystis* from artifact and from other nonspecific staining. A recent comparison of four staining methods found CW and GMS stains to have the best parameters for routine use in a clinical laboratory.[45]

Immunofluorescent Monoclonal Antibody Stains for Pneumocystis

Immunofluorescent antibody (IFA) stains, which use monoclonal antibodies (MAbs) directed against human *Pneumocystis*, are also available for the direct detection of this organism in clinical specimens. IFA stains have the advantage of being able to detect both the trophic and cyst forms of the organism. IFA staining is more expensive than conventional stains, however, and is also more time consuming. A recent study comparing histochemical staining with CW, GMS, or Diff-Quik to IFA staining with Merifluor *Pneumocystis* found the IFA stain to be the most sensitive, but also the least specific staining method.[45] These results led the authors to recommend that if the primary staining method in a clinical microbiology laboratory is IFA staining, then confirmation with a second method should be performed to increase the specificity and positive predictive value of the final test result.[45]

Patients who do not have AIDS who develop PCP have a significantly higher number of neutrophils and significantly fewer organisms in BAL fluid obtained during an episode of PCP.[35] It may therefore be more difficult to obtain organisms by induced sputum or BAL in patients who do not have AIDS. Although direct visualization of *Pneumocystis* life forms with the use of immunofluorescent or conventional stains has been the mainstay of PCP diagnosis, the diagnostic challenge of a small organism burden in patients who do not have AIDS has led to the development of more sensitive diagnostic technologies.

Diagnosis of Pneumocystis pneumonia by Polymerase Chain Reaction

Molecular methods for the detection of *P jirovecii* can offer diagnostic objectivity and the potential for increased sensitivity and specificity compared with microscopic identification of organisms (**Table 1**).[45–51] Several authors have described PCR assays for the detection of *Pneumocystis* from respiratory sources using various targets, detection methods, PCR platforms, qualitative versus quantitative assays, and patient populations.[52–57] Previously developed nested PCR methods tended to have low specificities resulting in high false-positive rates. Recently, real-time PCR has been used to detect *Pneumocystis* from respiratory sources and tissue.[46–49,58–62] The main advantages of real-time PCR are the rapid turnaround times (<3 hours), reduced possibility of run-to-run contamination, and higher specificity compared with conventional PCR techniques. In addition, real-time PCR allows accurate quantification of *P jirovecii* DNA, thereby allowing for the potential of identifying carriers of *Pneumocystis* who do not have pneumonia symptoms. A recent study comparing nested and quantitative real-time PCR methods for the amplification of the *P jirovecii* DHPS gene found the real-time PCR to have a statistically significant increased specificity compared with nested PCR (96% versus 81%; $P = .015$).[46]

Recently, the Mayo Clinic developed a rapid real-time PCR assay that detects a unique *Pneumocystis* target gene, cdc2.[47] This assay is performed on BAL fluid using the LightCycler PCR platform with fluorescence resonance energy transfer hybridization probes. This assay has been fully characterized using clinical specimens for routine use in a clinical microbiology laboratory. The LightCycler PCR assay was 21% more sensitive than CW staining and was highly specific demonstrating no cross-reactivity with other microbial pathogens or human DNA.[47]

Despite the increased sensitivity and specificity of PCR, the potential remains for this diagnostic approach to produce false-positive results. This potential has led some authors to recommend that PCR detection of *P jirovecii* be regarded in the same manner as detection of *Streptococcus pneumoniae* in the upper airway—a transient colonizer with the potential of causing pneumonia in immunocompromised individuals.[63]

Reverse Transcriptase Polymerase Chain Reaction Assay for Pneumocystis pneumonia

The detection of *Pneumocystis* nucleic acids by PCR can identify the presence of organisms. The detection of *Pneumocystis* DNA by PCR provides no information concerning the organism's viability or infectivity, however. Messenger RNA is much less stable than DNA, and its identification may serve as a surrogate for organism viability. Recent evidence suggests reverse transcriptase (RT)–PCR identification of *Pneumocystis* mRNA in BAL specimens yields a diagnostic sensitivity of 100% and specificity of 86%, and that this assay may become a useful tool for detecting and monitoring *P jirovecii* in minimally invasive clinical samples.[50]

Serum Indicators of Pneumocystis Infection

Great interest remains in the use of serum testing to diagnose PCP, particularly for patients who do not have AIDS who have respiratory failure and whose low organism burden decreases the diagnostic yield of noninvasive sputum analysis and in whom bronchoscopy portends increased risk. An elevated serum lactate dehydrogenase has been noted in patients who have PCP, although it is likely to be a reflection of the underlying lung inflammation and injury rather than a specific marker for the disease.[64] KL-6 antigen is a high molecular weight mucin-like glycoprotein strongly expressed on type 2 alveolar pneumocytes and bronchiolar epithelial cells. Serum KL-6 is an indicator of interstitial pneumonitis, and has been reportedly elevated in patients complicated with

Table 1
Diagnostic performance of contemporary tests for diagnosing pneumocystis pneumonia[a]

Method	Specimen	Sensitivity (%)	Specificity (%)	Comments
Microscopy[45]				
Conventional stains	BAL	49–79	99	Stains used in this study included CW, GMS, and Diff-Quik
IFA	BAL	91	95	IFA stain used in this study was Merifluor pneumocystis
RT-PCR[46–49]	BAL	94–100	96–100	*Pneumocystis* targets used in these studies included the cdc2, DHFR, DHPS, and HSP70 genes
RT-PCR[50]	BAL	100	86	Diagnostic performance declined with IS or OPW specimens
β-glucan[51]	Serum	92	86	Because of the study population, reported specificity may be higher than that expected in a population exposed to endemic fungi

Abbreviations: BAL, Bronchoalveolar lavage; β-glucan, (1 → 3) β-D-Glucan; cdc2, Cell division cycle 2; CW, Calcofluor white; DHFR, Dihydrofolate reductase; DHPS, Dihydropteroate synthase; GMS, Grocott-Gomori methenamine-silver; HSP70, Heat-shock protein 70; IFA, Immunofluorescent antibody; IS, Induced sputum; OPW, Oropharyngeal wash; PCP, Pneumocystis pneumonia; PCR, Polymerase chain reaction; RT-PCR, Reverse-transcriptase polymerase chain reaction.

[a] Sensitivity/specificity from author-selected recent publications studying performance of currently used diagnostic testing modalities for PCP.

PCP.[65,66] KL-6 elevation in PCP may not be as reliable as other serum markers, however, given its poor specificity.[51] (1 → 3) β-D-glucan (BDG), which is the major component of the cell wall of most fungi, has been used as a serologic marker for the diagnosis of candidiasis and aspergillosis. A recent study comparing serum indicators for the diagnosis of PCP found serum BDG to be a reliable marker with a sensitivity and specificity of 92.3% and 86.1%, respectively.[51] The clinician must keep in mind that BDG assays cannot always reliably differentiate the BDG release into the blood from *Pneumocystis* compared with other fungi. BDG levels have been used as a diagnostic adjunct for patients who have HIV who have newly identified symptoms consistent with PCP.[58,67,68] Other recent reports indicate that serial BDG levels decrease during treatment of PCP.[69–71] These preliminary studies suggest that serum BDG might be useful as an adjunctive noninvasive diagnostic test for PCP, although the diagnostic performance of this test must be further evaluated to determine its predictive values in various patient groups at risk for this infection.

PROPHYLAXIS AND TREATMENT OF *PNEUMOCYSTIS PNEUMONIA*

An official American Thoracic Society workshop was convened in 2006 to discuss recent advances and future directions in PCP.[42] Experts at the meeting agreed and reconfirmed that both patients infected with HIV and immunosuppressed patients who are HIV-negative need to receive prophylaxis to prevent disease depending on specific risks to the patient's immune system. In adults infected with HIV, primary prophylaxis against PCP should begin when the CD4+ count is less than 200 cells per cubic millimeter or if there is a history of oropharyngeal candidiasis.[72] Patients who have had previous episodes of PCP should receive lifelong secondary prophylaxis unless reconstitution of the immune system occurs in response to HAART. Primary or secondary prophylaxis may be discontinued in patients infected with HIV who have responded to HAART as manifested by an increase in the CD4+ cell count to greater than 200 cells per cubic millimeter for a period of 3 months. Conversely, prophylaxis should be reintroduced if the CD4+ count decreases to less than 200 cells per cubic millimeter.

Patients who are not infected with HIV but are receiving immunosuppressive medications or who have an underlying acquired or inherited immunodeficiency should receive PCP prophylaxis. In a retrospective series of 116 patients, a corticosteroid dose equivalent to 16 mg of prednisone or greater taken for a period of 8 weeks or more was associated with a significant risk for PCP in patients who did not have AIDS.[3] Similar observations have been noted in patients who have cancer or in patients who have connective

Table 2
Prophylactic medications for pneumocystis pneumonia

Medication	Dose	Route	Evidence for Resistance	Comments
Preferred regimen				
TMP-SMX	1 DS tablet daily or 1 SS tablet daily	Oral	DHPS mutations	First choice
	1 DS tablet 3 times per week	Oral		Alternate choice
Alternative regimens				
Dapsone	50 mg twice daily or 100 mg daily	Oral	None documented	Ensure patient does not have G6PD deficiency
Dapsone plus pyrimethamine plus leucovorin[a]	50 mg daily 50 mg weekly 25 mg weekly	Oral	None documented	—
Dapsone plus pyrimethamine plus leucovorin[a]	200 mg weekly 75 mg weekly 25 mg weekly	Oral	None documented	—
Pentamidine	300 mg monthly	Aerosol	Clinical resistance suspected	—
Atovaquone	1500 mg daily	Oral	Mutations of coenzyme Q binding site	For maximal absorption, take with high-fat meals

Abbreviations: DHPS, Dihydropteroate synthase; DS, Double strength; G6PD, Glucose-6 phosphate dehydrogenase; SS, Single strength.
[a] Recommended for patients who have HIV who are seropositive for toxoplasmosis with CD4+ count <100 cells per cubic millimeter or for patients who are HIV negative who have risk factors for toxoplasmosis.

Table 3
Medications for treatment of pneumocystis pneumonia

Medication	Dose	Route	Evidence for Resistance	Comments
TMP-SMX	TMP: 15–20 mg/kg SMX: 75–100 mg/kg Divided into three or four doses daily	Oral or Intravenous	DHPS mutations	First choice
Pentamidine	4 mg/kg daily	Intravenous	Clinical resistance suspected	Alternate choice
TMP plus dapsone	TMP: 5 mg/kg three times daily Dapsone: 100 mg/day once daily	Oral	DHPS mutations	Alternate choice
Atovaquone	750 mg two times daily	Oral	Mutations of coenzyme Q binding site	Alternate choice
Primaquine plus clindamycin	Primaquine: 30 mg daily Clindamycin: 600 mg three times daily	Oral	None documented	Alternate choice
Adjunctive glucocorticoids	Prednisone: 40 mg twice daily for 5 days 40 mg once daily for 5 days 20 mg once daily for 11 days	Oral	NA	Recommended for patients who have HIV with a room air $Pao_2 \leq 70$ mm Hg or alveolar–arterial oxygen gradient ≥ 35 mm Hg

Abbreviations: DHPS, Dihydropteroate synthase; NA, Not applicable; TMP, Trimethoprim, TMP-SMX, Trimethoprim-sulfamethoxazole.

tissue disease treated with corticosteroids.[2,4] Clinicians have been hesitant to use TMP-SMX for PCP prophylaxis in patients who have dermatologic or rheumatologic conditions receiving methotrexate because of the concern for myelosuppression. The safety of one single-strength tablet daily or one double-strength tablet three times per week concurrently with methotrexate has been proved in a trial of patients who had Wegener granulomatosis, without significant bone marrow suppression or other major side effects.[73] Medications recommended for prophylaxis are listed in **Table 2**.

Medications used to treat PCP are listed in **Table 3**. TMP-SMX is consistently the most useful and effective agent in treating severe PCP. The standard doses are trimethoprim (15–20 mg/kg) and sulfamethoxazole (75–100 mg/kg) intravenously (IV) or by mouth daily in four divided doses. Unfortunately, adverse effects are common and patients who have known allergies to sulfa cannot tolerate this medication. IV pentamidine (3–4 mg/kg IV daily) is as effective as TMP-SMX but is used less often because of its greater toxicities, including hypotension, hypoglycemia, and pancreatitis, and its required parenteral administration.[74,75] Other drugs for PCP include atovaquone, clindamycin and primaquine, trimetrexate, and trimethoprim and dapsone.[74–78] Preliminary evidence suggests that the addition of caspofungin to standard treatment with TMP-SMX may provide synergistic activity in severe PCP in patients who do not have HIV,[26] and may also have some efficacy in PCP in immunocompromised patients who do not have AIDS.[79]

The recommended duration of therapy differs in patients who have or do not have AIDS. In patients who have PCP who do not have AIDS, the typical duration of therapy is 14 days. Treatment should be individualized and extended if recovery is prolonged. Treatment of PCP in patients who have AIDS was increased from 14 to 21 days because of the risk for relapse after only 14 days of treatment. This increased risk for relapse is likely due in part to the greater organism burden and the slower clinical response time in patients who have PCP and AIDS.

Several studies have demonstrated the benefits of adjunctive corticosteroids in patients who have AIDS and symptoms of moderate to severe PCP. Specifically, corticosteroids are of benefit in patients infected with HIV who have hypoxemia manifest as a partial pressure of arterial oxygen under 70 mm Hg with the patient breathing room air or an alveolar–arteriolar gradient greater than 35. Such patients should receive prednisone at a dose of 40 mg twice daily for 5 days, then 40 mg daily on days 6 through 11, and then 20 mg daily on days 12 through 21.[80] This use improves clinical outcome and mortality without increasing the risk for other opportunistic infections and has become standard treatment.

The role for adjunctive corticosteroids in patients who do not have AIDS is less clear. A retrospective study of 31 patients who had PCP but not HIV demonstrated similar rates for intubation and death in patients receiving adjunctive corticosteroids compared with those who did not receive them. The steroid group did have a shorter duration of mechanical ventilation, shorter ICU stay, and less oxygen use.[6] A second retrospective study of 31 patients who had PCP but not HIV demonstrated no difference in mortality or need for mechanical ventilation in the steroid-treated group.[81] The available data do not clearly support routine use of adjunctive corticosteroids in patients who have PCP but not AIDS, and treatment must be individualized. Many clinicians opt to maintain a stable dose of corticosteroids while treating the infection with antimicrobial therapy.

EMERGING RESISTANCE

An additional concern regarding treatment of PCP is the worry of emerging drug resistance. Mutations in the dihydrofolate reductase enzyme, the target of trimethoprim and pyrimethamine, have been increasingly found in patients who have PCP.[24] Similarly, mutations in the cytochrome *b* gene have been demonstrated to confer resistance to atovaquone.[25] Mutations have also been discovered in the *Pneumocystis* DHPS gene, which encodes the enzyme that is inhibited by dapsone and sulfamethoxazole. These mutations result in alterations in the enzyme's active site.[21–23] Although several reports have connected these DHPS mutations with prophylaxis failure,[82] treatment failure,[83] increased mortality,[83] and selection by sulfa drug pressure,[83,84] treatment failures have not yet been consistently reported in all studies.[85] Further study is required to determine the significance of the DHPS mutations in various populations and in different geographic locations. Nonetheless, the presence of molecular resistance is being increasingly observed, and clinicians should closely monitor clinical responses to standard *Pneumocystis* treatment regimens. Furthermore, continued basic investigations to identify new drug targets are clearly warranted.

SUMMARY

PCP continues to be a devastating opportunistic infection for which care providers must continue to maintain a high index of suspicion in immuno-compromised patients at risk. These include patients (1) who have known HIV/AIDS, (2) who are receiving high doses of glucocorticoids, (3) who are receiving multiple immunosuppressive medications, including new biologic agents, (4) who have been diagnosed with malignancy, particularly hematologic in origin, (5) who are experiencing organ rejection, or (6) who have not received or have discontinued PCP prophylaxis. In these patients, laboratory specimens from clin-ically relevant sites, such as induced sputum or BAL, should be obtained. Given the increased sensitivity of molecular testing with PCR, in partic-ular RT-PCR, this diagnostic modality is recom-mended when available. For clinical laboratories not yet in possession of this technology, micro-scopic examination using the histochemical stain most familiar to local laboratory personnel is usually sufficient for establishing the diagnosis. TMP-SMX is most effective in treating severe PCP and remains the first-line recommended therapy.[1] Mutations to the therapeutic targets of TMP-SMX exist, however, and care providers must have a heightened suspicion for possible drug resistance in a patient not responding to treatment. The possibility of emerging resistance to TMP-SMX and other antimicrobial agents emphasizes the need to continue the study of this organism to support the development of novel treatment strategies for this important infection.

REFERENCES

1. Thomas CF Jr, Limper AH. Pneumocystis pneu-monia. N Engl J Med 2004;350:2487–98.
2. Sepkowitz KA, Brown AE, Telzak EE, et al. Pneumo-cystis carinii pneumonia among patients without AIDS at a cancer hospital. JAMA 1992;267:832–7.
3. Yale SH, Limper AH. Pneumocystis carinii pneu-monia in patients without acquired immunodefi-ciency syndrome: associated illness and prior corticosteroid therapy. Mayo Clin Proc 1996;71:5–13.
4. Sepkowitz KA. Opportunistic infections in patients with and patients without Acquired Immunodefi-ciency Syndrome. Clin Infect Dis 2002;34:1098–107.
5. Bollee G, Sarfati C, Thiery G, et al. Clinical picture of Pneumocystis jirovecii pneumonia in cancer patients. Chest 2007;132:1305–10.
6. Pareja JG, Garland R, Koziel H. Use of adjunctive corticosteroids in severe adult non-HIV Pneumocys-tis carinii pneumonia. Chest 1998;113:1215–24.
7. Thomas CF Jr, Limper AH. Current insights into the biology and pathogenesis of Pneumocystis pneu-monia. Nat Rev Microbiol 2007;5:298–308.
8. Edman JC, Kovacs JA, Masur H, et al. Ribosomal RNA sequence shows Pneumocystis carinii to be a member of the fungi. Nature 1988;334:519–22.
9. Stringer JR, Beard CB, Miller RF, et al. A new name (Pneumocystis jirovecii) for Pneumocystis from humans. Emerg Infect Dis 2002;8:891–6.
10. Miller RF, Ambrose HE, Wakefield AE. Pneumocystis carinii f. sp. hominis DNA in immunocompetent health care workers in contact with patients with P. carinii pneumonia. J Clin Microbiol 2001;39:3877–82.
11. Wakefield AE, Lindley AR, Ambrose HE, et al. Limited asymptomatic carriage of Pneumocystis jiro-vecii in human immunodeficiency virus-infected patients. J Infect Dis 2003;187:901–8.
12. Calderon EJ, Rivero L, Respaldiza N, et al. Systemic inflammation in patients with chronic obstructive pulmonary disease who are colonized with Pneumo-cystis jirovecii. Clin Infect Dis 2007;45:e17–9.
13. Montes-Cano MA, de la Horra C, Dapena FJ, et al. Dynamic colonisation by different Pneumocystis jiro-vecii genotypes in cystic fibrosis patients. Clin Microbiol Infect 2007;13:1008–11.
14. Morris A, Sciurba FC, Lebedeva IP, et al. Association of chronic obstructive pulmonary disease severity and Pneumocystis colonization. Am J Respir Crit Care Med 2004;170:408–13.
15. Sing A, Roggenkamp A, Autenrieth IB, et al. Pneumo-cystis carinii carriage in immunocompetent patients with primary pulmonary disorders as detected by single or nested PCR. J Clin Microbiol 1999;37:3409–10.
16. Vidal S, de la Horra C, Martin J, et al. Pneumocystis jirovecii colonisation in patients with interstitial lung disease. Clin Microbiol Infect 2006;12:231–5.
17. Limper AH, Thomas CF Jr, Anders RA, et al. Interac-tions of parasite and host epithelial cell cycle regula-tion during Pneumocystis carinii pneumonia. J Lab Clin Med 1997;130:132–8.
18. Limper AH, Martin WJ 2nd. Pneumocystis carinii: inhibition of lung cell growth mediated by parasite attachment. J Clin Invest 1990;85:391–6.
19. Afessa B, Green W, Chiao J, et al. Pulmonary complications of HIV infection: autopsy findings. Chest 1998;113:1225–9.
20. Matsumoto Y, Yoshida Y. Sporogony in Pneumocys-tis carinii: synaptonemal complexes and meiotic nuclear divisions observed in precysts. J Protozool 1984;31:420–8.
21. Beard CB, Fox MR, Lawrence GG, et al. Genetic differences in Pneumocystis isolates recovered from immunocompetent infants and from adults with AIDS: epidemiological implications. J Infect Dis 2005;192:1815–8.
22. Crothers K, Beard CB, Turner J, et al. Severity and outcome of HIV-associated Pneumocystis pneu-monia containing Pneumocystis jirovecii dihydropter-oate synthase gene mutations. AIDS 2005;19:801–5.

23. Huang L, Crothers K, Atzori C, et al. Dihydropteroate synthase gene mutations in *Pneumocystis* and sulfa resistance. Emerg Infect Dis 2004;10:1721–8.

24. Nahimana A, Rabodonirina M, Bille J, et al. Mutations of *Pneumocystis jirovecii* dihydrofolate reductase associated with failure of prophylaxis. Antimicrobial Agents Chemother 2004;48:4301–5.

25. Kessl JJ, Hill P, Lange BB, et al. Molecular basis for atovaquone resistance in *Pneumocystis jirovecii* modeled in the cytochrome bc(1) complex of *Saccharomyces cerevisiae*. J Biol Chem 2004;279:2817–24.

26. Utili R, Durante-Mangoni E, Basilico C, et al. Efficacy of caspofungin addition to trimethoprim-sulfamethoxazole treatment for severe *Pneumocystis pneumonia* in solid organ transplant recipients. Transplantation 2007;84:685–8.

27. Hanna DB, Gupta LS, Jones LE, et al. AIDS-defining opportunistic illnesses in the HAART era in New York City. AIDS Care 2007;19:264–72.

28. Sullivan PS, Denniston M, McNaghten A, et al. Use of a population-based survey to determine incidence of AIDS-defining opportunistic illnesses among HIV-positive persons receiving medical care in the United States. AIDS Res Ther 2007;4:17–22.

29. Dungarwalla M, Marsh JC, Tooze JA, et al. Lack of clinical efficacy of rituximab in the treatment of autoimmune neutropenia and pure red cell aplasia: implications for their pathophysiology. Ann Hematol 2007;86:191–7.

30. Harigai M, Koike R, Miyasaka N. *Pneumocystis pneumonia* associated with infliximab in Japan. N Engl J Med 2007;357:1874–6.

31. Kalyoncu U, Karadag O, Akdogan A, et al. *Pneumocystis carinii* pneumonia in a rheumatoid arthritis patient treated with adalimumab. Scand J Infect Dis 2007;39:475–8.

32. Kaur N, Mahl TC. *Pneumocystis jirovecii* (*carinii*) pneumonia after infliximab therapy: a review of 84 cases. Dig Dis Sci 2007;52:1481–4.

33. Kolstad A, Holte H, Fossa A, et al. *Pneumocystis jirovecii* pneumonia in B-cell lymphoma patients treated with the rituximab-CHOEP-14 regimen. Haematologica 2007;92:139–40.

34. Lahiff C, Khiaron OB, Nolan N, et al. *Pneumocystis carinii* pneumonia in a patient on etanercept for psoriatic arthritis. Ir J Med Sci 2007;176:309–11.

35. Limper AH, Offord KP, Smith TF, et al. *Pneumocystis carinii* pneumonia. Differences in lung parasite number and inflammation in patients with and without AIDS. Am Rev Respir Dis 1989;140:1204–9.

36. Walzer PD, Evans HE, Copas AJ, et al. Early predictors of mortality from *Pneumocystis jirovecii* pneumonia in HIV-infected patients: 1985–2006. Clin Infect Dis 2008;46:625–33.

37. Radhi S, Alexander T, Ukwu M, et al. Outcome of HIV-associated *Pneumocystis pneumonia* in hospitalized patients from 2000 through 2003. BMC Infect Dis 2008;8:118–9.

38. DeLorenzo LJ, Huang CT, Maguire GP, et al. Roentgenographic patterns of *Pneumocystis carinii* pneumonia in 104 patients with AIDS. Chest 1987;91:323–7.

39. Goodman PC. *Pneumocystis carinii* pneumonia. J Thorac Imaging 1991;6:16–21.

40. Cregan P, Yamamoto A, Lum A, et al. Comparison of four methods for rapid detection of *Pneumocystis carinii* in respiratory specimens. J Clin Microbiol 1990;28:2432–6.

41. Wolfson JS, Waldron MA, Sierra LS. Blinded comparison of a direct immunofluorescent monoclonal antibody staining method and a Giemsa staining method for identification of *Pneumocystis carinii* in induced sputum and bronchoalveolar lavage specimens of patients infected with human immunodeficiency virus. J Clin Microbiol 1990;28:2136–8.

42. Huang L, Morris A, Limper AH, et al. An Official ATS workshop summary: recent advances and future directions in *Pneumocystis pneumonia* (PCP). Proc Am Thorac Soc 2006;3:655–64.

43. Wang Y, Doucette S, Qian Q, et al. Yield of primary and repeat induced sputum testing for *Pneumocystis jiroveci* in human immunodeficiency virus-positive and -negative patients. Arch Pathol Lab Med 2007;131:1582–4.

44. Alvarez F, Bandi V, Stager C, et al. Detection of *Pneumocystis carinii* in tracheal aspirates of intubated patients using calcofluor-white (Fungi-Fluor) and immunofluorescence antibody (Genetic Systems) stains. Crit Care Med 1997;25:948–52.

45. Procop GW, Haddad S, Quinn J, et al. Detection of *Pneumocystis jiroveci* in respiratory specimens by four staining methods. J Clin Microbiol 2004;42:3333–5.

46. Alvarez-Martinez MJ, Miro JM, Valls ME, et al. Sensitivity and specificity of nested and real-time PCR for the detection of *Pneumocystis jirovecii* in clinical specimens. Diagn Microbiol Infect Dis 2006;56:153–60.

47. Arcenas RC, Uhl JR, Buckwalter SP, et al. A real-time polymerase chain reaction assay for detection of *Pneumocystis* from bronchoalveolar lavage fluid. Diagn Microbiol Infect Dis 2006;54:169–75.

48. Bandt D, Monecke S. Development and evaluation of a real-time PCR assay for detection of *Pneumocystis jirovecii*. Transpl Infect Dis 2007;9:196–202.

49. Huggett JF, Taylor MS, Kocjan G, et al. Development and evaluation of a real-time PCR assay for detection of *Pneumocystis jirovecii* DNA in bronchoalveolar lavage fluid of HIV-infected patients. Thorax 2007;63:154–9.

50. de Oliveira A, Unnasch TR, Crothers K, et al. Performance of a molecular viability assay for the diagnosis of *Pneumocystis pneumonia* in HIV-infected patients. Diagn Microbiol Infect Dis 2007;57:169–76.

51. Tasaka S, Hasegawa N, Kobayashi S, et al. Serum indicators for the diagnosis of *Pneumocystis pneumonia*. Chest 2007;131:1173–80.

52. Cartwright CP, Nelson NA, Gill VJ. Development and evaluation of a rapid and simple procedure for detection of *Pneumocystis carinii* by PCR. J Clin Microbiol 1994;32:1634–8.

53. Helweg-Larsen J, Jensen JS, Benfield T, et al. Diagnostic use of PCR for detection of *Pneumocystis carinii* in oral wash samples. J Clin Microbiol 1998;36:2068–72.

54. Lu JJ, Chen CH, Bartlett MS, et al. Comparison of six different PCR methods for detection of *Pneumocystis carinii*. J Clin Microbiol 1995;33:2785–8.

55. Peters SE, Wakefield AE, Banerji S, et al. Quantification of the detection of *Pneumocystis carinii* by DNA amplification. Mol Cell Probes 1992;6:115–7.

56. Ribes JA, Limper AH, Espy MJ, et al. PCR detection of *Pneumocystis carinii* in bronchoalveolar lavage specimens: analysis of sensitivity and specificity. J Clin Microbiol 1997;35:830–5.

57. Tamburrini E, Mencarini P, Visconti E, et al. Comparison of two PCR methods for detection of *Pneumocystis carinii* in bronchoalveolar lavage fluid. J Eukaryot Microbiol 1996;43:20S.

58. Cuetara MS, Alhambra A, Chaves F, et al. Use of a serum (1–>3)-beta-D-glucan assay for diagnosis and follow-up of *Pneumocystis jirovecii* pneumonia. Clin Infect Dis 2008;47:1364–6.

59. Fillaux J, Malvy S, Alvarez M, et al. Accuracy of a routine real-time PCR assay for the diagnosis of *Pneumocystis jirovecii* pneumonia. J Microbiol Methods 2008;75:258–61.

60. Flori P, Bellete B, Durand F, et al. Comparison between real-time PCR, conventional PCR and different staining techniques for diagnosing *Pneumocystis jirovecii* pneumonia from bronchoalveolar lavage specimens. J Med Microbiol 2004;53:603–7.

61. Larsen HH, Huang L, Kovacs JA, et al. A prospective, blinded study of quantitative touch-down polymerase chain reaction using oral-wash samples for diagnosis of *Pneumocystis pneumonia* in HIV-infected patients. J Infect Dis 2004;189:1679–83.

62. Larsen HH, Masur H, Kovacs JA, et al. Development and evaluation of a quantitative, touch-down, real-time PCR assay for diagnosing *Pneumocystis carinii* pneumonia. J Clin Microbiol 2002;40:490–4.

63. Robberts FJ, Liebowitz LD, Chalkley LJ. Polymerase chain reaction detection of *Pneumocystis jirovecii*: evaluation of 9 assays. Diagn Microbiol Infect Dis 2007;58:385–92.

64. Quist J, Hill AR. Serum lactate dehydrogenase (LDH) in *Pneumocystis carinii* pneumonia, tuberculosis, and bacterial pneumonia. Chest 1995;108:415–8.

65. Hamada H, Kohno N, Yokoyama A, et al. KL-6 as a serologic indicator of *Pneumocystis carinii* pneumonia in immunocompromised hosts. Intern Med 1998;37:307–10.

66. Tanaka M, Tanaka K, Fukahori S, et al. Elevation of serum KL-6 levels in patients with hematological malignancies associated with cytomegalovirus or *Pneumocystis carinii* pneumonia. Hematology 2002;7:105–8.

67. Fujii T, Nakamura T, Iwamoto A. *Pneumocystis pneumonia* in patients with HIV infection: clinical manifestations, laboratory findings, and radiological features. J Infect Chemother 2007;13:1–7.

68. Pisculli ML, Sax PE. Use of a serum beta-glucan assay for diagnosis of HIV-related *Pneumocystis jirovecii* pneumonia in patients with negative microscopic examination results. Clin Infect Dis 2008;46:1928–30.

69. Akamatsu N, Sugawara Y, Kaneko J, et al. Preemptive treatment of fungal infection based on plasma (1 -> 3)beta-D: -glucan levels after liver transplantation. Infection 2007;35:346–51.

70. Kawagishi N, Miyagi S, Satoh K, et al. Usefulness of beta-D glucan in diagnosing *Pneumocystis carinii* pneumonia and monitoring its treatment in a living-donor liver-transplant recipient. J Hepatobiliary Pancreat Surg 2007;14:308–11.

71. Marty FM, Koo S, Bryar J, et al. (1–>3)beta-D-glucan assay positivity in patients with *Pneumocystis (carinii) jirovecii* pneumonia. Ann Intern Med 2007;147:70–2.

72. Masur H, Kaplan JE, Holmes KK. Guidelines for preventing opportunistic infections among HIV-infected persons–2002. Recommendations of the U.S. Public Health Service and the Infectious Diseases Society of America. Ann Intern Med 2002;137:435–78.

73. Wegener's Granulomatosis Etanercept Trial (WGED) Research Group. Etanercept plus standard therapy for Wegener's granulomatosis. N Engl J Med 2005; 352:351–61.

74. Hughes WT. Prevention and treatment of *Pneumocystis carinii* pneumonia. Annu Rev Med 1991;42: 287–95.

75. Masur H. Prevention and treatment of *Pneumocystis pneumonia*. N Engl J Med 1992;327:1853–60.

76. Castro M. Treatment and prophylaxis of *Pneumocystis carinii* pneumonia. Semin Respir Infect 1998;13: 296–303.

77. Colby C, McAfee S, Sackstein R, et al. A prospective randomized trial comparing the toxicity and safety of atovaquone with trimethoprim/sulfamethoxazole as *Pneumocystis carinii* pneumonia prophylaxis following autologous peripheral blood stem cell transplantation. Bone Marrow Transplant 1999;24:897–902.

78. Wilkin A, Feinberg J. *Pneumocystis carinii* pneumonia: a clinical review. Am Fam Physician 1999; 60:1699–708.

79. Hof H, Schnulle P. *Pneumocystis jirovecii* pneumonia in a patient with Wegener's granulomatosis treated efficiently with caspofungin. Mycoses 2008; 51(Suppl 1):65–7.

80. Consensus statement on the use of corticosteroids as adjunctive therapy for pneumocystis pneumonia

in the acquired immunodeficiency syndrome. The National Institutes of Health-University of California Expert Panel for Corticosteroids as Adjunctive Therapy for *Pneumocystis pneumonia*. N Engl J Med 1990;323:1500–4.

81. Delclaux C, Zahar JR, Amraoui G, et al. Corticosteroids as adjunctive therapy for severe *Pneumocystis carinii* pneumonia in non-human immunodeficiency virus-infected patients: retrospective study of 31 patients. Clin Infect Dis 1999;29:670–2.

82. Hauser PM, Sudre P, Nahimana A, et al. Prophylaxis failure is associated with a specific *Pneumocystis carinii* genotype. Clin Infect Dis 2001;33:1080–2.

83. Helweg-Larsen J, Benfield TL, Eugen-Olsen J, et al. Effects of mutations in *Pneumocystis carinii* dihydropteroate synthase gene on outcome of AIDS-associated *P. carinii* pneumonia. Lancet 1999;354:1347–51.

84. Nahimana A, Rabodonirina M, Helweg-Larsen J, et al. Sulfa resistance and dihydropteroate synthase mutants in recurrent *Pneumocystis carinii* pneumonia. Emerg Infect Dis 2003;9:864–7.

85. Navin TR, Beard CB, Huang L, et al. Effect of mutations in *Pneumocystis carinii* dihydropteroate synthase gene on outcome of *P carinii* pneumonia in patients with HIV-1: a prospective study. Lancet 2001;358:545–9.

Invasive Fungal Infections in the Era of Biologics

Tamra M. Arnold, PharmD, BCPS[a], Catherine R. Sears, MD[b],
Chadi A. Hage, MD[c,d],*

KEYWORDS

- TNF-alpha • Invasive mycoses
- Histoplasmosis • Coccidioidomycosis
- Aspergillosis • Infliximab • Etanercept • Adalimumab

Antagonists of tumor necrosis factor-α (TNF-α) have revolutionized the treatment of select inflammatory diseases including rheumatoid arthritis and Crohn's disease. Currently three TNF-α antagonists—adalimumab, etanercept, and infliximab—have been approved worldwide for use for the treatment of various rheumatic diseases.[1] Although these three medications exhibit efficacy in the treatment of autoimmune disorders, they also seem to affect host resistance to infectious pathogens, particularly granulomatous infections.[2] The TNF-α antagonists have been associated with numerous adverse events, of which serious infections and malignancies are the most common.[3] Mycobacterium tuberculosis, histoplasmosis, aspergillosis, listeriosis, cytomegalovirus, coccidiomycosis, nocardiosis, and other serious bacterial infections have been reported in several series and case reports of patients receiving TNF-α antagonist therapy. This article focuses solely on fungal infections associated with the anti-TNF-α therapies.

ANTI-TUMOR NECROSIS FACTOR-α THERAPIES

Although anti-TNF-α factor therapies target the same cytokine, their mechanisms of action and therefore efficacy and side effects are different. Infliximab (Remicade) was the first agent approved for treatment of Crohn's disease. Initially, however, it was studied for treatment of rheumatic arthritis (RA). Infliximab is a chimeric molecule that combines the Fc region of human immunoglobulin G1 (IgG1) with the variable region of the mouse antibody against TNF-α. It binds to both membrane-bound and soluble TNF-α, interfering with the binding of TNF-α to its receptor. The loss of bioactivity is a result of binding to soluble TNF-α, whereas binding to membrane-bound TNF-α causes complement- and/or antibody-dependent lysis of cells that express TNF-α, such as lymphocytes and monocytes.[4,5] Infliximab does not inhibit TNF-β (lymphotoxin-α). Infliximab is approved for treatment of RA, Crohn's disease, ankylosing spondylitis, psoriatic arthritis, plaque psoriasis, and ulcerative colitis. The usual dose of infliximab is 3 to 5 mg/kg for RA and Crohn's disease, respectively, administered intravenously at weeks 0, 2, and 6 and followed by maintenance infusions every 8 weeks.[6] For patients who do not respond, doses may be escalated to 10 mg/kg.

Etanercept (Enbrel) is indicated for treatment of RA, psoriatic arthritis, ankylosing spondylitis, and polyarticular-course juvenile idiopathic arthritis.[7]

[a] Division of Clinical Pharmacy, Roudebush VA Medical Center, 1481 W. 10th Street, Indianapolis, IN 46202, USA
[b] Department of Medicine, Indiana University, 1481 W. 10th Street, 111P-IU, Indianapolis, IN 46202, USA
[c] Division of Pulmonary-Critical Care, Department of Medicine, Indiana University, Roudebush VA Medical Center, 1481 W. 10th Street, 111P-IU, Indianapolis, IN 46202, USA
[d] Division of Infectious Diseases, Department of Medicine, Indiana University, Roudebush VA Medical Center, 1481 W. 10th Street, 111P-IU, Indianapolis, IN 46202, USA
* Corresponding author.
E-mail address: chage@iupui.edu (C.A. Hage).

Clin Chest Med 30 (2009) 279–286
doi:10.1016/j.ccm.2009.02.007
0272-5231/09/$ – see front matter. Published by Elsevier Inc.

chestmed.theclinics.com

Etanercept is a soluble dimeric fusion protein that consists of the extracellular ligand-binding portion of the human 75-kDa (p75) TNF receptor linked to the Fc portion of human IgG1. The fusion protein binds to both TNF-α and TNF-β, interfering with their ability to interact with their receptors. Unlike infliximab, etanercept can interact only with soluble TNF-α.[4] The usual dose of etanercept is either 25 mg twice weekly or 50 mg once weekly administered subcutaneously.[7]

Adalimumab (Humira) is indicated for RA, Crohn's disease, juvenile idiopathic arthritis, psoriatic arthritis, ankylosing spondylitis, and plaque psoriasis. Adalimumab is a recombinant human IgG1 monoclonal antibody specific for TNF-α; it does not inhibit TNF-β. The usual dose is 40 mg administered subcutaneously every 2 weeks, but the dose may be increased to 40 mg every week if necessary.[8]

ROLE OF TUMOR NECROSIS FACTOR-α IN INFECTION

TNF-α plays a central role in the host immune response to infectious pathogens. Alveolar macrophages secrete large amounts of TNF-α in response to antigen presentation. T lymphocytes and natural killer cells produce it to a lesser extent. TNF-α is essential in the recruitment of inflammatory cells to the site of infection and in the formation and maintenance of infectious granulomas. Shortly after fungal or mycobacterial infection occurs, monocytes, dendritic cells, effector T cells, and B cells migrate to the site of infection and organize to form these granulomas. It is thought that the role of infectious granulomas is to contains the pathogen and prevent its spread beyond the original site of infection. If the integrity of the granuloma is disrupted, pathogen replication and dissemination may occur.[9]

Animal studies have demonstrated clearly the relationship between TNF-α, chemokine production, and granuloma formation. In TNF-α–deficient mice, chemokine levels lagged behind those in wild-type mice, leading to delayed or aberrant granuloma formation, increased bacterial replication, and destructive immunopathology.[9,10] In an experimental model of histoplasmosis, anti-TNF-α antibody blocked the T-helper (Th)-1 arm of cellular immunity[11] and prevented the development of a protective immune response.[12] For these reasons, it is not surprising that infections, including invasive fungal infections (IFIs), are a common side effect of the TNF-α inhibitor therapies.

INVASIVE FUNGAL INFECTIONS ASSOCIATED WITH TUMOR NECROSIS FACTOR-α INHIBITORS

The true incidence of IFIs associated with the TNF-α inhibitors is unknown for various reasons. Studies reporting on the emergent infections often lack the appropriate denominator, the recipients of anti-TNF agents. TNF-α inhibitors are prescribed commonly in conjunction with other immunosuppressants to help decrease the dose of these additional medications.[13–16] On the other hand, the disease states for which these medications are administered could predispose a patient to infection. For example, a patient suffering from RA is at increased risk of infection, probably because of underlying immune dysregulation.[17] Recently, however, a meta-analysis showed a significant association between TNF-α blockade and serious infections (the trial did not include etanercept). The rates of serious infections were low, on average 6 per 100 patient-years, and there seemed to be no significant difference in the rates of infection with infliximab, etanercept, or adalimumab.[3] Postmarketing studies suggest that the rate of serious infections complicating anti-TNF-α therapies might be much higher than reported in clinical trials evaluating TNF-α blockers.[18]

SPECIFIC INVASIVE FUNGAL INFECTIONS
Histoplasmosis

Histoplasmosis is the most common IFI associated with TNF-α inhibitors. In a recent survey of infectious diseases specialists, histoplasmosis was second only to *Staphylococcus aureus* as the cause of serious infection complicating anti-TNF and other biologic therapies.[19] In most reported cases, patients are from areas in which the fungus is endemic and have received concurrent immunosuppressants. To date 86 cases of histoplasmosis have been reported with some clinical information.[2,11,20–30] The two most common indications for anti-TNF therapy are RA and inflammatory bowel diseases. According to the FDA MedWatch, the complicating anti-TNF agent in most of the 240 patients who had histoplasmosis was infliximab (207 cases), followed by etanercept (17 cases) and adalumimab (16 cases).[31] The type of infection varied from acute pulmonary to extrapulmonary or progressive disseminated histoplasmosis; pulmonary involvement was reported in the majority of cases.[32] Typical presenting signs and symptoms included cough, fever, malaise, dyspnea, and interstitial pneumonitis on chest radiograph. Many of these signs and symptoms also could be caused by the patient's underlying disease state, resulting in a delay in recognition and therefore treatment of the histoplasmosis.[22] Rapid diagnosis can be achieved most reliably by the urine or serum *Histoplasma* antigen test[32] and cytopathologic analysis of bronchoalveolar lavage (BAL).[11] Most patients were treated with amphotericin B followed by itraconazole. Mortality was nearly 20% in the cases for which that information was available.

Coccidioidomycosis

To date 30 cases of coccidioidomycosis associated with anti-TNF therapy have been reported. Of these, 28 (93%) were associated with infliximab and 2 (7%) with etanercept.[33–38] Bergstrom and colleagues[33] estimated a relative risk of 5.23 for developing symptomatic coccidioidomycosis in patients residing in endemic areas receiving infliximab, as compared with those who are not taking an anti-TNF agent. Pneumonia was present in all cases, and five cases had evidence of disseminated infection. All patients were concomitantly taking methotrexate and/or corticosteroids. The diagnosis was made by positive serologic findings in 11 of the 15 cases for which such information is available. In four cases, the coccidioidomycosis was diagnosed by biopsy (lung, BAL, or skin) or from a culture.[33,34,37] The coccidioidal serology before anti-TNF therapy was negative in all six patients who were tested before initiation of infliximab. Of the 15 patients for whom information on treatment and outcome was available, 14 received antifungal therapy (amphotericin B, itraconazole, or fluconazole) with an attributable mortality of approximately 13% (2/15).[33,34,37]

Aspergillosis and Zygomycetes

Sixty-five cases of aspergillosis associated with TNF-α inhibitor use have been reported to date. Most cases were associated with infliximab (48 cases, 74%), followed by etanercept (15 cases, 23%) and adalimumab (2 cases, 3%).[27,28,39–50] Of the 25 patients for whom the indication was known, 18 received the TNF-α inhibitor for graft-versus-host disease (GVHD) following allogeneic bone marrow transplantation for a hematologic malignancy, 5 for rheumatologic diseases, and 2 for inflammatory bowel disease. Sixty-three of the 65 patients were receiving concomitant immunosuppressant medications. Most patients developed invasive pulmonary aspergillosis and were diagnosed by culture or by biopsy obtained through bronchoscopy. One case was determined by a positive BAL culture result plus positive antigen testing. The overall prognosis was grave: mortality reached 82% in patients who had GVHD.[43,46,47]

Four cases of Zygomycetes infection have been reported in the literature to date.[46,51,52] Three of the four cases were associated with infliximab use (in one patient who suffered from Crohn's disease and in two patients who had GVHD). The fourth case was a patient who had RA who developed orbital cellulitis along with disseminated Zygomycetes infection in association with adalimumab therapy.[52] No patient survived.

Candida Infections

Sixty-four cases of *Candida* infections associated with TNF-α inhibitor therapy have been identified. Of those cases, 84% (54/64) were associated with infliximab, 14% (9/64) with etanercept, and 2% (1/64) with adalimumab.[21,28,39,40,44,47,53–56] The indication for TNF-α therapy was known is 18 cases, 11 of which were GVHD, 5 were inflammatory bowel disease, and 2 were RA. The site of infection varied but included the bloodstream, abscesses, esophagus, oropharynx, and endovascular sites. These Candida infections were associated with 50% mortality (in cases for which outcome data were available). Of note, 75% of the patients who died were coinfected with additional organisms: *Pneumocystis* and *Aspergillus* in one case,[44] a mixed intra-abdominal abscess[21] in another, and a *Salmonella* species in the last case.[55]

Cryptococcus Infections

To date 28 cases of *Cryptococcus* infections associated with TNF-α inhibitor therapy have been reported.[28,57–64] Of the 28 cases, 17 (61%) have been associated with infliximab, 10 (36%) with etanercept, and 1 (3%) with adalimumab. Most patients presented with pneumonia. Additional clinical manifestations that have been noted include fungemia, involvement of the central nervous system, cutaneous infections, tenosynovitis requiring amputation of the involved fingers, and a rare case of *Cryptococcus albidus* infection. Typically *Cryptococcus* infections were diagnosed by biopsy. The infections responded to fluconazole or amphotericin B, and no patients died.

Blastomycosis

Two cases of blastomycosis have been reported in abstract form with very limited information.[38]

OTHER AGENTS

Although anti-TNF agents are considered essential in the treatment of RA, Crohn's disease, and other inflammatory diseases, other biologic agents now are being introduced in clinical use.

Rituximab (Rituxin) is a chimeric murine/human monoclonal antibody against CD20, which is found on mature and pre-B lymphocytes. Binding of rituximab to CD20 causes B-lymphocyte lysis and almost complete depletion of B-cell lineages.[65,66] B-cell depletion usually lasts 3 to 9 months but has been observed for up to 12 to 15 months.[65–67] Initially approved for treatment of certain B-cell non-Hodgkin's lymphomas, following or in combination with other chemotherapeutic regimens, rituximab also is approved for treatment of moderately to severely active RA in combination with methotrexate in adult patients who have had an inadequate response to one or more TNF-antagonist therapies.[65] It is being used increasingly for the treatment of other autoimmune diseases, including autoimmune-mediated thrombocytopenias and lupus.[67]

Although initial oncology trials did not show any increase in serious infections, later publications have suggested an increased risk of infections with rituximab. Although several cases of fungal infections have been reported in patients receiving rituximab for B-cell non-Hodgkin's lymphoma, it often is difficult to attribute these infections solely to rituximab because of concomitant or recent use of cytotoxic chemotherapeutic agents. In a review of 745 patients who had RA and who were receiving either rituximab or placebo, 17 serious infections were observed in the rituximab group compared with seven in the placebo group; none were fungal infections.[68]

Pneumocystis pneumonia has been reported in association with rituximab.[69–74] One case of fatal Pneumocystis pneumonia was diagnosed in a patient treated with rituximab in addition to methotrexate and low-dose prednisolone for RA. The diagnosis was made by polymerase chain reaction (PCR) on BAL fluid.[73] The increased risk of Pneumocystis infection with administration of rituximab was supported further by clinical trials that examined the addition of rituximab to standard chemotherapy for lymphomas. One study reported 10 cases (4.4%) of Pneumocystis jirovecii pneumonia in patients receiving rituximab, cytoxan, hydroxydaunorubicin (Adriamycin), vincristine (Oncovin), and prednisone/prednisolone or rituximab, cytoxan, hydroxydaunorubicin, vincristine (Oncovin), etoposide and prednisone, compared with three cases (0.8%) in patients receiving chemotherapeutic regimens that did not include rituximab.[71]

Aspergillosis has been attributed to the use of rituximab in patients who are otherwise immunocompromised because of an underlying lymphoma after solid-organ transplantation,[75] hematopoietic stem cell transplantation,[76] or autoimmune disease.[77] On the other hand, rituximab was given for more than a year to a patient who had chronic disseminated aspergillosis treated with voriconazole with no evidence of progression of the disease.[78] Disseminated histoplasmosis and mucormycosis also have been reported in association with rituximab use.[79,80]

Abatacept (Orencia) is a fusion protein that binds to CD80 and CD86 receptors on antigen-presenting cells, preventing their interaction with the CD28 receptor on T cells. It mimics the function of naturally occurring cytotoxic T-lymphocyte antigen-4, which results in a decrease in T-cell activation and proliferation. This decrease subsequently affects B-cell function, causing inhibition of TNF-a, interleukin (IL)-2, IL-6, and possibly interferon-gamma.[66,81] Abatacept has been approved for treatment of patients who have moderately to severely active RA and who have had an inadequate response to more than one disease-modifying anti-rheumatic drug (DMARD) or TNF antagonist. It can be used alone or in combination with DMARDs or TNF-α agonists.[81]

There are few reports of fungal infections related to abatacept therapy. Of 1960 patients who received abatacept, 49 had serious infections, and only one had a fungal infection (pulmonary aspergillosis). This patient had a history of tuberculosis and pulmonary fibrosis and died of aspergillosis and Pseudomonas septicemia.[68] Two other studies containing 1286 and 223 patients who had RA observed no fungal infections 6 months after starting abatacept therapy.[82,83]

Natalizumab (Tysabri) is a recombinant monoclonal antibody that competitively binds to alpha-4 integrin, a membrane protein on all leukocytes except neutrophils. It is involved in cell adhesion and leukocyte transmigration across endothelial cells and into peripheral tissues and may interfere with the activation of T lymphocytes.[84] It is approved for treatment of relapsing multiple sclerosis and in moderate to severe Crohn's disease with inflammation that has not responded to conventional therapy. Many of the reports of opportunistic infections associated with natalizumab therapy have focused on three patients in early trials of the agent who developed progressive multifocal leukoencephalopathy (PML), two of whom died. Since that time, larger studies have been performed, one of which showed a 0.1% risk of PML in the 3116 patients studied. Natalizumab was taken off the market for a short time and now carries a black box warning regarding the risk of developing PML.[84] The package insert notes that fewer than 1% of patients receiving natalizumab for Crohn's disease developed opportunistic infections, among which are listed Pneumocystis jirovecii pneumonia and bronchopulmonary aspergillosis. Subsequent studies did not observe any fungal infections.

Anakinra (Kineret) is an IL-1 receptor antagonist that contains a single methionine residue at its amino terminus. It is approved for adults who have RA rheumatoid arthritis and who have not responded to one or more DMARDs. It can be used alone or in combination with DMARDs or TNF inhibitors.[85] Four trials reviewed 2771 patients who had RA arthritis receiving anakinra compared with 729 patients who had similar characteristics receiving placebo. No cases of fungal infection were observed,[68] and no case studies reporting fungal infections were found.

SUMMARY

With the advent and widespread use of immuno-modulating biologic agents, emerging invasive fungal infections are reported increasingly. To date there is no reliable method to screen patients before starting anti-TNF therapy to predict their risk for acquiring fungal infections, partly because most of these infections are de novo infections. Patients should be counseled about avoiding high-risk activities that are associated with the endemic mycosis in their geographic areas. Physicians should maintain a high level of suspicion for endemic fungal infections when patients receiving anti-TNF therapy or other biologics present with pulmonary or systemic infections. Rapid diagnosis and initiation of antifungal therapy are of utmost importance.

REFERENCES

1. Rigby WF. Drug insight: different mechanisms of action of tumor necrosis factor antagonists—passive-aggressive behavior? Nat Clin Pract Rheumatol 2007;3:227–33.
2. Lee JH, Slifman NR, Gershon SK, et al. Life-threatening histoplasmosis complicating immunotherapy with tumor necrosis factor alpha antagonists infliximab and etanercept. Arthritis Rheum 2002;46:2565–70.
3. Bongartz T, Sutton AJ, Sweeting MJ, et al. Anti-TNF antibody therapy in rheumatoid arthritis and the risk of serious infections and malignancies: systematic review and meta-analysis of rare harmful effects in randomized controlled trials. JAMA 2006;295:2275–85.
4. Gaffo A, Saag KG, Curtis JR. Treatment of rheumatoid arthritis. Am J Health Syst Pharm 2006;63:2451–65.
5. Klinkhoff A. Biological agents for rheumatoid arthritis: targeting both physical function and structural damage. Drugs 2004;64:1267–83.
6. Remicade: [package insert]. Malvern (PA): Centocor, Inc.; 2008 [revised].
7. Etanercept [package insert]. Thousand Oaks (CA): Amgen, Wyeth; 2008. Available at: http://www.enbrel.com. Accessed December 30, 2008.
8. Humira [package insert]. Chicago: Abbott Laboratories; 2008 [revised].
9. Algood HM, Lin PL, Flynn JL. Tumor necrosis factor and chemokine interactions in the formation and maintenance of granulomas in tuberculosis. Clin Infect Dis 2005;41(Suppl 3):S189–93.
10. Mohan VP, Scanga CA, Yu K, et al. Effects of tumor necrosis factor alpha on host immune response in chronic persistent tuberculosis: possible role for limiting pathology. Infect Immun 2001;69(3):1847–55.
11. Wood KL, Hage CA, Knox KS, et al. Histoplasmosis after treatment with anti-tumor necrosis factor-alpha therapy. Am J Respir Crit Care Med 2003;167(9):1279–82.
12. Deepe GS Jr, Gibbons RS. T cells require tumor necrosis factor-alpha to provide protective immunity in mice infected with Histoplasma capsulatum. J Infect Dis 2006;193(2):322–30.
13. Filler SG, Yeaman MR, Sheppard DC. Tumor necrosis factor inhibition and invasive fungal infections. Clin Infect Dis 2005;41(Suppl 3):S208–12.
14. Maini R, St Clair EW, Breedveld F, et al. Infliximab (chimeric anti-tumour necrosis factor alpha monoclonal antibody) versus placebo in rheumatoid arthritis patients receiving concomitant methotrexate: a randomised phase III trial. ATTRACT Study Group. Lancet 1999;354(9194):1932–9.
15. Papadakis KA, Shaye OA, Vasiliauskas EA, et al. Safety and efficacy of adalimumab (D2E7) in Crohn's disease patients with an attenuated response to infliximab. Am J Gastroenterol 2005;100(1):75–9.
16. Witthoft T, Ludwig D. Effectiveness and tolerability of repeated treatment with infliximab in patients with Crohn's disease: a retrospective data analysis in Germany. Int J Colorectal Dis 2005;20(1):18–23.
17. Doran MF, Crowson CS, Pond GR, et al. Predictors of infection in rheumatoid arthritis. Arthritis Rheum 2002;46(9):2294–300.
18. Salliot C, Gossec L, Ruyssen-Witrand A, et al. Infections during tumour necrosis factor-alpha blocker therapy for rheumatic diseases in daily practice: a systematic retrospective study of 709 patients. Rheumatology (Oxford) 2007;46(2):327–34.
19. Winthrop KL, Yamashita S, Beekmann SE, et al. Mycobacterial and other serious infections in patients receiving anti-tumor necrosis factor and other newly approved biologic therapies: case finding through the Emerging Infections Network. Clin Infect Dis 2008;46(11):1738–40.

20. Asrani NS. Disseminated histoplasmosis associated with the treatment of rheumatoid arthritis with anticytokine therapy. Ann Intern Med 2008; 149:594–5.

21. Colombel JF, Loftus EV Jr, Tremaine WJ, et al. The safety profile of infliximab in patients with Crohn's disease: the Mayo Clinic experience in 500 patients. Gastroenterology 2004;126:19–31.

22. Galandiuk S, Davis BR. Infliximab-induced disseminated histoplasmosis in a patient with Crohn's disease. Nat Clin Pract Gastroenterol Hepatol 2008;5:283–7.

23. Goulet CJ, Moseley RH, Tonnerre C, et al. Clinical problem-solving. The unturned stone. N Engl J Med 2005;352:489–94.

24. Jain VV, Evans T, Peterson MW. Reactivation histoplasmosis after treatment with anti-tumor necrosis factor alpha in a patient from a nonendemic area. Respir Med 2006;100:1291–3.

25. Nakelchik M, Mangino JE. Reactivation of histoplasmosis after treatment with infliximab. Am J Med 2002;112:78.

26. Sawalha AH, Lutz BD, Chaudhary NA, et al. Panniculitis: a presenting manifestation of disseminated histoplasmosis in a patient with rheumatoid arthritis. J Clin Rheumatol 2003;9:259–62.

27. Schiff MH, Burmester GR, Kent JD, et al. Safety analyses of adalimumab (HUMIRA) in global clinical trials and US postmarketing surveillance of patients with rheumatoid arthritis. Ann Rheum Dis 2006;65: 889–94.

28. Wallis RS, Broder MS, Wong JY, et al. Granulomatous infectious diseases associated with tumor necrosis factor antagonists. Clin Infect Dis 2004; 38:1261–5.

29. Zaman R, Abbas M. Case report of fatal disseminated histoplasmosis in a patient with rheumatoid arthritis following therapy with etanercept and methotrexate Presented at the 40th annual meeting of the Infectious Diseases Society of America; Chicago, October 24–27, 2002 [abstract 378].

30. Zhang Z, Correa H, Begue RE. Tuberculosis and treatment with infliximab. N Engl J Med 2002;346:623–6.

31. Food and Drug Administration. FDA alert; information for healthcare professionals; Cimzia (certolizumab pegol), Enbrel (etanercept), Humira (adalimumab), and Remicade (infliximab). Available at: http://www.fda.gov/cder/drug/InfoSheets/HCP/TNF_blockersHCP.htm. Accessed December 30, 2008.

32. Tsiodras S, Samonis G, Boumpas DT, et al. Fungal infections complicating tumor necrosis factor alpha blockade therapy. Mayo Clin Proc 2008;83:181–94.

33. Bergstrom L, Yocum DE, Ampel NM, et al. Increased risk of coccidioidomycosis in patients treated with tumor necrosis factor alpha antagonists. Arthritis Rheum 2004;50:1959–66.

34. Dweik M, Baethge BA, Duarte AG. Coccidioidomycosis pneumonia in a nonendemic area associated with infliximab. South Med J 2007;100:517–8.

35. Maini RN, Breedveld FC, Kalden JR, et al. Sustained improvement over two years in physical function, structural damage, and signs and symptoms among patients with rheumatoid arthritis treated with infliximab and methotrexate. Arthritis Rheum 2004;50: 1051–65.

36. Mertz LE, Blair JE. Coccidioidomycosis in rheumatology patients: incidence and potential risk factors. Ann N Y Acad Sci 2007;1111:343–57.

37. Rogan MP, Thomas K. Fatal miliary coccidioidomycosis in a patient receiving infliximab therapy: a case report. J Med Case Reports 2007;1:79.

38. Ruderman E, Markenson J. Granulomatous infections and tumor necrosis factor antagonist therapies. Presented at the Proceedings of the Annual European Congress of Rheumatology EULAR; Lisbon, Portugal, June 19–21, 2003 [abstract THU0209].

39. Busca A, Locatelli F, Marmont F, et al. Recombinant human soluble tumor necrosis factor receptor fusion protein as treatment for steroid refractory graft-versus-host disease following allogeneic hematopoietic stem cell transplantation. Am J Hematol 2007;82:45–52.

40. Couriel D, Saliba R, Hicks K, et al. Tumor necrosis factor-alpha blockade for the treatment of acute GVHD. Blood 2004;104:649–54.

41. De Rosa FG, Shaz D, Campagna AC, et al. Invasive pulmonary aspergillosis soon after therapy with infliximab, a tumor necrosis factor-alpha-neutralizing antibody: a possible healthcare-associated case? Infect Control Hosp Epidemiol 2003;24:477–82.

42. Finn S, Bond J, McCarthy D, et al. Angioinvasive aspergillosis presenting as neutropenic colitis. Histopathology 2006;49:440–1.

43. Jacobsohn DA, Hallick J, Anders V, et al. Infliximab for steroid-refractory acute GVHD: a case series. Am J Hematol 2003;74:119–24.

44. Kaur N, Mahl TC. Pneumocystis carinii pneumonia with oral candidiasis after infliximab therapy for Crohn's disease. Dig Dis Sci 2004;49:1458–60.

45. Lassoued S, Sire S, Farny M, et al. Pulmonary aspergillosis in a patient with rheumatoid arthritis treated by etanercept. Clin Exp Rheumatol 2004; 22:267–8.

46. Marty FM, Lee SJ, Fahey MM, et al. Infliximab use in patients with severe graft-versus-host disease and other emerging risk factors of non-Candida invasive fungal infections in allogeneic hematopoietic stem cell transplant recipients: a cohort study. Blood 2003;102:2768–76.

47. Patriarca F, Sperotto A, Damiani D, et al. Infliximab treatment for steroid-refractory acute graft-versus-host disease. Haematologica 2004;89:1352–9.

48. Slusher JR, Maldonado ME, Mousavi F, et al. Central nervous system Aspergillus fumigatus presenting as

cranial nerve palsy in a patient with ankylosing spondylitis on anti-TNF therapy. Rheumatology (Oxford) 2008;47:739–40.

49. van der Klooster JM, Bosman RJ, Oudemans-van Straaten HM, et al. Disseminated tuberculosis, pulmonary aspergillosis and cutaneous herpes simplex infection in a patient with infliximab and methotrexate. Intensive Care Med 2003;29: 2327–9.

50. Warris A, Bjorneklett A, Gaustad P. Invasive pulmonary aspergillosis associated with infliximab therapy. N Engl J Med 2001;344:1099–100.

51. Devlin SM, Hu B, Ippoliti A. Mucormycosis presenting as recurrent gastric perforation in a patient with Crohn's disease on glucocorticoid, 6-mercaptopurine, and infliximab therapy. Dig Dis Sci 2007;52: 2078–81.

52. Singh P, Taylor SF, Murali R, et al. Disseminated mucormycosis and orbital ischaemia in combination immunosuppression with a tumour necrosis factor alpha inhibitor. Clin Experiment Ophthalmol 2007; 35:275–80.

53. Belda A, Hinojosa J, Serra B, et al. [Systemic candidiasis and infliximab therapy]. Gastroenterol Hepatol 2004;27:365–7 [in Spanish].

54. Burmester G, Mariette X, Montecucco C, et al. Adalimumab alone and in combination with disease-modifying antirheumatic drugs for the treatment of rheumatoid arthritis in clinical practice: the Research in Active Rheumatoid Arthritis (ReAct) trial. Ann Rheum Dis 2007;66:732–9.

55. Netea MG, Radstake T, Joosten LA, et al. Salmonella septicemia in rheumatoid arthritis patients receiving anti-tumor necrosis factor therapy: association with decreased interferon-gamma production and toll-like receptor 4 expression. Arthritis Rheum 2003; 48:1853–7.

56. Ricart E, Panaccione R, Loftus EV, et al. Infliximab for Crohn's disease in clinical practice at the Mayo Clinic: the first 100 patients. Am J Gastroenterol 2001;96:722–9.

57. Arend SM, Kuijper EJ, Allaart CF, et al. Cavitating pneumonia after treatment with infliximab and prednisone. Eur J Clin Microbiol Infect Dis 2004;23: 638–41.

58. Chavez-Lopez M, Marquez-Diaz F, Aguayo-Leytte G. [Cerebral cryptococcosis associated with etanercept]. Enferm Infecc Microbiol Clin 2006;24: 288 [in Spanish].

59. Hage CA, Wood KL, Winer-Muram HT, et al. Pulmonary cryptococcosis after initiation of anti-tumor necrosis factor-alpha therapy. Chest 2003;124: 2395–7.

60. Hoang JK, Burruss J. Localized cutaneous Cryptococcus albidus infection in a 14-year-old boy on etanercept therapy. Pediatr Dermatol 2007;24: 285–8.

61. Horcajada JP, Pena JL, Martinez-Taboada VM, et al. Invasive cryptococcosis and adalimumab treatment. Emerg Infect Dis 2007;13:953–5.

62. Shrestha RK, Stoller JK, Honari G, et al. Pneumonia due to Cryptococcus neoformans in a patient receiving infliximab: possible zoonotic transmission from a pet cockatiel. Respir Care 2004;49:606–8.

63. Starrett W, Czachor J, Dallal M, et al. Cryptococcal pneumonia following treatment with infliximab for rheumatoid arthritis. Presented at the 40th annual meeting of the Infectious Diseases Society of America; Chicago, October 24–27, 2002 [abstract 374:110].

64. True DG, Penmetcha M, Peckham SJ. Disseminated cryptococcal infection in rheumatoid arthritis treated with methotrexate and infliximab. J Rheumatol 2002; 29:1561–3.

65. Rituximab: (Rituxin) [package insert]. San Francisco (CA): Genentech, Inc.; 2008.

66. Saketkoo LA, Espinoza LR. Impact of biologic agents on infectious diseases. Infect Dis Clin North Am 2006;20:931–61.

67. Gea-Banacloche JC, Weinberg GA. Monoclonal antibody therapeutics and risk for infection. Pediatr Infect Dis J 2007;26:1049–52.

68. Salliot C, Dougados M, Gossec L. Risk of serious infections during rituximab, abatacept and anakinra treatments for rheumatoid arthritis: meta-analyses of randomised placebo-controlled trials. Ann Rheum Dis 2009;68:25–32.

69. Ennishi D, Terui Y, Yokoyama M, et al. Increased incidence of interstitial pneumonia by CHOP combined with rituximab. Int J Hematol 2008;87: 393–7.

70. Hatoum HH, Sarosi GA, Knox KS, et al. Acute respiratory failure and diffuse pulmonary infiltrates four weeks after rituximab therapy. Respiratory Medicine CME, in press.

71. Kolstad A, Holte H, Fossa A, et al. Pneumocystis jirovecii pneumonia in B-cell lymphoma patients treated with the rituximab-CHOEP-14 regimen. Haematologica 2007;92:139–40.

72. Spina M, Jaeger U, Sparano JA, et al. Rituximab plus infusional cyclophosphamide, doxorubicin, and etoposide in HIV-associated non-Hodgkin lymphoma: pooled results from 3 phase 2 trials. Blood 2005;105:1891–7.

73. Teichmann LL, Woenckhaus M, Vogel C, et al. Fatal Pneumocystis pneumonia following rituximab administration for rheumatoid arthritis. Rheumatology (Oxford) 2008;47:1256–7.

74. Venhuizen AC, Hustinx WN, van Houte AJ, et al. Three cases of Pneumocystis jirovecii pneumonia (PCP) during first-line treatment with rituximab in combination with CHOP-14 for aggressive B-cell non-Hodgkin's lymphoma. Eur J Haematol 2008;80: 275–6.

75. Verschuuren EA, Stevens SJ, van Imhoff GW, et al. Treatment of posttransplant lymphoproliferative disease with rituximab: the remission, the relapse, and the complication. Transplantation 2002;73:100–4.

76. Fianchi L, Rossi E, Murri R, et al. Severe infectious complications in a patient treated with rituximab for idiopathic thrombocytopenic purpura. Ann Hematol 2007;86:225–6.

77. Helbig G, Stella-Holowiecka B, Krawczyk-Kulis M, et al. Successful treatment of pure red cell aplasia with repeated, low doses of rituximab in two patients after ABO-incompatible allogeneic haematopoietic stem cell transplantation for acute myeloid leukaemia. Haematologica 2005;90(Suppl:ECR33).

78. Jung N, Owczarczyk K, Hellmann M, et al. Efficacy and safety of rituximab in a patient with active rheumatoid arthritis and chronic disseminated pulmonary aspergillosis and history of tuberculosis. Rheumatology (Oxford) 2008;47:932–3.

79. Vieira CA, Agarwal A, Book BK, et al. Rituximab for reduction of anti-HLA antibodies in patients awaiting renal transplantation: 1. Safety, pharmacodynamics, and pharmacokinetics. Transplantation 2004;77:542–8.

80. Vigna-Perez M, Hernandez-Castro B, Paredes-Saharopulos O, et al. Clinical and immunological effects of Rituximab in patients with lupus nephritis refractory to conventional therapy: a pilot study. Arthritis Res Ther 2006;8:R83.

81. Abatacept: (Orencia) [package insert]. Princeton (NJ): Bristol-Myers squibb; 2008.

82. Genovese MC, Becker JC, Schiff M, et al. Abatacept for rheumatoid arthritis refractory to tumor necrosis factor alpha inhibition. N Engl J Med 2005;353:1114–23.

83. Schiff MH, Pritchard C, Huffstutter JE, et al. The 6-month safety and efficacy of abatacept in patients with rheumatoid arthritis who underwent a washout after anti-TNF therapy or were directly switched to abatacept: the ARRIVE trial. Ann Rheum Dis 2008.

84. Stuve O, Bennett JL. Pharmacological properties, toxicology and scientific rationale for the use of natalizumab (Tysabri) in inflammatory diseases. CNS Drug Rev 2007;13:79–95.

85. Anakinra: (Kineret) [package insert]. Thousand Oaks (CA): Amgen; 2008.

Candida in the ICU

Rabih O. Darouiche, MD[a,b,c],*

KEYWORDS
- *Candida* • Candidemia • Invasive infection
- Deep-seated infection • Candidiasis • ICU

The past two decades have marked a dramatic rise in the frequency of infections caused by *Candida* species. Although invasive *Candida* infections can affect any hospitalized patient, they are more common and have unique attributes in certain populations, including patients who have cancer or a critical illness. Whereas only 1% to 8% of patients residing in the hospital develop invasive candidiasis (which is synonymous with invasive or deep-seated *Candida* infections), about 10% of patients residing in ICUs suffer from this serious infection.[1] Although both ICU and non-ICU patients share well-recognized risks for invasive candidiasis, such as the use of broad-spectrum antibacterial agents, vascular access, and total parenteral nutrition, the former group of patients is more likely to have had recent surgery but less likely to have malignancy, neutropenia, or immunosuppression.[2] Likewise, critically ill patients who have invasive *Candida* infections tend to have a less favorable response to antifungal treatment and a higher all-cause mortality than other hospitalized patients.[2]

Invasive candidiasis accounts for up to 15%[1] or 30%[3] of all nosocomial infections in critically ill patients. The rising incidence and distinguishing features of invasive candidiasis in patients in ICUs prompted the writing of this article, which addresses both documented and suspected deep-seated *Candida* infections, compares the clinical efficacy of antifungal agents, and assesses particularly challenging scenarios in this patient population.

INVASIVE CANDIDIASIS

Invasive candidiasis in critically ill patients commonly presents in one of two forms: documented fungal infection in nonneutropenic patients and suspected fungal infection in febrile patients.

Documented Invasive Candida Infections

Although a substantial proportion of patients become colonized with *Candida* species during hospitalization, only few subsequently develop invasive *Candida* infection.[1] Most cases of documented invasive *Candida* infections in patients in the ICU are associated with candidemia, but some patients present, in the presence or absence of candidemia, with endocarditis, peritonitis, pyelonephritis, myositis, ostomyelitis, discitis, or meningitis, or with an abscess in deep-seated tissues, including the abdomen, brain, kidneys, and heart. The growth of *Candida* species from respiratory samples is almost always indicative of colonization unless a lung biopsy demonstrates histopathologic evidence of fungal invasion of tissues. About 80% of cases of candidemia arise from or evolve in the presence of a vascular access, including access related to central venous catheters, hemodialysis catheters, peripherally inserted central catheters, and implanted ports.[4]

Candida species are the fourth most common cause of nosocomial bloodstream infections in North America, and they have a higher crude mortality rate (up to 40%) than any type of bacteremia, including that of *Staphylococcus aureus*, the most common cause of nosocomial bloodstream infection (with a crude mortality of 25%).[5] Blood cultures from almost a quarter of patients who have candidemia also yield bacterial growth.[5] Not only is the overall incidence of nosocomial bloodstream infection several-fold higher in

[a] Michael E. Debakey Veterans Affairs Medical Center, Infectious Disease Section (Room 4B-370), 2002 Holcome Boulevard, Houston, TX 77030, USA
[b] Baylor College of Medicine, Department of Medicine, Infectious Disease Section (BCM 286, Room N1319), One Baylor Plaza, Houston, TX 77030, USA
[c] Center for Prostheses Infection, Department of Physical Medicine and Rehabilitation, Baylor College of Medicine, 1333 Moursund Avenue, Suite A221, Houston, TX 77030, USA
* Michael E. Debakey Veterans Affairs Medical Center, Houston, TX.
E-mail address: rdarouiche@aol.com

Clin Chest Med 30 (2009) 287–293
doi:10.1016/j.ccm.2009.02.013
0272-5231/09/$ – see front matter. Published by Elsevier Inc.

patients in the ICU than in those in other hospital units[6] but candidemia also is more prevalent in the former group. An estimated 33% to 55% of all episodes of candidemia occur in patients in the ICU, and the associated mortality rates range from 5% to 71%.[7] Risk factors for candidemia in patients in the ICU include the use of intravascular catheters, parenteral nutrition, prior abdominal surgery, the use of broad-spectrum antibacterial therapy, the use of corticosteroids, acute renal failure, a prolonged stay in the ICU, and *Candida* colonization, particularly if it is multifocal.[7]

Although *Candida albicans* was and still is the most common cause of *Candida* bloodstream infections, *Candida* species other than albicans account for a growing proportion of instances that represents one third to one half of all episodes of candidemia.[7–10] The most common non-*albicans* species is *C parapsilosis*, which accounts for about one third of *Candida* infections, followed by *C glabrata*, *C tropicalis*, and *C krusei* (which is less frequently isolated from patients who are critically ill than from patients who have cancer), and much less frequently by *C lusitaniae*, *C guilliermondii,* and *C rugosa*.[9] The receipt of fluconazole and presence of a vascular access are associated with an increased risk of bloodstream infection by the collective group of non-*albicans Candida* strains rather than by *C albicans*.[8] There are also specific risk factors for infection by particular non-*albicans* strains. These risk factors include in-dwelling devices, hyperalimentation, and being a neonate for *C parapsilosis*; surgery, the use of urinary or vascular catheters, and the receipt of azoles for *C glabrata*; neutropenia and bone marrow transplant for *C tropicalis*; azole prophylaxis, neutropenia, and bone marrow transplant for *C kruzei*; the intake of amphotericin B for *C lusitaniae* and *C guilliermondii*; and having burns for *C rugosa*.[9] The mortality rate from bloodstream infection due to non-*albicans Candida* strains is collectively as high[9,11] or higher[10] than that caused by *C albicans*. Regardless of the causative strain, candidemia in patients in the ICU is associated with a considerable increase in the length of hospital stay (from 10 to 21 days) and hospital charges (from $39,000 to $92,000) in adults and children.[7,12]

Since the last Infectious Disease Society of America guidelines for treatment of invasive candidiasis and candidemia were published,[13,14] several new antifungal agents with excellent activity against *Candida* species and favorable safety profiles have become available for patient care. Some of those newer agents have been incorporated into the soon-to-be reported new Infectious Disease Society of America guidelines.

At the time this article was written, available antifungal agents for treatment of invasive *Candida* infections include the azoles (fluconazole, itraconazole, and voriconazole), echinocandins (caspofungin, micafungin, and anidulafungin), and polyenes (amphotericin B, amphotericin B lipid complex, and liposomal amphotericin B).

A total of seven published prospective, randomized clinical trials have compared the efficacy and safety of various antifungal agents that belong to the same or different classes of antifungal agents for treatment of invasive candidiasis with or without candidemia in nonneutropenic patients. In cases of patients who had candidemia, antifungal therapy was given for 14 days after the last positive blood culture. As shown in **Table 1**,[15–21] neither the type nor the dose of the antifungal agent significantly enhanced efficacy. However, the azoles and echinocandins were generally safer than amphotericin B and even lipid formulations of amphotericin B. Excluded from **Table 1** because of the inclusion of some patients with neutropenia was a prospective, randomized clinical trial that demonstrated a comparable efficacy but less toxicity when treating presumed invasive *Candida* infections using fluconazole (400 mg/d) or amphotericin B (20–50 mg/d; 0.67 mg/Kg/d in neutropenic patients).[22]

Timely removal of the vascular catheter responsible for candidemia shortens the duration of bloodstream infection[23] and improves clinical outcome.[24,25] In patients who have candidemia and who happen to have an in-dwelling vascular catheter, clinical characteristics that suggest that the catheter is not the source of the bloodstream infection include disseminated infection, the previous receipt of chemotherapy or corticosteroids, and poor response to antifungal therapy.[24] A time-to-positivity of peripheral blood cultures that is greater than 30 hours was found to be a sensitive (100%) but nonspecific (specificity 51%) marker for catheter-related candidemia.[4] Rapid clinical response and prompt resolution of candidemia after removal of the potentially infected vascular catheter suggest but do not confirm that the vascular access was the source of the bloodstream infection and that endocarditis does not exist. Clinical judgment based on patient history and a physical examination should dictate whether to perform a workup for endocarditis (including cardiac echocardiographic and retinal examination) in patients who have candidemia. In patients who have catheter-related candidemia, it is generally recommended to remove the infected vascular catheter and treat the patient for 2 weeks after resolution of positive cultures and the symptoms of infection.[13,23]

Table 1
Results of prospective, randomized clinical trials of invasive candidiasis with or without candidemia in nonneutropenic subjects

First Author (Ref)	Type of Infection	Efficacy Outcome	Safety
Rex[15]	Candidemia	Fluconazole (400 mg/d) not inferior to amphotericin B (0.5–0.6 mg/Kg/d)	Amphotericin B more toxic
Rex[16]	Candidemia	Fluconazole (800 mg/d) not inferior to fluconazole (800 mg/d) plus amphotericin B (0.7 mg/Kg/d)	Amphotericin B more toxic
Kullberg[17]	Candidemia	Voriconazole (6 mg/Kg Q 12 hours, first day, then 3 mg/Kg Q 12 hours) not inferior to amphotericin B (0.7–1 mg/Kg/d) followed by fluconazole (400 mg/d) after 3–7 days	Amphotericin B more toxic
Mora-Duarte[18]	Invasive candidiasis, including candidemia	Caspofungin (70 mg, first day, then 50 mg/d) reportedly superior to amphotericin B (0.6–1.0 mg/Kg/d)[a]	Amphotericin B more toxic
Reboli[19]	Invasive candidiasis, including candidemia	Anidulafungin (200 mg, first day, then 100 mg/d) not inferior to fluconazole (800 mg, first day, then 400 mg/d)	Comparable rates of adverse events
Kuse[20]	Invasive candidiasis, including candidemia	Micafungin (100 mg/d) not inferior to liposomal amphotericin B (3 mg/Kg/d)	Liposomal amphotericin B more toxic
Pappas[21]	Invasive candidiasis, including candidemia	Micafungin (100 mg/d or 150 mg/d) not inferior to caspofungin (70 mg, first day, then 50 mg/d)	Comparable rates of adverse events

[a] The difference in the response rates to caspofungin and amphotericin B could be explained by the differences in withdrawal from the study because of drug toxicity. (Patients who withdrew because of drug toxicity were considered as having failed to respond.)

Suspected Invasive Candida Infections

Although in clinical practice there may be more cases of suspected than documented invasive fungal infections in patients in the ICU, there are much less clinical data to guide the management of unproven infections.[26] An invasive *Candida* infection is typically considered when a febrile, nonneutropenic patient in the ICU who has some risk factors for *Candida* infection (eg, vascular access, administration of total parenteral nutrition, the receipt of corticosteroids, therapy using broad-spectrum antimicrobial agents, recent surgery, a prolonged stay in the ICU, colonization with *Candida*) fails to respond to broad-spectrum antibacterial therapy. It is essential that this undocumented infection be suspected, if indicated, because of two important two reasons:

(a) Difficulty or delay in diagnosing deep-seated infections. Not only are the clinical manifestations of *Candida* and bacterial infections in patients in the ICU generally indistinguishable but laboratory tests that could diagnose *Candida* infection also are not practical or optimal. For instance, serologic markers and molecular-based tests are not universally available (the topic of nonmicrobiologic diagnosis of invasive candidiasis is discussed in a separate article in this issue), and a bleeding diathesis may preclude the performance of a tissue biopsy—the gold standard technique for diagnosing invasive infection. Furthermore, it is not sufficient to rely on blood cultures because premortem blood cultures indicated the growth of *Candida* in only one third to one half of patients who showed autopsy findings of disseminated candidiasis.

(b) Rapid progression of invasive *Candida* infections. This is reflected by the robust, direct relationship between hospital mortality and the number of days from onset of candidemia to the initiation of antifungal therapy. The hospital mortality rates in patients who had candidemia were reported to be 15% if fluconazole was started when blood cultures were obtained, 24% if fluconazole was initiated one day later, 37% if fluconazole was started 2 days later, and at least 41% if fluconazole was initiated 3 or more days later.[27] Multivariate analysis indicated that delay in starting antifungal therapy is an independent determinant of hospital mortality in patients who have candidemia.[28]

A single prospective, randomized clinical trial assessed the efficacy of empiric antifungal therapy (fluconazole 800 mg/d) compared with placebo in patients in the ICU suspected to have invasive fungal infection.[29] This study failed to show clinical benefit from empiric therapy using fluconazole, perhaps because fewer fungal infections than anticipated occurred in the control group. Future studies should focus on patients in the ICU who have numerous strong risk factors for *Candida* infection, which could include, for example, colonization by *Candida* of multiple sites rather than just one bodily site. In that regard, empiric antifungal therapy among selected patients in the ICU who are at high risk for infection has been shown to be cost-effective in reducing mortality.[30,31] Additionally, because some undocumented episodes of invasive *Candida* infection could be caused by species other than *C albicans* and *C parapsilosis*, it would be reasonable to conduct a future placebo-controlled, comparative study to assess the efficacy of an antifungal agent that possesses activity against non-*albicans* *Candida* species that exceeds that of fluconazole for empiric treatment of suspected invasive *Candida* infections in patients in the ICU.

CHALLENGING SCENARIOS

In addition to invasive *Candida* infections that have been comprehensively assessed in prospective, randomized clinical trials, clinicians frequently face challenging conditions for which no established guidelines exist. Particularly challenging scenarios include infections by non-*albicans* *Candida* species.

Certain non-*albicans* *Candida* strains require special attention, particularly *C glabrata* because of reduced susceptibility to fluconazole and *C parapsilosis* owing to its diminished response to echinocandins. This is particularly problematic in patients in whom the results of cultures are pending because clinical features do not accurately predict the fungal pathogenesis of bloodstream infection.[32]

Most strains of *C glabrata* are not inherently resistant to fluconazole but exhibit reduced susceptibility to this drug.[33] However, because tests for antifungal susceptibilities are not routinely available in hospital laboratories and do not have a robust evidence of clinical relevance, it is preferable not to take the risk of treating bloodstream infection or serious invasive infections due to *C glabrata* by using a high dosage of fluconazole (400–800 mg/d) because of the high reported rate of mortality.[34] Available options would include treatment using other azoles (eg, voriconazole) or any echinocandin or amphotericin B-based preparation (**Table 2**).

In cases of infection by *C parapsilosis*, candidemia has been reported to either evolve or fail to resolve after the patient receives echinocandin therapy.[35] In contrast, *C parapsilosis* is usually responsive to all azoles and polyenes (see **Table 2**). The minimum inhibitory concentrations of echinocandins for *C parapsilosis* are generally about fourfold higher than the minimum inhibitory concentrations for other *Candida* species. *C parapsilosis* causes about one third of all episodes of *Candida* infection of in-dwelling devices,[36] so this infectious scenario will become even more challenging in the future because both the number of devices used and the proportion of device-related infections that are caused by *Candida* species are escalating.[37] Although some antifungal agents may be more active than others against biofilm-embedded *Candida* organisms in vitro[38] and in vivo,[39,40] there has been no comprehensive effort to clinically eradicate biofilm-based infections. That is why it is still recommended that *Candida* infection of not just vascular catheters but also of surgical implants be treated using both antifungal agents and removal of the infected device.[41] Because preliminary reports indicated that some combinations of antibiofilm and antimicrobial agents can help salvage catheters associated with bacteremia, it would be reasonable to assess their ability to cure candidemia when judiciously leaving the infected catheter in place.

Table 2
Comparison of in vitro activity of antifungal agents against *Candida* species

Class/Drug	*Candida* Species			
	C Albicans	*C Glabrata*	*C Parapsilosis*	*C Krusei*
Azoles				
Fluconazole	++	+	++	−
Itraconazole	++	±	++	+
Voriconazole	++	+	++	++
Echinocandins				
Caspofungin	++	++	±	++
Micafungin	++	++	±	++
Anidulafungin	++	++	±	++
Polyenes				
Amphotericin B	++	++	++	++
Amphotericin B lipid complex	++	++	++	++
Liposomal amphotericin B	++	++	++	++

C krusei is inherently resistant to fluconazole and may have reduced susceptibility to itraconazole, but it is responsive to voriconazole and all echinocandin and polyene agents.[9] Fortunately, *C krusei* is less frequently a pathogen in patients who are critically ill than in patients who have cancer. Although amphotericin B is not as active against *C lusitaniae* and *C guilliermondii* as it is against other species of *Candida*, these two fungal species collectively account for a small portion (less than 5%) of *Candida* infections in patients in the ICU. Furthermore, other classes of antifungal agents possess good activity against *C lusitaniae* and *C guilliermondii*.

SUMMARY

Invasive candidiasis, a common nosocomial infection in critically ill patients, is associated with serious medical complications and tremendous economic consequences. Although newer antifungal agents are safer than the traditionally used amphotericin B, they may or may not offer distinct advantages in terms of efficacy. Early diagnosis and, consequently, prompt treatment of deep-seated infections have the potential of improving outcome. Although the clinical benefit from giving empiric antifungal therapy for suspected but undocumented invasive *Candida* infection has not been proved, it has been suggested that this therapeutic approach is cost-effective. Despite encouraging in vitro and in vivo results, there is no established clinical protocol for attempting the salvage of devices infected by *Candida* species. There is a critical need to further assess the following three issues: (1) the role of antifungal agents other than fluconazole for empiric treatment of suspected but undocumented deep-seated *Candida* infections in patients who are critically ill and at high risk for *Candida* infection, (2) the ability of novel approaches to be used to salvage devices infected by *Candida* species while ensuring a cure of the infection, and (3) the utility of nonmicrobiologic diagnosis of invasive candidiasis to grant the opportunity to clinicians to properly intervene earlier in the disease course, if indicated.

REFERENCES

1. Eggimann P, Garbino J, Pittet D. Epidemiology of *Candida* species infections in critically ill non-immunosuppressed patients. Lancet Infect Dis 2003; 3(11):685–702.
2. DiNubille MJ, Lupinacci RJ, Strohmaier KM, et al. Invasive candidiasis treated in the intensive care unit: observations from a randomized clinical trial. J Crit Care 2007;22(3):237–44.
3. Magnason S, Kristinsson KG, Stefansson T, et al. Risk factors and outcome in ICU-acquired infections. Acta Anaesthesiol Scand 2008;52(9): 1238–45.
4. Ben-Ami R, Weinberger M, Orni-Wasserlauff R, et al. Time to blood culture positivity as a marker for catheter-related candidemia. J Clin Microbiol 2008;46(7): 2222–6.
5. Klotz SA, Chasin BS, Powell B, et al. Polymicrobial bloodstream infections involving *Candida* species: analysis of patients and review of the literature. Diagn Microbiol Infect Dis 2007;59(4):401–6.

6. Suljagić V, Cobeljić M, Mirović V, et al. Nosocomial bloodstream infections in ICU and non-ICU patients. Am J Infect Control 2005;33(6):333–40.

7. Bouza E, Munoz P. Epidemiology of candidemia in intensive care units. Int J Antimicrob Agents 2008; 32(Suppl 2):S87–91.

8. Chow JK, Golan Y, Ruthazer R, et al. Factors associated with candidemia caused by non-*albicans* Candida species versus *Candida albicans* in the intensive care unit. Clin Infect Dis 2008;46(8): 1206–13.

9. Krmercy V, Barnes AJ. Non-*albicans* Candida spp. causing fungaemia: pathogenicity and antifungal resistance. J Hosp Infect 2002;50(4):243–60.

10. Playford EG, Marriott D, Nguyen Q, et al. Candidemia in nonneutropenic critically ill patients: risk factors for non-*albicans* Candida spp. Crit Care Med 2008;36(7):2034–9.

11. Dimopoulos G, Ntziora F, Rachiotis G, et al. *Candida albicans* versus non-*albicans* intensive care unit–acquired bloodstream infections: differences in risk factors and outcome. Anesth Analg 2008;106(2): 523–9.

12. Zaoutis TE, Argon J, Chu J, et al. The epidemiology and attributable outcomes of candidemia in adults and children hospitalized in the United States: a propensity analysis. Clin Infect Dis 2005;41(9): 1232–9.

13. Rex JH, Walsh TJ, Sobel JD, et al. Practice guidelines for the treatment of candidiasis. Infectious Diseases Society of America. Clin Infect Dis 2000; 30(4):662–78.

14. Pappas PG, Rex JH, Sobel JD, et al. Guidelines for treatment of candidiasis. Clin Infect Dis 2004;38(2): 161–89.

15. Rex JH, Bennett JE, Sugar AM, et al. A randomized trial comparing fluconazole with amphotericin B for the treatment of candidemia in patients without neutropenia. Candidemia Study Group and the National Institute. N Engl J Med 1994;331(20):1325–30.

16. Rex JH, Pappas PG, Karchmer AW, et al. A randomized and blinded multicenter trial of high-dose fluconazole plus placebo versus fluconazole plus amphotericin B as therapy for candidemia and its consequences in nonneutropenic subjects. Clin Infect Dis 2003;36(10):1221–8.

17. Kullberg BJ, Sobel JD, Ruhnke M, et al. Voriconazole versus a regimen of amphotericin B followed by fluconazole for candidaemia in non-neutropenic patients: a randomised non-inferiority trial. Lancet 2005;366(9495):1435–42.

18. Mora-Duarte J, Betts R, Rotstein C, et al. Comparison of caspofungin and amphotericin B for invasive candidiasis. N Engl J Med 2002;347(25):2020–9.

19. Reboli AC, Rotstein C, Pappas PG, et al. Anidulafungin versus fluconazole for invasive candidiasis. N Engl J Med 2007;356(24):2472–82.

20. Kuse ER, Chetchotisakd P, de Cunha CA, et al. Micafungin versus liposomal amphotericin B for candidemia and invasive candidosis: a phase III randomised double-blind trial. Lancet 2007;369(9572): 1519–27.

21. Pappas PG, Rotstein CM, Betts RF, et al. Micafungin versus caspofungin for treatment of candidemia and other forms of invasive candidiasis. Clin Infect Dis 2007;45(7):883–93.

22. Anaissie EJ, Darouiche RO, Abi-Said D, et al. Management of invasive candidal infections: results of a prospective, randomized, multicenter study of fluconazole versus amphotericin B and review of the literature. Clin Infect Dis 1996;23(5):964–72.

23. Rex JH, Bennett JE, Sugar AM, et al. Intravascular catheter exchange and duration of candidemia. NIAID Mycosis Study Group and the Candidemia Study Group. Clin Infect Dis 1995;21(4):994–6.

24. Raad I, Hanna H, Boktour M, et al. Management of central venous catheters in patients with cancer and candidemia. Clin Infect Dis 2004;38(8): 1119–27.

25. Pasqualotto AC, de Moraes AB, Zanini RR, et al. Analysis of independent risk factors for death among pediatric patients with candidemia and a central venous catheter in place. Infect Control Hosp Epidemiol 2007;28(7):799–804.

26. De Pauw BE, Walsh TJ, Donnelly JP, et al. Revised definitions of invasive fungal disease from the European Organization for Research and Treatment of Cancer/Invasive Fungal Infections Cooperative Group and the National Institute of Allergy and Infectious Diseases Mycosis Study Group (EORTC/MSG) Consensus Group. Clin Infect Dis 2008;45(12): 1813–21.

27. Garey KW, Rege M, Pai MP, et al. Time to initiation of fluconazole therapy impacts mortality in patients with candidemia: a multi-institutional study. Clin Infect Dis 2006;43(1):25–31.

28. Morrell M, Fraser VJ, Kollef MH. Delaying the empiric treatment of *Candida* bloodstream infection until positive blood culture results are obtained: a potential risk for hospital mortality. Antimicrobial Agents Chemother 2005;49(9):3640–5.

29. Schuster MG, Edwards JE Jr, Sobel JD, et al. Empirical fluconazole versus placebo for intensive care unit patients: a randomized trial. Ann Intern Med 2008;149(2):83–90.

30. Golan Y, Wolf MP, Pauker SG, et al. Empirical anti-*Candida* therapy among selected patients in the intensive care unit: a cost-effectiveness analysis. Ann Intern Med 2005;143(12):857–69.

31. Chen H, Suda KJ, Turpin RS, et al. High- versus low-dose fluconazole therapy for empiric treatment of suspected invasive candidiasis among high-risk patients in the intensive care unit: cost-effectiveness analysis. Curr Med Res Opin 2007;23(5):1057–65.

32. Shorr AF, Lazarus DR, Sherner JH, et al. Do clinical features allow for accurate prediction of fungal pathogenesis in bloodstream infections? Potential implications of the increasing prevalence of non-*albicans* candidemia. Crit Care Med 2007;35(4): 1077–83.

33. Klevay MJ, Ernst EJ, Hollanbaugh JL, et al. Therapy and outcome of *Candida glabrata* versus *Candida albicans* bloodstream infection. Diagn Microbiol Infect Dis 2008;60(3):273–7.

34. Tumbarello M, Sanguinetti M, Trecarichi EM, et al. Fungaemia caused by *Candida glabrata* with reduced susceptibility to fluconazole due to altered gene expression: risk factors, antifungal treatment and outcome. J Antimicrob Chemother 2008;62(6): 1379–85.

35. Cheung C, Guo Y, Gialanella P, et al. Development of candidemia on caspofungin therapy: a case report. Infection 2006;34(6):345–8.

36. Kojic EM, Darouiche RO. Comparison of adherence of *Candida albicans* and *Candida parapsilosis* to silicone catheters in vitro and in vivo. Clin Microbiol Infect 2003;9(7):684–90.

37. Kojic EM, Darouiche RO. *Candida* infections of medical devices. Clin Microbiol Rev 2004;17(2):255–67.

38. Lewis RE, Kontoyiannis DP, Darouiche RO, et al. Antifungal activity of amphotericin B, fluconazole, and voriconazole in an in vitro model of *Candida* catheter-related bloodstream infection. Antimicrobial Agents Chemother 2002;46(11):3499–505.

39. Mukherjee PK, Long L, Kim HG, et al. Amphotericin B lipid complex is efficacious in the treatment of *Candida albicans* biofilms using a model of catheter-associated *Candida* biofilms. Int J Antimicrob Agents 2009;33(2):149–53.

40. Schinabeck MK, Long LA, Hossain MA, et al. Rabbit model of *Candida albicans* biofilm infection: liposomal amphotericin B antifungal lock therapy. Antimicrobial Agents Chemother 2004;48(5):1727–32.

41. Darouiche RO. Treatment of infections associated with surgical implants. N Engl J Med 2004;350(14): 1422–9.

Fungal Infections in Hematopoietic Stem Cell Transplantation and Solid-Organ Transplantation—Focus on Aspergillosis

Marcio Nucci, MD[a], Elias Anaissie, MD[b],*

KEYWORDS

- Fungal infection • Transplantation • Aspergillosis
- Stem cell transplantation • Solid organ transplantation

Invasive fungal infections (IFIs) represent a major complication in recipients of hematopoietic stem cell transplantation (HSCT) and solid-organ transplantation (SOT). The incidence of IFIs in transplant recipients has increased over the past 20 years, and these infections continue to be associated with high morbidity and mortality.[1]

This article reviews the important concepts guiding the management of IFIs in HSCT and SOT recipients, including epidemiologic trends, new risk factors, and a timetable of infections, pathogens, therapy, and prevention of these infections. An emphasis is given to invasive aspergillosis (IA).

Recipients of HSCT and SOT differ significantly in the risks and epidemiology of IFI. Because SOT involves a surgical procedure, the immediate period post transplant is associated with a risk of invasive candidiasis in those transplants involving organs in the abdominal cavity, especially the liver, pancreas, and intestine. IA, however, occurs in a significant proportion of lung transplant recipients and less frequently in other transplants.[2] Another aspect that distinguishes SOT from HSCT is that because immunosuppression is maintained for life, SOT recipients are at risk for infections associated with chronic suppression of T cell–mediated immunity (CMI), such as cryptococcosis and histoplasmosis. These infections occur late after transplant. By contrast, HSCT recipients are at high risk of developing IA, and invasive candidiasis is uncommon in patients receiving fluconazole prophylaxis. Cryptococcosis and histoplasmosis are rarely reported.[3]

FUNGAL INFECTIONS IN RECIPIENTS OF HEMATOPOIETIC STEM CELL TRANSPLANTATION
Epidemiology

The incidence of IFIs in HSCT recipients varies according to the type of transplant (autologous or allogeneic), HLA matching (matched or mismatched), relatedness of the donor (related or unrelated), conditioning regimen (myeloablative or nonmyeloablative), and source of stem cells (bone marrow, peripheral blood, or cord blood).[3]

HSCT recipients are at increased risk of invasive candidiasis and invasive mold infections (IMIs), especially aspergillosis. In addition, infections caused by less common fungi have been reported,

[a] Mycology Laboratory, Department of Internal Medicine, University Hospital, Universidade Federal do Rio de Janeiro, Rua Professor Rodolpho Paulo Rocco, 255 Sala 4A 12, 21941-913 Rio de Janeiro, Brazil
[b] Myeloma Institute for Research and Therapy, University of Arkansas for Medical Sciences, 4301 West Markham, Slot 776, Little Rock, AR 72205, USA
* Corresponding author.
E-mail address: anaissieeliasj@exchange.uams.edu (E. Anaissie).

Clin Chest Med 30 (2009) 295–306
doi:10.1016/j.ccm.2009.03.001
0272-5231/09/$ – see front matter © 2009 Published by Elsevier Inc.

including *Fusarium* spp, *Trichosporon* spp, and others.[4]

The changing landscape of invasive fungal infections in recipients of hematopoietic stem cell transplantation

Fluconazole is now routinely used as prophylaxis among HSCT recipients because it has been shown to reduce the incidence of invasive candidiasis and fungal-related death in this patient population. Fluconazole prophylaxis has resulted in a steady decrease in the incidence of candidemia, at least partly attributed to a reduction in infections by susceptible species (*Candida albicans, C tropicalis,* and others), with occasional emergence of infections by non-"albicans" *Candida* spp (*C glabrata* and *C krusei*).[5]

This decrease in candidiasis has been associated with a relative increase in aspergillosis (caused by *Aspergillus fumigatus* and other *Aspergillus* spp)[6] and in IMIs caused by non-*Aspergillus* molds such as *Fusarium* spp and the agents of zygomycosis (mucormycosis).[4]

Risk of invasive fungal infections in recipients of hematopoietic stem cell transplantation

The risk of IFIs results from the interactions between the host and the pathogen and environmental exposure. IFIs develop when an imbalance develops between the weakened protective defense mechanisms of the host and the virulence factors of the offending pathogen.

An important host factor is the net state of immunosuppression; that is, the cumulative effect of various immunosuppressive factors including the underlying disease, prior and current therapies, comorbidities, infections with immunomodulating viruses (cytomegalovirus [CMV], HIV, and others), iron overload, and the presence of severe graft-versus-host disease (GVHD) and its therapy. These factors impair different host defenses, predisposing patients to various fungal pathogens.[7]

A role for the patient's immunogenetics and the pharmacogenomics of the different drugs used in the conditioning regimen is being increasingly recognized, whereas the role of host response to opportunistic fungi has been explored in relatively small studies. Single nucleotide polymorphisms of different host genes are thought to represent potential risk factors for the development of IA, including Toll-like receptor (TLR)-1, TLR-4, interleukin (IL)-10 promoter, IL-10 1082*G allele and G/G genotype, IL-15 +13,689*A allele and A/A genotype, transforming growth factor β +869 and T/T genotype, tumor necrosis factor α −308*A/A and variable number of tandem repeats at position −322 in promoter region of *TNR2* gene, mannose-binding lectin (MBL), MBL-associated protein 2, and lung surfactant protein SPA-2.[8–12]

Other risk factors for IFI include severe damage to the gut mucosa following chemotherapy, radiation therapy, or GVHD; hyperglycemia; and renal, hepatic, or respiratory failure.[13] Iron overload may also contribute to dysfunction of various organs.[14]

Gut mucosal colonization is a requirement for invasive candidiasis, which usually develops following translocation of *Candida* from the gut into the bloodstream.[15] Any condition leading to a breach of the integrity of the intestinal mucosa (as previously mentioned) increases the risk of invasive candidiasis. Disruption of skin integrity (eg, indwelling catheters) may occasionally play a role in predisposing patients to this infection.

Environmental exposures to *Aspergillus* spp or *Fusarium* spp through contaminated heating/cooling systems or hospital water systems, and to *Candida* spp from health care workers have been associated with sporadic cases and outbreaks of IFIs among HSCT recipients.[16]

Timetable of invasive fungal infections in recipients of hematopoietic stem cell transplantation

The posttransplant timetable of IFIs in allogeneic HSCT recipients may be divided into three periods that correspond broadly to the pattern of immune deficiency and organ damage following therapy: pre-engraftment, immediate postengraftment, and late postengraftment (**Table 1**).

Pre-engraftment The most common pathogens during this period are *Candida* spp, *Aspergillus* spp, and molds (*Fusarium* spp, Zygomycetes, and others). The latter IFIs occur in the setting of profound (<100/μL) and prolonged (>2 weeks) neutropenia, such as in patients who received stem cells obtained from bone marrow or cord blood. By contrast, transplantation with stem cells derived from the peripheral blood and transplants with reduced-intensity conditioning regimens (nonmyeloablative) have neutropenia of short duration and are therefore at lower risk for IFIs in the early posttransplant period. Among recipients of autologous HSCT, IMIs are rare.[17]

Immediate postengraftment The risk factors for IFIs during this period are mucosal damage, deficiency in CMI, and reactivation of immunomodulating viruses such as CMV. For allogeneic HSCT recipients, additional risk factors include severe acute GVHD and its therapy. During this period, patients are at risk for IMIs (especially aspergillosis).[18]

Table 1
Timetable and clinical syndromes of invasive fungal infections in hematopoietic stem cell transplant recipients

Infection and Time of Occurrence	Setting, Risk Factors	Clinical Manifestations
Pre-engraftment		
Acute disseminated candidiasis	Severe (<100/mm^3) neutropenia, mucositis, no azole prophylaxis	Fever ± hypotension, myalgias, skin lesions
Mold pneumonia[a]	Severe (<100/mm^3) and prolonged (>14 d) neutropenia	Fever ± dry cough, pleuritic chest pain
Mold sinusitis[a]	Severe (<100/mm^3) and prolonged (>14 days) neutropenia	Fever + nasal discharge, headache, epistaxis
Invasive fusariosis	Severe (<100/mm^3) and prolonged (>14 d) neutropenia ± skin breakdown ± onychomycosis	Fever + nodular skin lesions, with ecthyma gangrenosum-like appearance, target lesions, and so forth
Immediate and late postengraftment		
Chronic disseminated candidiasis (only immediate phase)	Prior severe neutropenia, mucositis, no azole prophylaxis	Fever, ↑ alkaline phosphatase, right upper quadrant pain, hepatosplenomegaly
Mold pneumonia[a]	Severe GVHD, high-dose corticosteroids	Fever, cough
Mold sinusitis[a]	Reactivation of immunomodulating viruses (CMV, others)	Fever, cough, nasal discharge, headache
Any period		
Catheter-related fungal infection (usually *Candida* spp)	Venous catheter	Fever ± rigors after manipulation of the venous catheter

[a] Caused by *Aspergillus* spp in most cases. Other molds include *Fusarium* spp, Zygomycetes, and others.

Late postengraftment Aspergillosis and other IMIs continue to occur during this period and may develop sometimes very late (>1 year) after allogeneic HSCT.[19] The main risk factor for IMIs in this period is severe deficiency in CMI caused by chronic GVHD and its treatment.

Invasive Aspergillosis in Recipients of Hematopoietic Stem Cell Transplantation

IA is now the leading cause of IFI in HSCT recipients and probably the most common cause of infection-related death. Risk factors include prolonged and profound neutropenia and severe defects in CMI, typically resulting from severe GVHD and its therapy with high doses of corticosteroids and other immunosuppressive agents.[20]

The incidence of aspergillosis varies according to the type of HSCT. In a study involving 19 United States sites during 22 months, the cumulative incidence of IA at 12 months post transplant was 0.5% after autologous HSCT, 2.3% after allogeneic HSCT from an HLA-matched donor, 3.2% after transplantation from an HLA-mismatched related donor, and 3.9% after transplantation from an unrelated donor.[17]

Clinical manifestations
Sinusitis and pneumonia are the most common forms of aspergillosis, and their clinical manifestations are determined by the host immune status.

Early in the posttransplant period, invasive pulmonary aspergillosis (IPA) is characterized by angioinvasion, with intra-alveolar hemorrhage and pulmonary infarction.[21] By contrast, angioinvasion is less commonly seen following engraftment and resolution of neutropenia. Despite myeloid recovery, with normal number of neutrophils, there is a paucity of inflammatory cells in lung tissue, indicating that these patients are functionally neutropenic.[22]

During neutropenia, the classic clinical picture of IPA is that of persistent or recurrent fever associated with signs of pulmonary infarction: dry cough and pleuritic chest pain.[23] Shortness of breath and dyspnea may also develop. Hemoptysis is more frequently reported after bone marrow recovery and occasionally evolves to death as a consequence of invasion of a large blood vessel. Spontaneous pneumothorax or pneumomediastinum associated with sharp chest pain and dyspnea is very rare.[24]

These clinical manifestations of IPA contrast with the subtle findings in nonneutropenic HSCT recipients. In a series of 22 cases of IMI (18 cases caused by *Aspergillus* spp), shortness of breath was present in 64% of patients, but only 32% had fever; cough and chest pain were noted in 23% and 14%, respectively.[25]

Sinusitis caused by *Aspergillus* spp occurs more frequently during the early posttransplant period, during neutropenia. Fever is a prominent feature, occurring in virtually all cases. Periorbital swelling, nasal congestion, headache, cough, and epistaxis are frequently observed, whereas nasal discharge occurs later in the course of the disease. Extension to the palate and orbit may rarely occur.[26]

Aspergillosis of the central nervous system (CNS) most commonly results from dissemination from a remote focus (usually the lungs) and is characterized by vascular thrombosis and cerebral infarction. The sudden development of CNS changes (headache, seizures, neurologic deficits, confusion, behavioral changes, or reduced consciousness) should alert the clinician to the possible diagnosis of cerebral aspergillosis.[27]

Radiology

The radiologic features of IPA in the early posttransplant period reflect the angioinvasive nature of the disease. Although often abnormal, the chest radiograph is rarely useful because the infiltrates are nonspecific, with patchy segmental or lobar consolidations and less frequently nodular opacities.[28] Later in the course of the disease, when neutropenia resolves, the chest radiograph may demonstrate the air crescent sign, a nodular opacity with a crescent or circumferential cavitation that is formed as a consequence of the retraction of the infarcted lung. The air crescent sign, although not specific of IPA, is highly characteristic of the condition in the proper clinical setting.[29]

The chest CT scan is very useful in the early diagnosis of IPA. The typical image is the halo sign, a nodule surrounded by a ground-glass opacity, representing pulmonary edema and hemorrhage surrounding an area of coagulative necrosis.[30] The halo sign, in the context of patients who have prolonged neutropenia, is not exclusive of IPA and may be observed with other conditions, including other IMIs such as zygomycosis.[31] The halo sign is usually transient and is rapidly replaced by nonspecific infiltrates.[32] Later in the course of the infection, the air crescent sign appears, usually when the patient recovers from neutropenia.

A rapid immune reconstitution following resolution of neutropenia may be associated with transient clinical and radiologic deterioration. The pulmonary immune reconstitution inflammatory syndrome of IPA was typically but incorrectly considered evidence of progressive infection. These patients are achieving control of their infection and do not require treatment modifications.[33]

IPA in nonneutropenic allogeneic HSCT recipients may be characterized by angioinvasion (as in neutropenic patients) or by airway invasion. In the latter form, the radiologic picture is that of a bronchopneumonia. Lung imaging by radiograph or CT scan shows air space consolidations with or without nodules, whereas the halo sign is less commonly seen.[34] Ground-glass opacities, bronchiolitis-bronchopneumonia pattern, and pleural, pericardial, hilar, and mediastinal lesions also occur in patients who have IPA, although they have no discriminative power.

The radiologic appearance of cerebral aspergillosis is variable, depending on the degree of immunosuppression. During neutropenia, multiple areas of cortical and subcortical hypodensity on CT and hyperintensity on MRI are consistent with infarction. If the infarctions become hemorrhagic (which is frequent), they exhibit increased density on CT and increased T1 signal on MRI. With neutrophil recovery, these lesions evolve into abscesses with ring enhancement.[35]

Serology

Detection of serum *Aspergillus* galactomannan has gained widespread acceptance as a sensitive method for the early diagnosis of aspergillosis and is now included in the consensus criteria for defining IFIs in cancer patients and HSCT recipients (European Organization for Research and Treatment of Cancer/Mycosis Study Group criteria).[36] The test has excellent performance characteristics in profoundly neutropenic patients provided it is performed at least two or three times a week and supported by chest CT scan findings (usually obtained in patients who have longer than 4 to 5 days of persistent fever).[37] Limitations of the test include reduced sensitivity during receipt of mold-active antifungal agents and false-positive results with the use of some semi-synthetic β-lactam antibiotics (including ampicillin, amoxicillin-clavulanate, and piperacillin-tazobactam). Gluconate-containing plasma expanders may also cause false-positive results when the test is performed on serum and bronchoalveolar lavage fluid.[38] Despite these limitations, the excellent test performance of serum galactomannan in neutropenic patients makes it a particularly useful diagnostic test for aspergillosis. Furthermore, the kinetics of the galactomannan test correlate with aspergillosis outcome[39] and may allow differentiation of progressive aspergillosis from pulmonary immune reconstitution inflammatory syndrome.[33]

In nonneutropenic HSCT recipients, the serum galactomannan test does not appear to perform as well. In a retrospective study that evaluated 157 adult allogeneic HSCT recipients, the positive predictive value of serum galactomannan testing was low during the first 100 days post transplant, and gastrointestinal chronic GVHD was the only factor associated with false-positive results.[40]

β-D-glucan (BDG) assays are widely used in Japan, and the Fungitell assay (Associates of Cape Cod, Inc., East Falmouth, Massachusetts) has recently been approved by the United States Food and Drug Administration based on studies in patients who have acute leukemia.[41] The test measures the amount of BDG released from the fungal cell wall into the circulation during invasive infection. The negative predictive value of twice-weekly BDG sampling is 100%, and unlike with serum galactomannan, BDG test results are not influenced by the use of mold-active antifungal agents; however, false-positive readings may result from the infusion of albumin or immunoglobulins, exposure to glucan-containing gauze, hemodialysis, and the use of amoxicillin-clavulanate.[41] Of note, the βDG assay can detect a much broader spectrum of fungal species than the Aspergillus galactomannan, including Candida, Aspergillus, Fusarium, and other fungi but not Cryptococcus neoformans or the agents of zygomycosis, because the latter two have very low βDG content in their cell wall.

Microbiologic tests

Identification of fungal pathogens by culture or molecular tools is critical because of the difficulties in distinguishing infections caused by fungi that have similar properties, such as the angioinvasive molds, and because they may require different management strategies. Indeed, it is practically impossible to distinguish infection with Aspergillus spp from infection by any of the angioinvasive molds such as Fusarium, Scopulariopsis, and Scedosporium spp, and to a lesser extent, infections caused by the agents of zygomycosis.

The genus Aspergillus comprises several hundred species, and 38 have been reported to cause disease in humans. Most infections, however, are caused by five species: A fumigatus (~90% of cases), A flavus, A niger, A terreus, and A nidulans. The interpretation of the growth of Aspergillus spp from different biologic materials depends on the clinical context. In allogeneic HSCT recipients, the predictive value of a culture yielding Aspergillus spp from respiratory secretions is between 60% and 80%.[42] Confirmation of the diagnosis is made by histopathology. Blood culture is a limited diagnostic tool for IA because Aspergillus fungemia is rarely encountered, even in disseminated disease.

Management of Invasive Fungal Infections in Recipients of Hematopoietic Stem Cell Transplantation

Prophylaxis
Primary prophylaxis is best applied to patients at high risk for IFI and in whom the consequences of IFI are severe, even with proper therapy.[43]

Prophylaxis for yeasts Fluconazole (400 mg/d) is considered the drug of choice for prophylaxis against Candida spp in allogeneic HSCT recipients.[44] Other agents including itraconazole oral solution (but not capsules),[45] voriconazole,[46] and micafungin[47] effectively prevent the occurrence of invasive candidiasis in HSCT recipients during the pre-engraftment period. Itraconazole is less well tolerated than the other azoles.[45]

Prophylaxis for yeasts and molds In addition to preventing candidiasis, micafungin prophylaxis was associated with a strong trend suggesting its effectiveness at preventing aspergillosis in HSCT recipients.[47]

In neutropenic patients who had acute myelogenous leukemia or myelodysplasia who received remission induction therapy, posaconazole prophylaxis was well tolerated and was as effective as fluconazole at preventing candidiasis. Posaconazole also reduced the incidence of aspergillosis and fungal-related mortality.[48] Although these results are not necessarily applicable to the early posttransplant neutropenic period following allogeneic HSCT, they suggest that patients at high risk for IA may benefit from prophylaxis with posaconazole. Compared with fluconazole in allogeneic HSCT recipients who had GVHD, posaconazole reduced the incidence of IA.[49] Similarly, itraconazole oral solution reduced the incidence of IA in two trials of allogeneic HSCT recipients, but the drug was discontinued in almost one fourth of the patients because of gastrointestinal side effects.[45] The results of a recent meta-analysis suggest that oral itraconazole solution effectively reduces *Aspergillus* infections when a threshold of bioavailable drug dosing is used.[50]

Secondary prophylaxis Because the risk of reactivation of aspergillosis is high following resumption of immunosuppression, secondary prophylaxis is indicated in such patients.[51] Among allogeneic HSCT patients who have a history of aspergillosis, the risk of reactivation was found to be lower when antifungal treatment was given for longer than 30 days and when radiographic abnormalities resolved before HSCT.[52] Options for secondary prophylaxis include intravenous amphotericin B (AMB) and its lipid formulations, caspofungin, itraconazole, voriconazole, and lipid AMB followed by voriconazole.[53]

Empiric antifungal therapy

Empiric antifungal therapy has been the standard of care in the management of the febrile neutropenic cancer patient since the 1980s.[54] The strategy consists of starting an antifungal agent in neutropenic patients after 4 to 7 days of persistent fever without apparent cause despite the use of appropriate antibacterial agents. Different drugs have been tested, including deoxycholate (d)-AMB, fluconazole, the lipid formulations of AMB, itraconazole, voriconazole, and caspofungin.[55] Despite problems in study design[56] and concerns about cost and toxicity, empiric therapy remains the most frequently used strategy in neutropenic patients. Starting antifungal therapy on the basis of persistent fever as the sole criterion, however, results in overtreatment of a significant number of patients, particularly among those receiving fluconazole prophylaxis. Among the latter patients, persistent fever is most commonly due to various factors such as uncontrolled occult bacterial infection, viral infection, drug fever, and others. Empiric therapy should therefore be reserved for patients at intermediate risk for IFI, when serodiagnostic markers are not readily available and when fluconazole prophylaxis is not given.

Diagnostic-based preemptive therapy

This strategy relies on the administration of antifungal therapy to patients who have early evidence of IFI,[55] such as persistent fever plus any of the following: pleuritic chest pain; pleural rub; positive serum galactomannan, BDG, or polymerase chain reaction; or new and suggestive pulmonary infiltrates on chest CT scans.[57] Diagnostic-based preemptive therapy has been successfully tested

in neutropenic patients,[37] although no standard recommendations exist. This strategy significantly decreases the risks associated with broad antifungal prophylaxis and empiric therapy, as discussed previously.

Treatment of documented infection

The drugs available for the treatment of IFIs include d-AMB; the three lipid formulations of AMB: AMB in lipid complex (ABLC), in liposome (L-AMB), and in colloidal dispersion; the azoles fluconazole, itraconazole, voriconazole, and posaconazole; and the echinocandins caspofungin, micafungin, and anidulafungin.

The selection of the antifungal agent must take several factors into consideration. For example, allogeneic HSCT recipients are at great risk for d-AMB–related nephrotoxicity.[58] Therefore, this drug should be avoided and an AMB lipid preparation used instead because these agents are at least as efficacious and much less nephrotoxic than the parent compound.

Invasive candidiasis There are eight published randomized trials in the treatment of candidemia and invasive candidiasis.[59] A minority of patients in these trials were HSCT recipients, making it difficult to select "a drug of choice." The first consideration in selecting an appropriate drug is recent exposure to fluconazole, which increases the likelihood of *C glabrata* or *C krusei* infection.[60] In such a setting, an echinocandin or a lipid AMB formulation would be more appropriate. Voriconazole is a viable option for *C krusei* infections. Another consideration is whether the patient is hemodynamically unstable, in which case an echinocandin would be preferable to an azole.

Catheter management in candidemia is controversial, but in neutropenic patients, its removal is less likely to have an impact on the outcome, because the gut is the most likely source of infection.[61]

Invasive aspergillosis The guidelines of the Infectious Disease Society of America (IDSA Guidelines) recommend voriconazole as the drug of choice for primary treatment of IA on the basis of a randomized trial that showed superior response and better survival compared with d-AMB.[62] An alternative option is L-AMB, at a dose of 3 mg/kg/d.[63] For salvage therapy, an AMB lipid formulation is preferred. Alternatives include itraconazole or posaconazole and an echinocandin (caspofungin). For patients who develop voriconazole-refractory aspergillosis, considerations include a change of class to an AMB product, an echinocandin (caspofungin), or a combination of agents. Combinations of voriconazole and an echinocandin have been evaluated in limited studies, with variable results.[64]

Other mycoses A lipid formulation of AMB remains the drug of choice for the treatment of zygomycosis.[65] Posaconazole, an oral azole active against some agents of zygomycosis, may be considered as follow-up therapy when the species causing the infection is known to be susceptible.[66] Surgical treatment and the reversal of immunosuppression and ketoacidosis are critical components of therapy.[65]

Fusariosis is probably best treated with an AMB lipid formulation, although successes have been reported with voriconazole and posaconazole.[67]

FUNGAL INFECTIONS IN RECIPIENTS OF SOLID-ORGAN TRANSPLANTATION

Most of the concepts presented for HSCT recipients, including diagnosis and therapy, are applicable to SOT recipients. Therefore, only the aspects that are specific to SOT recipients are presented.

Epidemiology

The incidence of IFIs differs according to the type of transplant. Liver transplant recipients have the highest incidence of invasive candidiasis, whereas aspergillosis is most commonly seen following lung transplantation. A multicenter epidemiologic study in 19 United States centers showed that the 12-month cumulative incidence of IA was 2.4% after lung transplantation, 0.8% after heart transplantation, 0.3% after liver transplantation, and 0.1% after kidney transplantation.[17] Because the occurrence of invasive candidiasis in SOT recipients is associated with complications of surgery, improvements in transplant surgical methods have resulted in a sharp reduction in the incidence of this infection.[2] By contrast, the incidence of IFIs caused by *Aspergillus* and other molds has increased with changes in underlying diseases and the use of more-severe immunosuppression after SOT.[68]

Risk of invasive fungal infections in recipients of solid-organ transplantation

The risk of IFIs in SOT recipients is determined by the interaction of three factors: epidemiologic exposure, the net state of immunosuppression, and anatomic alterations that impair mucosal barriers. Specific to SOT recipients is the reactivation of geographically related mycoses such as histoplasmosis and coccidioidomycosis. Patients living or visiting endemic regions are at high risk for developing these infections. The net state of immunosuppression is determined by the underlying condition; immunosuppressive therapies; metabolic factors such as malnutrition, uremia, and hyperglycemia; and infections with immunomodulating viruses (CMV, HIV, Epstein-Barr virus, hepatitis B and C, and others). Finally, of great importance are the technical/anatomic aspects of the transplant, including the type of organ transplanted, technical difficulties, device-associated risks (catheters, drains, endotracheal tubes), and devitalized tissue.[68]

Timetable of invasive fungal infections in recipients of solid-organ transplantation

The posttransplant timetable of IFIs in SOT recipients can be divided into three periods that correspond broadly to the pattern of immune deficiency and organ damage following therapy: early (first month after transplant), intermediate (1–6 months post transplant), and late (>6 months after transplant) (**Table 2**).

Early During this period, most IFIs occur as a result of complications of the surgical procedure. Invasive candidiasis is the most frequent IFI in this period. Occasionally patients may reactivate a pre-existing fungal infection or develop an IFI carried with the allograft.

Intermediate Immunosuppression caused by the antirejection treatment and the reactivation of immunomodulating viruses (particularly CMV) are the main determinants of the occurrence of IFIs during this period. Rejection is a major risk factor because high-dose corticosteroids and other agents are frequently required to treat it. IA typically occurs during this period, whereas geographically restricted IFIs are rare.

Late Late after transplantation, IFIs occur almost exclusively in patients who have a history of impaired allograft function, receipt of intense immunosuppression, and reactivation of immunomodulatory viruses such as CMV. IFIs during this period include aspergillosis, disseminated cryptococcosis, histoplasmosis, and others. Patients who have good allograft function are at very low risk of developing IFI, except following excessive environmental exposure.

Invasive Aspergillosis in Recipients of Solid-organ Transplantation

Among SOT, the incidence of IA is highest among lung transplant recipients, occurring in 3% to 15% of cases.[69]

In a review of 159 cases of IA in lung transplant recipients, IPA occurred at a median of 3.2 months post transplant, with 72% of the cases diagnosed

Table 2
Timetable and clinical syndromes of invasive fungal infections in solid organ transplant recipients

Infection and Time of Occurrence	Setting, Risk Factors	Clinical Manifestations
Early (first month)		
Acute disseminated candidiasis	Complications of surgery, no azole prophylaxis	Fever ± hypotension
Intermediate (1–6 mo)		
Invasive aspergillosis[a]	Immunosuppression for the prevention or treatment of rejection; reactivation of immunomodulating viruses (CMV, others)	Fever (may be absent), dry cough, dyspnea
Late (>6 mo)		
Cryptococcosis	Chronic immunosuppression; risk increases with chronic rejection	Headache, fever, mental status changes, skin lesions
Endemic mycoses	Chronic immunosuppression; risk increases in chronic rejection	Fever of insidious onset, respiratory complaints, signs of metastatic infection (manifestations depend on the organs involved)

[a] Less frequently caused by other molds such as *Fusarium* spp, Zygomycetes, and others.

within 6 months post transplant. Infections included tracheobronchitis (37%), invasive pulmonary disease (32%), and bronchial anastomotic infections (21%), and 10% had disseminated aspergillosis.[70]

Tracheobronchitis is characterized by ulceration, cartilage invasion, and pseudomembrane formation. Fever is insidious or absent. Other clinical findings include dry cough and dyspnea. CT scan findings are usually subtle, with focal plaques along the tracheal wall, with or without thickening of the tracheal mucosa.[71]

Complications involving the anastomosis site, infection of airway stenoses, and development of a bronchial-pulmonary artery fistula have been described.[72]

When IPA develops following lung transplantation, patients may remain asymptomatic, although up to a third may present with fever. CT scan of the chest may reveal nodules or cavitary lesions.

A remarkable finding in lung transplant recipients is the high frequency of airway colonization of by *Aspergillus* spp.[69]

Among liver transplant recipients, IPA occurs in 1% to 8%, with most infections developing within 1 month after transplant. Risk factors include renal dysfunction and retransplantation.[69] Clinical presentation is nonspecific, with fever (which may be absent), cough, and dyspnea. Patients may also remain asymptomatic. Nodules are frequently present on thoracic CT scan examination.

Serum *Aspergillus* galactomannan has been evaluated in SOT recipients. A meta-analysis of the few studies of galactomannan conducted in SOT recipients reported a sensitivity and specificity of 22% and 84%, respectively.[73] Among 70 lung transplant recipients (12 of whom developed IPA), 30% sensitivity and 93% specificity were noted.[74] Among 154 liver transplant recipients, positive galactomannan tests were documented in 21 patients, but only 1 patient developed proven aspergillosis. Patients who have autoimmune diseases and those requiring dialysis were more likely to have false-positive galactomannan tests.[75] In another study of 85 liver transplant recipients, serum galactomannan was obtained once a week during the first month following transplantation. False-positive results were observed in 9.6% of 414 serum samples. The number of false-positive results was significantly higher in the first week post transplant, and exposure to ampicillin was the only independent factor associated with false-positive results.[76]

Management of Invasive Fungal Infections in Recipients of Solid-Organ Transplantation

Prophylaxis
Anti-*Candida* prophylaxis is indicated for liver transplant recipients who have more than two risk factors such as retransplantation, renal failure (serum creatinine >2 mg/dL), prolonged

intraoperative time (>1 h), choledocojejunostomy, and intraoperative use of more than 40 units of blood products. Fluconazole (200–400 mg/d) or L-AMB (1–2 mg/kg/d) are the drugs of choice. Although no data from randomized trials exist to support the use of fluconazole prophylaxis in recipients of pancreas and small bowel transplants, the authors recommend instituting fluconazole prophylaxis (200–400 mg/d) because of the high rates of invasive candidiasis in these recipients.[59]

Prophylaxis for IA is appealing in lung transplant recipients because of the high incidence of this infection in such patients; however, no formal recommendations can be made because of the limited evidence. One study evaluated the safety of d-AMB and ABLC given in aerosol. Recipients of ABLC experienced less adverse events. IA occurred infrequently in both study arms, but the study was not powered to assess efficacy.[77]

Empiric antifungal therapy
According to the recent IDSA Guidelines for the management of invasive candidiasis, empiric therapy should be considered in critically ill patients who have risks factors for invasive candidiasis and no other known cause of their fever.[59] On the basis of these guidelines, many SOT recipients would be potential candidates for empiric therapy in the early posttransplant period, although formal recommendations cannot be made because of a lack of supporting evidence.

Treatment of documented infection
General principles of the therapy of specific fungal infections in the HSCT setting are applicable to SOT recipients. A cardinal rule of treating infections in these patients is the reduction of immunosuppressive therapies. Clinicians must also take into consideration not only the potential of drug interactions between the antifungal agents and different immunosuppressive regimens but also the toxicity of the antifungal agents that may compromise the allograft.

SUMMARY

IFIs remain a major cause of morbidity and mortality among transplant recipients and are associated with increased morbidity, resource use, and mortality. The epidemiology of IFIs is rapidly changing. The prevention of and therapy for these infections need to be individualized, which can be achieved by using different strategies including infection-control measures, improvement of the immune status, and antifungal prophylaxis and therapy.

REFERENCES

1. Wingard JR. New approaches to invasive fungal infections in acute leukemia and hematopoietic stem cell transplant patients. Best Pract Res Clin Haematol 2007;20:99–107.
2. Silveira FP, Husain S. Fungal infections in solid organ transplantation. Med Mycol 2007;45:305–20.
3. Marr KA. Fungal infections in hematopoietic stem cell transplant recipients. Med Mycol 2008;46: 293–302.
4. Nucci M. Emerging moulds: Fusarium, Scedosporium and Zygomycetes in transplant recipients. Curr Opin Infect Dis 2003;16:607–12.
5. Abi-Said D, Anaissie E, Uzun O, et al. The epidemiology of hematogenous candidiasis caused by different Candida species. Clin Infect Dis 1997;24: 1122–8.
6. Wingard JR. The changing face of invasive fungal infections in hematopoietic cell transplant recipients. Curr Opin Oncol 2005;17:89–92.
7. Thursky K, Byrnes G, Grigg A, et al. Risk factors for post-engraftment invasive aspergillosis in allogeneic stem cell transplantation. Bone Marrow Transplant 2004;34:115–21.
8. Zaas AK, Liao G, Chien JW, et al. Plasminogen alleles influence susceptibility to invasive aspergillosis. PLoS Genet 2008;4:e1000101.
9. Sambatakou H, Pravica V, Hutchinson IV, et al. Cytokine profiling of pulmonary aspergillosis. Int J Immunogenet 2006;33:297–302.
10. Sainz J, Perez E, Gomez-Lopera S, et al. IL1 gene cluster polymorphisms and its haplotypes may predict the risk to develop invasive pulmonary aspergillosis and modulate C-reactive protein level. J Clin Immunol 2008;28:473–85.
11. Granell M, Urbano-Ispizua A, Suarez B, et al. Mannan-binding lectin pathway deficiencies and invasive fungal infections following allogeneic stem cell transplantation. Exp Hematol 2006;34:1435–41.
12. Bochud PY, Chien JW, Marr KA, et al. Toll-like receptor 4 polymorphisms and aspergillosis in stem-cell transplantation. N Engl J Med 2008;359: 1766–77.
13. Kobayashi R, Kaneda M, Sato T, et al. Evaluation of risk factors for invasive fungal infection after allogeneic stem cell transplantation in pediatric patients. J Pediatr Hematol Oncol 2007;29:786–91.
14. Pietrangelo A. Iron chelation beyond transfusion iron overload. Am J Hematol 2007;82:1142–6.
15. Nucci M, Anaissie E. Revisiting the source of candidemia: skin or gut? Clin Infect Dis 2001;33:1959–67.
16. Anaissie EJ, Stratton SL, Dignani MC, et al. Pathogenic molds (including Aspergillus species) in hospital water distribution systems: a 3-year prospective study and clinical implications for patients with hematologic malignancies. Blood 2003;101:2542–6.

17. Morgan J, Wannemuehler KA, Marr KA, et al. Incidence of invasive aspergillosis following hematopoietic stem cell and solid organ transplantation: interim results of a prospective multicenter surveillance program. Med Mycol 2005;43(Suppl 1):S49–58.

18. Wald A, Leisenring W, Van Burik JA, et al. Epidemiology of *Aspergillus* infections in a large cohort of patients undergoing bone marrow transplantation. J Infect Dis 1997;175:1459–66.

19. Marr KA, Carter RA, Crippa F, et al. Epidemiology and outcome of mould infections in hematopoietic stem cell transplant recipients. Clin Infect Dis 2002;34:909–17.

20. Marr KA, Carter RA, Boeckh M, et al. Invasive aspergillosis in allogeneic stem cell transplant recipients: changes in epidemiology and risk factors. Blood 2002;100:4358–66.

21. Berenguer J, Allende MC, Lee JW, et al. Pathogenesis of pulmonary aspergillosis. Granulocytopenia versus cyclosporine and methylprednisolone-induced immunosuppression. Am J Respir Crit Care Med 1995;152:1079–86.

22. Stergiopoulou T, Meletiadis J, Roilides E, et al. Host-dependent patterns of tissue injury in invasive pulmonary aspergillosis. Am J Clin Pathol 2007; 127:349–55.

23. Gerson SL, Talbot GH, Lusk E, et al. Invasive pulmonary aspergillosis in adult acute leukemia: clinical clues to its diagnosis. J Clin Oncol 1985;3:1109–16.

24. Martino P, Girmenia C, Venditti M, et al. Spontaneous pneumothorax complicating pulmonary mycetoma in patients with acute leukemia. Rev Infect Dis 1990;12:611–7.

25. Shaukat A, Bakri F, Young P, et al. Invasive filamentous fungal infections in allogeneic hematopoietic stem cell transplant recipients after recovery from neutropenia: clinical, radiologic, and pathologic characteristics. Mycopathologia 2005;159:181–8.

26. Talbot GH, Huang A, Provencher M. Invasive aspergillus rhinosinusitis in patients with acute leukemia. Rev Infect Dis 1991;13:219–32.

27. Kleinschmidt-DeMasters BK. Central nervous system aspergillosis: a 20-year retrospective series. Hum Pathol 2002;33:116–24.

28. Thompson BH, Stanford W, Galvin JR, et al. Varied radiologic appearances of pulmonary aspergillosis. Radiographics 1995;15:1273–84.

29. Gefter WB, Albelda SM, Talbot GH, et al. Invasive pulmonary aspergillosis and acute leukemia. Limitations in the diagnostic utility of the air crescent sign. Radiology 1985;157:605–10.

30. Hruban RH, Meziane MA, Zerhouni EA, et al. Radiologic-pathologic correlation of the CT halo sign in invasive pulmonary aspergillosis. J Comput Assist Tomogr 1987;11:534–6.

31. Chamilos G, Marom EM, Lewis RE, et al. Predictors of pulmonary zygomycosis versus invasive pulmonary aspergillosis in patients with cancer. Clin Infect Dis 2005;41:60–6.

32. Caillot D, Couaillier JF, Bernard A, et al. Increasing volume and changing characteristics of invasive pulmonary aspergillosis on sequential thoracic computed tomography scans in patients with neutropenia. J Clin Oncol 2001;19:253–9.

33. Miceli MH, Maertens J, Buve K, et al. Immune reconstitution inflammatory syndrome in cancer patients with pulmonary aspergillosis recovering from neutropenia: proof of principle, description, and clinical and research implications. Cancer 2007;110:112–20.

34. Kojima R, Tateishi U, Kami M, et al. Chest computed tomography of late invasive aspergillosis after allogeneic hematopoietic stem cell transplantation. Biol Blood Marrow Transplant 2005;11:506–11.

35. Ashdown BC, Tien RD, Felsberg GJ. Aspergillosis of the brain and paranasal sinuses in immunocompromised patients: CT and MR imaging findings. AJR Am J Roentgenol 1994;162:155–9.

36. De PB, Walsh TJ, Donnelly JP, et al. Revised definitions of invasive fungal disease from the European Organization for Research and Treatment of Cancer/ Invasive Fungal Infections Cooperative Group and the National Institute of Allergy and Infectious Diseases Mycoses Study Group (EORTC/MSG) Consensus Group. Clin Infect Dis 2008;46:1813–21.

37. Maertens J, Theunissen K, Verhoef G, et al. Galactomannan and computed tomography-based preemptive antifungal therapy in neutropenic patients at high risk for invasive fungal infection: a prospective feasibility study. Clin Infect Dis 2005;41:1242–50.

38. Aquino VR, Goldani LZ, Pasqualotto AC. Update on the contribution of galactomannan for the diagnosis of invasive aspergillosis. Mycopathologia 2007;163: 191–202.

39. Miceli MH, Grazziutti ML, Woods G, et al. Strong correlation between serum aspergillus galactomannan index and outcome of aspergillosis in patients with hematological cancer: clinical and research implications. Clin Infect Dis 2008;46: 1412–22.

40. Asano-Mori Y, Kanda Y, Oshima K, et al. False-positive *Aspergillus* galactomannan antigenaemia after haematopoietic stem cell transplantation. J Antimicrob Chemother 2008;61:411–6.

41. Ostrosky-Zeichner L, Alexander BD, Kett DH, et al. Multicenter clinical evaluation of the (1→3) beta-D-glucan assay as an aid to diagnosis of fungal infections in humans. Clin Infect Dis 2005;41:654–9.

42. Perfect JR, Cox GM, Lee JY, et al. The impact of culture isolation of *Aspergillus* species: a hospital-based survey of aspergillosis. Clin Infect Dis 2001; 33:1824–33.

43. Mahfouz T, Anaissie E. Prevention of fungal infections in the immunocompromised host. Curr Opin Investig Drugs 2003;4:974–90.

44. Goodman JL, Winston DJ, Greenfield RA, et al. A controlled trial of fluconazole to prevent fungal infections in patients undergoing bone marrow transplantation. N Engl J Med 1992;326:845–51.

45. Marr KA, Crippa F, Leisenring W, et al. Itraconazole versus fluconazole for prevention of fungal infections in patients receiving allogeneic stem cell transplants. Blood 2004;103:1527–33.

46. Wingard JR, Carter SL, Walsh TJ, et al. Results of a randomized, double-blind trial of fluconazole (FLU) vs. voriconazole (VORI) for the prevention of invasive fungal infections (IFI) in 600 allogeneic blood and marrow transplant (BMT) patients. Blood 2007;110:163.

47. Van Burik JA, Ratanatharathorn V, Stepan DE, et al. Micafungin versus fluconazole for prophylaxis against invasive fungal infections during neutropenia in patients undergoing hematopoietic stem cell transplantation. Clin Infect Dis 2004;39:1407–16.

48. Cornely OA, Maertens J, Winston DJ, et al. Posaconazole vs. fluconazole or itraconazole prophylaxis in patients with neutropenia. N Engl J Med 2007;356:348–59.

49. Ullmann AJ, Lipton JH, Vesole DH, et al. Posaconazole or fluconazole for prophylaxis in severe graft-versus-host disease. N Engl J Med 2007;356:335–47.

50. Glasmacher A, Prentice A, Gorschluter M, et al. Itraconazole prevents invasive fungal infections in neutropenic patients treated for hematologic malignancies: evidence from a meta-analysis of 3,597 patients. J Clin Oncol 2003;21:4615–26.

51. Offner F, Cordonnier C, Ljungman P, et al. Impact of previous aspergillosis on the outcome of bone marrow transplantation. Clin Infect Dis 1998;26:1098–103.

52. Fukuda T, Boeckh M, Carter RA, et al. Risks and outcomes of invasive fungal infections in recipients of allogeneic hematopoietic stem cell transplants after nonmyeloablative conditioning. Blood 2003;102:827–33.

53. de FP, Spagnoli A, Di BP, et al. Efficacy of caspofungin as secondary prophylaxis in patients undergoing allogeneic stem cell transplantation with prior pulmonary and/or systemic fungal infection. Bone Marrow Transplant 2007;40:245–9.

54. Pizzo PA, Robichaud KJ, Gill FA, et al. Empiric antibiotic and antifungal therapy for cancer patients with prolonged fever and granulocytopenia. Am J Med 1982;72:101–11.

55. Segal BH, Almyroudis NG, Battiwalla M, et al. Prevention and early treatment of invasive fungal infection in patients with cancer and neutropenia and in stem cell transplant recipients in the era of newer broad-spectrum antifungal agents and diagnostic adjuncts. Clin Infect Dis 2007;44:402–9.

56. Sobel JD. Design of clinical trials of empiric antifungal therapy in patients with persistent febrile neutropenia: considerations and critiques. Pharmacotherapy 2006;26:47S–54S.

57. Senn L, Robinson JO, Schmidt S, et al. 1,3-Beta-D-glucan antigenemia for early diagnosis of invasive fungal infections in neutropenic patients with acute leukemia. Clin Infect Dis 2008;46:878–85.

58. Gubbins PO, Penzak SR, Polston S, et al. Characterizing and predicting amphotericin B-associated nephrotoxicity in bone marrow or peripheral blood stem cell transplant recipients. Pharmacotherapy 2002;22:961–71.

59. Pappas PG, Kauffman CA, Andes D, et al. Clinical practice guidelines for the management of candidiasis: 2009 update by the Infectious Diseases Society of America. Clin Infect Dis 2009;48:503–35.

60. Marr KA, Seidel K, White TC, et al. Candidemia in allogeneic blood and marrow transplant recipients: evolution of risk factors after the adoption of prophylactic fluconazole. J Infect Dis 2000;181:309–16.

61. Nucci M, Anaissie E. Should vascular catheters be removed from all patients with candidemia? An evidence-based review. Clin Infect Dis 2002;34:591–9.

62. Herbrecht R, Denning DW, Patterson TF, et al. Voriconazole versus amphotericin B for primary therapy of invasive aspergillosis. N Engl J Med 2002;347:408–15.

63. Cornely OA, Maertens J, Bresnik M, et al. Liposomal amphotericin B as initial therapy for invasive mold infection: a randomized trial comparing a high-loading dose regimen with standard dosing (AmBiLoad trial). Clin Infect Dis 2007;44:1289–97.

64. Marr KA, Boeckh M, Carter RA, et al. Combination antifungal therapy for invasive aspergillosis. Clin Infect Dis 2004;39:797–802.

65. Spellberg B, Edwards J Jr, Ibrahim A. Novel perspectives on mucormycosis: pathophysiology, presentation, and management. Clin Microbiol Rev 2005;18:556–69.

66. Van Burik JA, Hare RS, Solomon HF, et al. Posaconazole is effective as salvage therapy in zygomycosis: a retrospective summary of 91 cases. Clin Infect Dis 2006;42:e61–5.

67. Nucci M, Anaissie E. *Fusarium* infections in immunocompromised patients. Clin Microbiol Rev 2007;20:695–704.

68. Singh N. Fungal infections in the recipients of solid organ transplantation. Infect Dis Clin North Am 2003;17:113–34, viii.

69. Singh N, Paterson DL. *Aspergillus* infections in transplant recipients. Clin Microbiol Rev 2005;18:44–69.

70. Singh N, Husain S. *Aspergillus* infections after lung transplantation: clinical differences in type of transplant and implications for management. J Heart Lung Transplant 2003;22:258–66.

71. Gotway MB, Dawn SK, Caoili EM, et al. The radiologic spectrum of pulmonary *Aspergillus* infections. J Comput Assist Tomogr 2002;26:159–73.

72. Gordon SM, Avery RK. Aspergillosis in lung transplantation: incidence, risk factors, and prophylactic strategies. Transpl Infect Dis 2001;3:161–7.

73. Pfeiffer CD, Fine JP, Safdar N. Diagnosis of invasive aspergillosis using a galactomannan assay: a meta-analysis. Clin Infect Dis 2006;42:1417–27.

74. Husain S, Kwak EJ, Obman A, et al. Prospective assessment of Platelia Aspergillus galactomannan antigen for the diagnosis of invasive aspergillosis in lung transplant recipients. Am J Transplant 2004;4:796–802.

75. Kwak EJ, Husain S, Obman A, et al. Efficacy of galactomannan antigen in the Platelia Aspergillus enzyme immunoassay for diagnosis of invasive aspergillosis in liver transplant recipients. J Clin Microbiol 2004;42:435–8.

76. Fortun J, Martin-Davila P, Alvarez ME, et al. False-positive results of *Aspergillus* galactomannan antigenemia in liver transplant recipients. Transplantation 2009;87:256–60.

77. Drew RH, Dodds AE, Benjamin DK Jr, et al. Comparative safety of amphotericin B lipid complex and amphotericin B deoxycholate as aerosolized antifungal prophylaxis in lung-transplant recipients. Transplantation 2004;77:232–7.

Unique Characteristics of Fungal Infections in Lung Transplant Recipients

Shahid Husain, MD, MS

KEYWORDS

- Lung transplant • Fungal • Aspergillus • *Candida*
- Prophylaxis

Lung transplantation is an established mode of therapy for end-stage lung disease. More than 1478 lung transplants were performed in United States in 2008.[1] The International Society for Heart and Lung Transplantation reports that the lung transplant average 1-year survival rate is approximately 85%, with a 5-year survival rate of 53%.[2] Although bronchiolitis obliterans syndrome or obliterative bronchiolitis remains the major impediment of long-term survival, short-term survival is predominantly affected by infectious syndromes in lung transplant recipients.[3] Of these syndromes, fungal infections contribute significantly to patient morbidity and mortality.

Among solid-organ transplant recipients, lung transplant recipients appear to have a higher incidence of fungal infection. In a retrospective review of fungal infection in lung transplant recipients, the overall incidence of fungal infections ranged from 14% to 35%, and of those, 60% of cases were due to *Aspergillus* species, followed by *Candida* and *Cryptococcus* species.[4] This article focuses primarily on the unique clinical features of fungal infections and their management implications in lung transplant recipients. A detailed description of fungal infections in lung transplant recipients is reported elsewhere.[5]

UNIQUE SUSCEPTIBILITY OF LUNG TRANSPLANTS TO INFECTIONS

The two solid organs that are in direct continuity to the environment include the lung and the small intestine. Lungs are unique, however, because not only are they directly exposed to the environment but also their transplantation results in the impairment of host defenses of the organ. As a result of transplantation, denervation and impairment of lymphatic drainage ensue. These factors coupled with blunted cough reflex and defective mucociliary clearance contribute to the milieu of microbial growth in the transplanted lung (**Fig. 1**).[6]

EPIDEMIOLOGY AND RISK FACTORS
Aspergillus

The incidence and timing of invasive aspergillosis (IA) in lung transplant recipients has changed over time. Earlier reports had reported the incidence to be as high as 23% during the first year after transplantation.[7–9] Recent data, however, suggest a much lower incidence during the first year (cumulative incidence of 2.4%).[10] Thirty percent of the cases in this series occurred after 6 months. In one center, with universal azole prophylaxis, the median time to onset of IA was noted to be 483 days, which was in accordance with the data reported by the Prospective Antifungal Therapy Alliance.[11]

Higher risks of IA in lung transplant recipients have been noted in cases of relative ischemia at the site of anastomosis (**Box 1**).[12] In addition, single-lung transplant recipients have been noted to have a higher incidence of IA compared with double-lung transplants due to the presence of a structurally abnormal native lung, which

Multiorgan Transplant Infectious Diseases, University Health Network, University of Toronto, NCSB 11C-1206, 200 Elizabeth Street, Toronto, Ontario M5G 2C4, Canada
E-mail address: shahid.husain@uhn.on.ca

Clin Chest Med 30 (2009) 307–313
doi:10.1016/j.ccm.2009.03.002
0272-5231/09/$ – see front matter © 2009 Elsevier Inc. All rights reserved.

chestmed.theclinics.com

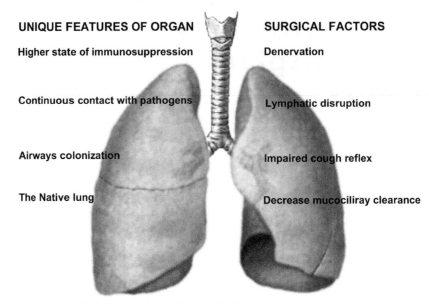

UNIQUE FEATURES OF ORGAN

Higher state of immunosuppression

Continuous contact with pathogens

Airways colonization

The Native lung

SURGICAL FACTORS

Denervation

Lymphatic disruption

Impaired cough reflex

Decrease mucociliray clearance

Fig. 1. Surgical and nonsurgical risk factors for fungal infections in lung transplant recipients.

serves as a reservoir.[9,13] In another study, immunoglobulin G levels lower than 400 mg/dL were associated with a significantly higher risk of infections including *Aspergillus* infections.[14] Similarly, another study showed that placement of a bronchial stent showed improvement in forced expiratory flow (midexpiratory phase) or forced expiratory volume in 1 second (FEV_1) but resulted in a higher incidence of *Aspergillus* colonization and IA.[15] Of all the factors studied, colonization of airways with *Aspergillus* (pre- or posttransplantation) has been consistently found to be associated with the subsequent development of IA.[13]

Candida, Cryptococcus, and Non-Aspergillus Molds

Candida species are a rare cause of invasive disease in lung transplant recipients. There have been no documented cases of invasive pulmonary candidiasis in adult lung transplant recipients, although in pediatric pulmonary transplants, 5% of the proven fungal infection cases were noted to be due to *Candida* species.[16] The most common presentation was candidemia, which accounted for 18% of the cases of blood stream infections in one study.[17] The risk factors for the development of candidemia in lung transplant recipients have not been specifically studied.

The true incidence of *Cryptococcus* infection in lung transplant recipients is not known. One study reported an incidence of 2.8% (range, 0.3%–5%),[18] and another reported an incidence of 13.7 to 14 per 1000 patients.[19]

UNIQUE FUNGAL CLINICAL SYNDROMES IN LUNG TRANSPLANTS
Colonization

Aspergillus
The true predictive value of *Aspergillus* colonization is hard to discern because in most case series, adequate data for prophylaxis has not been provided.[5] Pretransplant colonization with *Aspergillus* organisms was noted in 22% to 58% of cystic fibrosis patients and in 28% of non–cystic fibrosis patients undergoing transplantation.[20,21] Of those cystic fibrosis patients who had pretransplant colonization, 25% to 42% subsequently developed *Aspergillus* tracheobronchitis within 6 months of transplantation.[20,21] In one study, 34% of non–cystic fibrosis patients who had pretransplant colonization with *Aspergillus* organisms developed IA.[20] Earlier studies have reported that

---

Box 1
Unique risk factors for invasive aspergillosis in lung transplant recipients

Airway ischemia

Reperfusion injury

Single-lung transplant

Bronchial stents

Acquired hypogammaglobulinemia (<400 mg/dL)

Pretransplant *Aspergillus* colonization

Posttransplant *Aspergillus* colonization

up to 46% of lung transplant recipients had post-transplant *Aspergillus* colonization.[21] Patients were 11 times more likely to develop invasive disease if they were colonized with *Aspergillus* organisms within 6 months of transplantation in the absence of any prophylaxis.[21] In another study, the incidence of *Aspergillus* colonization was 0.24 per person-year in a universal prophylaxis group compared with 0.4 per person-year in a targeted prophylaxis group ($P = .21$).[22] *A fumigatus* was the most common species of *Aspergillus* in both groups. The median time to onset of *Aspergillus* colonization was 248 days in the universal prophylaxis group compared with 71 days ($P = .05$) in the targeted prophylaxis group.[22] *Aspergillus* colonization within a year of transplant was associated with a sixfold higher risk of developing IA. The use of universal azole prophylaxis had no impact on the incidence rate of *Aspergillus* colonization at 1 year.[22]

Candida

Candida species are frequently isolated from the respiratory secretions of lung transplant recipients. In one study, the incidence of *Candida* colonization was 0.53 per person-year in the universal prophylaxis group compared with 0.16 per person-year in the targeted prophylaxis group ($P = .006$). Sixty-six percent (23/35) of *Candida* colonization in the universal azole prophylaxis group was due to *Candida albicans*, whereas 100% of *Candida* colonization in the targeted prophylaxis group was due to *C albicans*. No case of invasive candidiasis was noted in this study.[22] It is reasonable to conclude that *Candida* species are infrequent pathogens unless concomitant bacterial infection or multisystem organ failure is present.[23]

Non-Aspergillus molds

In one retrospective review of lung transplant recipients, 14% of the isolates were due to non-*Aspergillus* molds. The median time to onset of colonization was 451 days. The most common isolate was *Cladosporium* species (41%), followed by *Phialemonium* species (17%) and zygomycetes (14%). Only one case of probable invasive fungal infection with *Mucor* species was reported in the study.[24]

Tracheobronchitis

Aspergillus

In an earlier literature review, tracheobronchitis was the most common presentation of IA in lung transplant recipients, accounting for 37% of cases.[13] Due to the recent widespread use of antifungal prophylaxis, the prevalence of pulmonary aspergillosis is now 61%.[22,25]

Tracheobronchitis typically involves the airways without involvement of lung parenchyma. The lesions are primarily multiple and ulcerative, with occasional formation of pseudomembranes initially restricted to the anastomatic site (**Fig. 2**).[26] Chest radiographs are usually normal. Tracheobronchitis usually occurs within the first 3 months following transplantation in patients who do not have stent placement. Patients are usually asymptomatic, and routine surveillance bronchoscopy is essential for early diagnosis.

The mortality rate in *Aspergillus* tracheobronchitis has been reported to be approximately 23% to 29%.[13]

Candida

Candida tracheobronchitis of the anastomatic site was reported in earlier case series;[27,28] however, the use of antifungal prophylaxis in the early transplant period has almost eliminated this problem.

Non-*Aspergillus* mold can theoretically cause the syndrome, but no occurrences have been reported.

Pneumonia

Aspergillus

Aspergillus pneumonia in lung transplant recipients distinctively lacks the characteristic halo

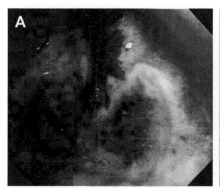
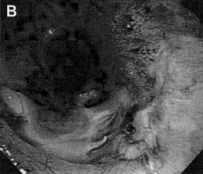

Fig. 2. (*A*) Tracheobronchitis secondary to *Aspergillus* infection in a lung transplant recipient. (*B*) Healed anastomosis of same patient after treatment.

sign noted in neutropenic stem cell transplant recipients.[13,29] There is no specific radiologic pattern, but most cases have a nodular density with focal areas of consolidation. *Aspergillus* pneumonia may also present as a cavitatory lesion.[30] The halo sign is rarely observed in organ transplant recipients.[30]

Candida

Candida pneumonia is very rare in adult lung transplant recipients. In one case series of pediatric lung transplant recipients, half of the cases of proven fungal infections were due to *Candida* species.[16] The isolation of *Candida* organisms from a lung transplant recipient who has pulmonary infiltrates may warrant further workup to rule out invasive disease.

GALACTOMANNAN FOR THE DIAGNOSIS OF INVASIVE ASPERGILLOSIS IN LUNG TRANSPLANT RECIPIENTS

Galactomannan is a polysaccharide cell wall component that is released by *Aspergillus* organisms during fungal growth. Detection of galactomannan by sandwich enzyme immunoassay is approved for use in hematopoietic stem cell transplant recipients. Few studies have evaluated the utility of galactomannan in the diagnosis of IA in lung transplants recipients. In one study of 70 lung transplant recipients that used 0.5 as a cut-off value for positive test, the sensitivity of the test in the serum was only 30%. Moreover, none of the cases of tracheobronchitis was positive.[31] When bronchoalveolar lavage (BAL) of lung transplant recipients was used for the diagnosis of IA, the sensitivity was 60% and the specificity was 95%, with positive and negative likelihood ratios of 14 and 0.41, respectively.[32] In another study, the sensitivity was 81.8% in patients who had aspergillosis, and the specificity was 95.8% in lung transplant patients who underwent BAL for surveillance for infection or rejection.[33] These findings suggest that the detection of galactomannan in the BAL of a lung transplant recipient who has a compatible clinical illness is highly suggestive of IA.

Polymerase chain reaction–based methods for the diagnosis appears promising; however, standardization of the primers precludes its widespread use.

ANTIFUNGAL PROPHYLAXIS IN LUNG TRANSPLANT RECIPIENTS
Amphotericin and Its Lipid Preparations

The ideal prophylactic strategy would be efficacious, convenient, devoid of side effects, and cost-effective. Because *Aspergillus* organisms are ubiquitous in nature and are inhaled into the small airways and bronchioles, causing the disease, delivery of the drug to the respiratory system by aerosolization to prevent IA is theoretically desirable. An optimal antifungal prophylactic strategy in lung transplant recipients still remains to be determined. A wide variation in the practice of antifungal prophylaxis in lung transplant recipients in terms of time of initiation, duration, and type of antifungal drug used has been noted in two surveys.[34,35]

Current practices of antifungal prophylaxis in lung transplant recipients are derived from nonrandomized clinical trails that have inadequate sample sizes, single-center noncomparative case series, or case-control studies.

Studies in lung transplant recipients have reported varying success rates with nebulized preparations of amphotericin B deoxycholate (AMB-D). In 49 lung or heart-lung transplant recipients who received antifungal prophylaxis with inhaled amphotericin B (20 mg, three times a day) during their initial hospital stay, the incidence of IA dropped from 12% to 0% at 3 months.[36] The incidence of IA continued to be lower (2% versus 12%) at 1 year.[36] In another study of 55 lung transplant recipients, however, prophylaxis with nebulized amphotericin B (6 mg every 8 hours for 120 days, followed by 6 mg/d for the rest of life) resulted in the development of IA in 33% of patients.[37] In contrast, another Spanish group noted a 0% rate of fungal infection at more than 1-year follow-up. Their regimen consisted of administering aerosolized amphotericin (0.2 mg/kg/every 8 hours) and fluconazole (400 mg/d) to 52 lung transplant recipients for a minimum of 1 month.[38]

The use of a lipid complex preparation of amphotericin B (ABLC) has been reported in two studies. In one study, subjects received 50 mg of ABLC by way of nebulizer from day 1 to day 4, followed by weekly administration of drugs for 7 weeks. This trial was not designed to determine the efficacy of the nebulized ABLC, but the reported rate of fungal infections at the end of study period was 12%. ABLC, however, was tolerated in 98% of patients. Pulmonary mechanics worsened in fewer than 5% of patients.[39] In another study involving 60 lung transplant recipients, each subject received 50 mg of nebulized ABLC every other day for 2 weeks, followed by weekly administration of nebulized ABLC with fluconazole for 3 weeks. IA was noted in only 1 patient (1.7%) at 6 months after transplantation.[40] One study reported the use of an inhaled liposomal preparation of amphotericin in 27 lung transplant recipients. These patients received inhaled AmBisome (25 mg, 6 mL) three times per week up to day 60 post transplantation, 25 mg once per week between day 60 and day 180, and 25 mg once every 2 weeks thereafter for life. Only one case of *Scedosporium* infection was reported.[41] The mean FEV_1 did not change significantly after the drug administration.

Side effects resulting in discontinuation of the drug are a major concern with the use of inhaled AMB-D.[42] The side effects are primarily attributed to the inhalation of the deoxycholate carrier of amphotericin. The lipid preparation of amphotericin has been reported to have fewer side effects. As shown in **Table 1**, the discontinuation rate due to the side effects was 12.2% in patients receiving inhaled AMB-D. The rate of discontinuation was merely 2.5% to 5.9% in patients receiving lipid preparations of amphotericin B.

Several factors may explain the variability of results in these studies; namely, the deposition characteristics of drugs, inadequate dosing, the duration of prophylaxis, the use of different nebulizers, and the evaluation of outcome at different time points. It is to be noted, however, that there are certain limitations associated with the use of inhaled preparations of amphotericin. It has been reported that distribution in single-lung transplant recipients occurs preferentially in the allograft, with unreliable distribution in the native lung, which could remain as a source of infection.[43,44] Although the short-term data on the pulmonary mechanics of lung transplant recipients appears to be to promising, the long-term effects of the administration of lipid preparations of the drug are not known. It would be prudent to assess the long-term effects of the drug on the pulmonary function of lung transplant recipients before the assessment of effectiveness of these therapies.

Triazoles

Triazoles, including itraconazole and voriconazole, have been shown to decrease the rate of IA in lung transplant recipients.[22,44]

In a retrospective review of solid-organ transplant recipients at a tertiary center, it was noted that the use of inhaled amphotericin (5–10 mg, twice daily), followed by oral itraconazole reduced the incidence rate of IA from 49.7/1000 patient-years to 31.6/1000 patient-years. The side effects of the drug were not reported in the study.[44] The safety and effectiveness of voriconazole in preventing fungal infections following lung transplantation was evaluated in a single-center, nonrandomized, retrospective, sequential study that included 95 patients.[22] Of these patients, 65 received voriconazole prophylaxis (two intravenous doses of 6 mg/kg) starting immediately after transplantation, followed by 200 mg orally twice daily for a minimum of 4 months. The control group consisted of 30 patients who received targeted prophylaxis with itraconazole with or without inhaled amphotericin. The universal prophylaxis with voriconazole not only decreased the rate of IA in lung transplant recipients to 1.5%, but the overall rate of non-*Aspergillus* fungal infections was only 3%. Only 27% of voriconazole recipients, however, had normal liver enzymes throughout the study. The values of alanine aminotransferases and aspartate aminotransferases were significantly higher in patients receiving voriconazole compared with those receiving itraconazole in this study. Routine monitoring of liver enzymes and calcineurin inhibitor levels is necessary to avoid hepatotoxicity and nephrotoxicity in patients receiving voriconazole prophylaxis.

Table 1
Side effect profile of various inhaled preparations of amphotericin

Side Effect	L-AMB (n = 118) (%)	ABLC (n = 51) (%)	AMB-D (n = 49) (%)
Wheezing	4	4.2	6.4
Cough	10	2.1	10.6
Shortness of breath	NR	2.1	20
Nausea	7	2.1	8.5
Decline in FEV_1	0	11.1	10.6
>1 AE	NR	27.5	42.9
Discontinuation rate	2.5	5.9	12.2

Abbreviations: AE, adverse events; L-AMB, liposomal amphotericin B; NR, not reported.
Data from Drew RH, Dodds AE, Benjamin Jr. DK, et al. Comparative safety of amphotericin B lipid complex and amphotericin B deoxycholate as aerosolized antifungal prophylaxis in lung-transplant recipients. Transplantation 2004; 77:232–7; and Monforte V, Roman A, Gavalda J, et al. Nebulized liposomal amphotericin B (n-LAB) prophylaxis for *Aspergillus* infection in lung transplantation (LT): pharmacokinetics, safety and efficacy. J Heart Lung Transplant 2009; 24(2):S108–9.

SUMMARY

The landscape of fungal infection in lung transplant recipients is changing. Fungal infections in lung transplant recipients exhibit unique clinical features, including colonization and tracheobronchitis that require distinct management challenges. The risk stratification and the optimal prophylactic strategy still remain to be defined. Galactomannan measurement in the BAL appears promising for the diagnosis of IA. The efficacy and long-term safety of inhaled amphotericin for prophylaxis remains to be explored. Azole use for prophylaxis is complicated by its interaction with immunosuppressive drugs and side effects. Finally, the long-term sequel of antifungal prophylaxis in terms of development of resistant strains and emergence of newer fungal species remains to be seen. In summary, the field of fungal infection in lung transplantation continues to be exciting and full of opportunities.

REFERENCES

1. National Data on Lung transplant, 2009.
2. Christie JD, Edwards LB, Aurora P, et al. Registry of the International Society for Heart and Lung Transplantation: twenty-fifth official adult lung and heart/lung transplantation report–2008. J Heart Lung Transplant 2008;27:957–69.
3. Trulock EP, Edwards LB, Taylor DO, et al. The registry of the International Society for Heart and Lung Transplantation: twenty-first official adult heart transplant report–2004. J Heart Lung Transplant 2004;23:804–15.
4. Kubak BM. Fungal infection in lung transplantation. Transpl Infect Dis 2002;4(Suppl 3):24–31.
5. Silveira FP, Husain S. Fungal infections in lung transplant recipients. Curr Opin Pulm Med 2008;14:211–8.
6. Chan KM. Approach towards infectious pulmonary complications in lung transplant recipients. In: Singh N, Aguado JM, editors. Infectious complications in transplant patients. Semin Respir Infect 2002;17(4):291–302.
7. Yeldandi V, Laghi F, McCabe MA, et al. Aspergillus and lung transplantation. J Heart Lung Transplant 1995;14:883–90.
8. Kanj SS, Tapson V, Davis RD, et al. Infections in patients with cystic fibrosis following lung transplantation. Chest 1997;112:924–30.
9. Westney GE, Kesten S, De Hoyos A, et al. Aspergillus infection in single and double lung transplant recipients. Transplantation 1996;61:915–9.
10. Morgan J, Wannemuehler KA, Marr KA, et al. Incidence of invasive aspergillosis following hematopoietic stem cell and solid organ transplantation: interim results of a prospective multicenter surveillance program. Med Mycol 2005;43(Suppl 1):S49–58.
11. Husain S. Differences in invasive aspergillosis in solid organ transplant recipients, 2008. Available at: http://www.aspergillus.org.uk/indexhome.htm?secure/conferences/confabstracts/inputform.php~main. Accessed January 10, 2009.
12. Higgins R, McNeil K, Dennis C, et al. Airway stenoses after lung transplantation: management with expanding metal stents. J Heart Lung Transplant 1994;13:774–8.
13. Singh N, Husain S. Aspergillus infections after lung transplantation: clinical differences in type of transplant and implications for management. J Heart Lung Transplant 2003;22:258–66.
14. Goldfarb NS, Avery RK, Goormastic M, et al. Hypogammaglobulinemia in lung transplant recipients. Transplantation 2001;71:242–6.
15. Crespo M, Raza K, Studer S, et al. Risk of pulmonary aspergillosis after bronchial stent placement in lung transplant (LTx) recipients. Presented at the 26th Annual Meeting and Scientific Sessions of the International Society of Heart and Lung Transplantation. Madrid, Spain, April 5-6, 2006.
16. Danziger-Isakov LA, Worley S, Arrigain S, et al. Increased mortality after pulmonary fungal infection within the first year after pediatric lung transplantation. J Heart Lung Transplant 2008;27:655–61.
17. Palmer SM, Alexander BD, Sanders LL, et al. Significance of blood stream infection after lung transplantation: analysis in 176 consecutive patients. Transplantation 2000;69:2360–6.
18. Husain S, Wagener MM, Singh N. Cryptococcus neoformans infection in organ transplant recipients: variables influencing clinical characteristics and outcome. Emerg Infect Dis 2001;7:375–81.
19. Vilchez R, Shapiro R, McCurry KR, et al. Longitudinal study of cryptococcosis in adult solid-organ transplant recipients. Transpl Int 2003;16(5):336–40.
20. Helmi M, Love RB, Welter D, et al. Aspergillus infection in lung transplant recipients with cystic fibrosis: risk factors and outcomes comparison to other types of transplant recipients. Chest 2003;123:800–8.
21. Nunley DR, Ohori P, Grgurich WF, et al. Pulmonary aspergillosis in cystic fibrosis lung transplant recipients. Chest 1998;114:1321–9.
22. Husain S, Paterson DL, Studer S, et al. Voriconazole prophylaxis in lung transplant recipients. Am J Transplant 2006;6:3008–16.
23. Chaparro C, Kesten S. Infections in lung transplant recipients. Clin Chest Med 1997;18:339–51.
24. Silveira FP, Kwak EJ, Paterson DL, et al. Post-transplant colonization with non-Aspergillus molds and risk of development of invasive fungal disease in lung transplant recipients. J Heart Lung Transplant 2008;27:850–5.
25. Sole A, Morant P, Salavert M, et al. Aspergillus infections in lung transplant recipients: risk factors

and outcome. Clin Microbiol Infect 2005;11: 359–65.

26. Kramer MR, Denning DW, Marshall SE, et al. Ulcerative tracheobronchitis after lung transplantation. A new form of invasive aspergillosis. Am Rev Respir Dis 1991;144:552–6.

27. Hadjiliadis D, Howell DN, Davis RD, et al. Anastomotic infections in lung transplant recipients. Ann Transplant 2000;5:13–9.

28. Palmer SM, Perfect JR, Howell DN, et al. Candidal anastomotic infection in lung transplant recipients: successful treatment with a combination of systemic and inhaled antifungal agents. J Heart Lung Transplant 1998;17:1029–33.

29. Paterson DL, Singh N. Invasive aspergillosis in transplant recipients. Medicine (Baltimore) 1999; 78:123–38.

30. Singh N, Paterson DL. *Aspergillus* infections in transplant recipients. Clin Microbiol Rev 2005;18:44–69.

31. Husain S, Kwak EJ, Obman A, et al. Prospective assessment of Platelia *Aspergillus* galactomannan antigen for the diagnosis of invasive aspergillosis in lung transplant recipients. Am J Transplant 2004;4:796–802.

32. Husain S, Paterson DL, Studer SM, et al. *Aspergillus* galactomannan antigen in the bronchoalveolar lavage fluid for the diagnosis of invasive aspergillosis in lung transplant recipients. Transplantation 2007;83:1330–6.

33. Husain S, Clancy CJ, Nguyen MH, et al. Performance characteristics of the Platelia *Aspergillus* enzyme immunoassay for detection of *Aspergillus* galactomannan antigen in bronchoalveolar lavage fluid. Clin Vaccine Immunol 2008;15:1760–3.

34. Husain S, Zaldonis D, Kusne S, et al. Variation in antifungal prophylaxis strategies in lung transplantation. Transpl Infect Dis 2006;8(4):213–8.

35. Dummer JS, Lazariashvilli N, Barnes J, et al. A survey of anti-fungal management in lung transplantation. J Heart Lung Transplant 2004;23:1376–81.

36. Reichenspurner H, Gamberg P, Nitschke M, et al. Significant reduction in the number of fungal infections after lung-, heart-lung, and heart transplantation using aerosolized amphotericin B prophylaxis. Transplant Proc 1997;29:627–8.

37. Monforte V, Roman A, Gavalda J, et al. Nebulized amphotericin B prophylaxis for *Aspergillus* infection in lung transplantation: study of risk factors. J Heart Lung Transplant 2001;20:1274–81.

38. Calvo V, Borro JM, Morales P, et al. Antifungal prophylaxis during the early postoperative period of lung transplantation. Valencia Lung Transplant Group. Chest 1999;115:1301–4.

39. Drew RH, Dodds AE, Benjamin DK Jr, et al. Comparative safety of amphotericin B lipid complex and amphotericin B deoxycholate as aerosolized antifungal prophylaxis in lung-transplant recipients. Transplantation 2004;77:232–7.

40. Borro JM, Sole A, de la TM, et al. Efficiency and safety of inhaled amphotericin B lipid complex (Abelcet) in the prophylaxis of invasive fungal infections following lung transplantation. Transplant Proc 2008;40:3090–3.

41. Monforte V, Roman A, Gavalda J, et al. Nebulized liposomal amphotericin B (n-LAB) prophylaxis for *Aspergillus* infection in lung transplantation (LT): pharmacokinetics, safety and efficacy. J Heart Lung Transplant 2005;24(Suppl 2):S108–9.

42. Corcoran TE, Venkataramanan R, Mihelc KM, et al. Aerosol deposition of lipid complex amphotericin-B (Abelcet) in lung transplant recipients. Am J Transplant 2006;6:2765–73.

43. Monforte V, Roman A, Gavalda J, et al. Nebulized amphotericin B concentration and distribution in the respiratory tract of lung-transplanted patients. Transplantation 2003;75:1571–4.

44. Minari A, Husni R, Avery RK, et al. The incidence of invasive aspergillosis among solid organ transplant recipients and implications for prophylaxis in lung transplants. Transpl Infect Dis 2002;4:195–200.

Noninvasive Pulmonary *Aspergillus* Infections

Brent P. Riscili, MD, Karen L. Wood, MD*

KEYWORDS

- *Aspergillus* • Allergic bronchopulmonary aspergillosis
- Chronic • Necrotizing • Aspergilloma

Aspergillus is a spore-forming fungus that can be found in warm or cold environments, indoors and outdoors. It is thermotolerant (grows at 15°C–53°C) and can thrive in the human respiratory tract. It obtains nutrients from decaying matter and is a common inhabitant of soil, water, compost, and damp areas, such as basements. Numerous species of *Aspergillus* exist; however, only approximately 20 species cause disease in humans, with *Aspergillus fumigatus* being the most commonly isolated (90%). *Aspergillus flavus, Aspergillus terreus, Aspergillus niger,* and *Aspergillus nidulans* can also cause human illness.[1] *Aspergillus* grows as septate dichotomous branching hyphae at acute (45°) angles. The hyphae contain conidiophores, which harbor hundreds of conidia or spores. These spores are 2 to 3 μm in diameter and can have an impact on the terminal airways.[2] They are easily dispersed by physical contact or air currents.[2] Air quality studies have shown that humans may inhale hundreds of these spores daily, making them a common inhabitant of the airway, yet only some develop disease from *Aspergillus*.[2] Thus, colonization must be separated from infection when these organisms are present.

Once inhaled, *Aspergillus* can cause several types of disease, which depends, in large part, on the underlying immune function of the host (**Table 1**). The immune system normally clears fungal spores, and colonization does not usually cause any significant problems. In patients who have underlying lung disease, especially previous cavitary disease as seen in tuberculosis (TB), a fungus ball or aspergilloma may form. Patients who have impaired immunity or chronic lung disease, such as chronic obstructive pulmonary disease (COPD), can develop semi-invasive or chronic pulmonary aspergillosis (CPA). For those severely immunocompromised, invasive disease can develop and has the potential to disseminate systemically. Other patients can have an exaggerated immune response to *Aspergillus* antigens in the airways and develop allergic bronchopulmonary aspergillosis (ABPA). This is most commonly reported in those who have steroid-dependent asthma or cystic fibrosis (CF).[3]

ALLERGIC BRONCHOPULMONARY ASPERGILLOSIS

ABPA is caused by an exaggerated hypersensitivity reaction to antigens produced by *Aspergillus* species, most commonly *A fumigatus*. It was first described by Hinson and colleagues[4] in 1952. The pathogenesis of the disease is complex and is thought to be attributable to several immunologic and genetic predisposing host factors. Although *A fumigatus* is the most common cause of ABPA, other fungi have been implicated, giving rise to the term *allergic bronchopulmonary mycosis* (ABPM).[5] ABPA is most commonly seen in immunocompetent hosts who have underlying steroid-dependent asthma or CF, and the incidence in these diseases can range from 1% to 2%[6–10] and from 5% to 15%,[6,11] respectively. It has been reported in patients who do not have asthma; however, this is rare.[12] Most healthy persons are able to clear these organisms from the respiratory tract and do not develop disease; therefore, it seems that exposure alone is not likely to cause ABPA.

Division of Pulmonary, Allergy, Critical Care, and Sleep Medicine, The Ohio State University Medical Center, 201 Davis Heart and Lung Research Institute, 473 West 12th Avenue, Columbus, OH 43210, USA
* Corresponding author.
E-mail address: karen.wood@osumc.edu (K.L. Wood).

Clin Chest Med 30 (2009) 315–335
doi:10.1016/j.ccm.2009.02.008

Table 1
Spectrum of diseases caused by Aspergillus

Disease	No Disease	Aspergilloma	Chronic Pulmonary Aspergillosis	Invasive Aspergillosis	ABPA
Host factors	Normal immunocompetent host	Most commonly occurs in previously abnormal lung tissue, such as old cavities from TB	Usually seen in chronic lung disease, such as chronic obstructive pulmonary disease, or in patients with mild immunocompromise, such as those on chronic steroids	Typically seen in immunocompromised hosts, especially those who have undergone bone marrow transplantation or are on chronic immunosuppressive therapy. Tissue invasion seen and dissemination possible	Results from hypersensitivity to Aspergillus species (most often A fumigatus) Manifests as severe asthma, pulmonary infiltrates, and pulmonary and peripheral eosinophilia

Risk Factors

ABPA is most commonly seen in patients who have underlying asthma or CF.[13] The obstructive nature, high incidence of atopy, and impaired mucous clearance seen in these conditions may play a role in the pathogenesis; however, ABPA is not always seen in patients who have the most severe underlying disease.[14,15] Host susceptibility may also be important. Cases of familial inheritance have been identified.[16,17] Other genetic variables, including human leukocyte antigen (HLA)-restricted phenotypes, mutations in the cystic fibrosis transmembrane receptor (CFTR), and polymorphisms in surfactant proteins, have also been implicated.[18–26]

Type I diabetes mellitus and ankylosing spondylitis have been genetically linked to specific HLA alleles.[20–22] Chauhan and colleagues[19,23] have published several articles suggesting that HLA-DR alleles (subtypes of HLA-DR2 and HLA-DR5) may be involved in susceptibility to ABPA in much the same way. The mechanism is thought to be through antigen presentation and the production of major histocompatibility complex class II HLA-restricted CD4+ T helper (Th) 2 lymphocytes important in disease pathogenesis.[18,19,23,27] Other HLA phenotypes (HLA-DQ2) have been associated with resistance to developing ABPA.[19] It seems that the combination of HLA-DQ2 and HLA-DR2/5 alleles present may determine a particular patient's risk for developing ABPA.[18,19]

Mutations in the CFTR may be an important risk factor. One study examined 11 asthmatic patients who had ABPA and normal sweat chloride. They found that 6 of 11 had a mutation in the CFTR, suggesting that mutations in this gene may be associated with increased risk for developing ABPA independent of having CF.[24] In a similar study, Marchand and colleagues[25] compared 21 patients who had ABPA and 143 patients who had various disorders in a genetics clinic. Screening for 13 mutations in the CFTR gene, they demonstrated that 28.5% of patients who had ABPA had at least 1 mutation compared with 4.6% of asthmatic controls and 4.2% of patients who had other genetic disorders.

Polymorphisms in the collagen region of pulmonary surfactant protein (SP)-A2 have also been described and linked to increased levels of serum IgE and eosinophilia, which are important contributors in the pathogenesis of ABPA.[26]

ABPA has been reported in diseases other than asthma or CF, including bronchocentric granulomatosis, hyper-IgE syndrome, and chronic granulomatous disease.[12,28] Another condition that is thought to be similar to and sometimes associated with ABPA is allergic fungal sinusitis (AFS).[29] This condition is an inflammatory allergic response to fungal antigens, including *Aspergillus*, in the sinuses. There have been reported incidences of the two diseases occurring concomitantly or separated by some temporal duration. Patients who have AFS are characterized by chronic rhinosinusitis, atopy, and having a history of asthma. In addition, they can share some other features with patients who have ABPA, including pulmonary infiltrates, central bronchiectasis (CB), eosinophilia, total and *A fumigatus*-specific IgE, *Aspergillus*-specific IgG, and a positive skin prick test result to *Aspergillus*. The treatment consists of corticosteroids and sinus surgery.[30] It is thought that some of the same mechanisms may be responsible in both diseases.[31–33]

Immunopathogenesis

The pathogenesis of ABPA is complex and not completely understood. An abnormal exaggerated local and systemic immune response to *Aspergillus* antigens seems to be responsible.[13] *Aspergillus* and other fungi are inhaled from the environment and colonize the airways. They are able to germinate, resulting in the growth of fungal hyphae, typically without tissue invasion. This source of constant antigen exposure sustains a local and systemic inflammatory response that can lead to bronchospasm. Obstructive airway disease and impaired mucociliary clearance may also play a role in airway colonization, especially in CF.[34] The amount of spore exposure has not been found to correlate with *Aspergillus* antigen hypersensitivity.[35] Normal persons typically clear these organisms, suggesting that colonization may result from fungal impairment of the immune system or defects in host defenses. *Aspergillus* spores have been shown to impair complement activation and evade phagocytosis despite attachment of phagocytes to the spores.[36,37] In addition, patients on chronic steroid therapy have been found to have decreased response of phagocytic cells to fungal antigens.[38]

Locally, fungal products, including proteolytic enzymes, such as elastase, collagenase, and trypsin, are released.[39,40] These products damage the airway matrix, resulting in more inflammation and release of proinflammatory cytokines, further propagating the inflammatory response (**Fig. 1**).[41] *Aspergillus* extracts have been shown to cause desquamation of epithelial cells, which may facilitate fungal invasion and stimulate further inflammatory cytokine release.[40,42,43]

A type I immune response involving cell-bound IgE causes mast cell and eosinophil degranulation.[15,44,45] These cells release major basic protein, cationic protein, histamine, and matrix metalloproteinase-9, which have all been implicated in tissue destruction.[14,46] As the inflammatory process progresses, a type III response involving the influx of IgG and complement activation causes further tissue destruction.[13,47–49] With time, the milieu of growth factors and cytokines promotes bronchial wall thickening, airway remodeling, and bronchiectasis and can eventually lead to fibrosis (see **Fig. 1**).[41] Sputum from patients who have APBA has been shown to have increased numbers of eosinophils and neutrophils, which has been found to correlate with bronchiectasis.[50]

The systemic response involves activation of *Aspergillus*-specific T and B lymphocytes. A major contributor is thought to be the Th2 CD4+ T-cell response. Through cytokine interaction with interleukin (IL)-4, IL-5, IL-13, and interferon gamma (INF) T cells promote B-cell stimulation and production of IgE, in addition to eosinophil influx and degranulation (see **Fig. 1**).[51–54] People who have atopy generally have an exaggerated Th2 response. IL-4 has been shown to play a central role in this process, driving the Th2 response in an autocrine fashion, stimulating eosinophils and promoting production of nonspecific IgE. Studies have found that patients who have ABPA have increased sensitivity to IL-4 compared with patients who do not have APBA and those who are simply atopic.[45,55–57]

The humoral response also plays an important role in pathogenesis. B lymphocytes produce polyclonal *Aspergillus*-specific IgE, IgA, and IgG, which is not seen in patients who are only sensitized to *Aspergillus* (see **Fig. 1**).[58] Although *Aspergillus*-specific and non–*Aspergillus*-specific IgE is present, most of the IgE circulating in the blood is nonspecific, produced peripherally, and IL-4 driven. *Aspergillus*-specific IgE and IgA seem to be produced locally by bronchoalveolar lymphoid tissue, suggesting that the immune response to airway colonization and constant antigen exposure is important.[7,59,60] *Aspergillus*-specific IgG is primarily produced by peripheral lymphoid tissue.[60] B lymphocytes also undergo IL-4–induced changes that may exaggerate the humoral response, including an increase in CD86 costimulatory ligand, increased CD23 expression, and increased IL-4 sensitivity, which are all indicative of an exaggerated response toward *Aspergillus* antigens.[56,61] Cytokines play a pivotal role in the pathogenesis of ABPA, and as outlined previously, IL-4, IL-5, IL-13, and INF have all been implicated.[41,43,53,62] In a mouse model of ABPA, which closely approximates human disease, monocyte chemoattractant protein-1,

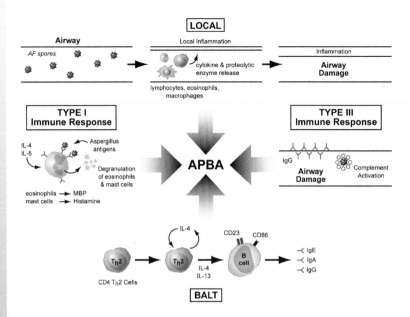

Fig. 1. Schematic diagram of the mechanisms involved in the immunopathogenesis of ABPA. MPB, major basic protein. (*Courtesy of* T. Eubank, PhD, Columbus, OH.)

CCL2, eotaxin, regulated on activation normal T-cell expressed and secreted (RANTES)/CCl5, and IL-8 were also found to be important in the disease process.[51,62,63]

Pathologic Findings

Gross lung specimens from patients who have ABPA typically demonstrate airways filled with thick tenacious sputum and fibrous material that may consist of fungal hyphae. Charcot-Leyden crystals (byproducts of eosinophil breakdown), Curschmann's spirals (desquamated epithelium associated with eosinophilic infiltration), and inflammatory cells (macrophages, eosinophils, and lymphocytes) are often seen.[64,65] Examination of the airway shows bronchial wall inflammation with eosinophils, neutrophils, and lymphocytes.[14,64,65] There is degranulation of inflammatory cell exoproducts, such as eosinophil major basic protein, which results in damage to the basement membrane and underlying cellular matrix proteins.[39,40] Bronchiectasis is the most common pathologic change in the airways and commonly occurs in a central location. Other pathologic findings are less common but may be present, including bronchocentric granulomatosis, mononuclear and lymphocytic infiltrates, eosinophilic pneumonitis, exudative and obliterative bronchiolitis, interstitial pneumonitis, vasculitis, microabscesses, and desquamation.[14,39,66] The presence of *Aspergillus* in microabscesses is thought to bridge the boundary between ABPA and semi-invasive disease, as seen in CPA.[14,39,66] The underlying changes consistent with asthma may also be present and include eosinophilic, lymphocytic, and

plasma cell infiltrates; goblet cell hyperplasia; and basement membrane thickening.[67]

Clinical Features

Diagnosis can be a dilemma in patients who have asthma or CF, because the results of serum studies and radiographic appearances may overlap with ABPA in both diseases. Patients who have asthma may have mild or severe disease. It is not uncommon for these patients to present with frequent and recurrent exacerbations requiring corticosteroids. In addition, they may have atopy with positive results of allergy testing and other associated conditions, such as allergic rhinitis.[13] Most patients present with poorly controlled asthma at the time of an ABPA exacerbation, Common findings include wheezing, cough, fatigue, fever, chest pain, and copious thick sputum production that may contain brown plugs or specks often containing fungal debris.[3,6,68] In some cases, hemoptysis has been reported.[69] Infiltrates on chest radiographs, fevers, or evidence of bronchiectasis in an asthmatic patient may be a clue. Infiltrates may be fleeting and are often found in the upper and middle lung fields. In some instances, patients can be asymptomatic and the only manifestation of their disease may be silent pulmonary infiltrates.[70] For patients who have CF, increased sputum production, cough, fatigue, weight loss, or hemoptysis may be the initial presentation.[6] ABPA should be considered in patients who fail to improve with antibiotic therapy for a CF exacerbation.[6,71] It may be especially difficult to differentiate symptoms attributable to ABPA compared with those of an underlying CF exacerbation. The Cystic Fibrosis Foundation has set forth guidelines and minimal diagnostic criteria to help establish the diagnosis in these patients.[6]

Laboratory Findings

Laboratory findings in patients who have ABPA result from the exaggerated immune response to *Aspergillus* antigens in susceptible individuals and are key in making the diagnosis. Essentially, all patients have positive immediate skin test reactivity to *Aspergillus*. Positive sputum cultures are found in approximately half.[71] Patients can have local and systemic eosinophilia, which may wax and wane on steroid therapy or between flares.[7,72,73] Nonspecific IgE is markedly elevated, but this finding may be seen in asthmatics and atopic individuals who do not have ABPA as well. In addition, *Aspergillus*-specific IgE, IgG, and IgA are usually present. *Aspergillus* precipitins are usually present and are caused by precipitating IgG antibody directed at *Aspergillus* antigens.[7,47,58–60,72,73] Asthmatics who do not have APBA can have positive skin test results and positive serum precipitins to *Aspergillus* in up to 20% to 30% and 10% of cases, respectively.[8,45,74,75]

Radiology

Fig. 2 outlines the most common chest radiographic and CT findings associated with ABPA.[13,76–82] High-resolution CT is superior to plain radiographs for identifying bronchiectasis and atelectasis and other subtle abnormalities.[83,84] CB involving the inner two thirds of the lung fields is common but not specific and may be seen in patients who do not have APBA, including those who have asthma and CF.[80,81] Most asthmatics have a relatively normal-appearing chest radiograph, and abnormalities associated with ABPA in these patients are usually easier to appreciate. In CF, however, many of the underlying radiographic findings, including bronchiectasis, infiltrates, mucoid impaction, and even fibrosis, may mimic those found in ABPA.[85] **Figs. 3** and **4** demonstrate a typical chest radiograph and CT scan from a patient who has ABPA.

Pulmonary Function Tests

Several studies have looked at the results of pulmonary function tests of patients who have ABPA during and between exacerbations. Most patients demonstrate obstructive lung disease with some degree of reversibility. In one study, Pepys and McCarthy found patients who had ABPA to have severe reversible obstructive airways disease with forced expiratory volume in 1 second declines of 40% to 50%.[45,47] Patients who have chronic disease and fibrosis may also demonstrate a restrictive pattern and fixed airway obstruction on their pulmonary function tests.[44,47,86,87]

Diagnosis

The goal is to identify the disease early and prevent end-stage complications. To make the diagnosis, patients must fulfill the clinical, radiographic, and laboratory criteria.[88,89] The current diagnostic criteria for asthmatics include a history of asthma, CB on chest CT, immediate positive result of skin test to *Aspergillus*, total serum IgE greater than 1000 ng/mL, elevated serum IgE or IgG specific for *A fumigatus*, infiltrates on chest radiographs, precipitating antibodies to *A fumigatus*, peripheral eosinophilia, and tenacious mucous plugs.[88,89] Patients who meet the first five criteria listed are classified as having ABPA with CB (ABPA-CB). Those fulfilling these criteria without evidence of bronchiectasis are categorized as having ABPA-seropositive (ABPA-S) **(Fig. 5)**.[90] The remaining criteria support the diagnosis but are not essential. Patients who have APBA-S have been found to have lower levels of IgE and IgG to *A fumigatus*, fewer exacerbations, and less likelihood to progress to end-stage fibrosis when compared with patients who have ABPA-CB. Greenberger and colleagues[90] concluded that ABPA-S is an earlier stage of disease or possibly a less aggressive form.

In patients who fulfill the clinical and radiographic criteria for ABPA, assessment should begin with a skin prick test. This test has excellent negative predictive value, and patients with a negative test result can essentially be ruled out.[73] One study demonstrated that 20% of asthmatics of 255 consecutive patients tested in an asthma clinic had a positive skin pin prick test result.[8] Others have shown that a positive test result can be present in up to 20% to 30% of patients who have persistent asthma and is only indicative of reactivity toward *Aspergillus* but not necessarily ABPA.[8,45,74,75] Those with a positive skin test result should have total serum IgE (also commonly elevated in asthma) and *Aspergillus*-specific IgE and IgG tested. If these test results are both positive, the diagnosis of ABPA can be made.[13,47,72,73] If only one of these test results is positive, patients require close follow-up and possibly repeat testing if suspicion is still high **(Fig. 6)**.[73] Serum precipitins against *Aspergillus* are also usually elevated but, again, may be positive in 10% of asthmatics who do not have ABPA.[8,45,75] Serum precipitins can also be found in

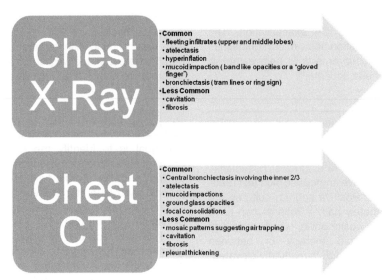

Chest X-Ray
- **Common**
  - fleeting infiltrates (upper and middle lobes)
  - atelectasis
  - hyperinflation
  - mucoid impaction (band like opacities or a "gloved finger")
  - bronchiectasis (tram lines or ring sign)
- **Less Common**
  - cavitation
  - fibrosis

Chest CT
- **Common**
  - Central bronchiectasis involving the inner 2/3
  - atelectasis
  - mucoid impactions
  - ground glass opacities
  - focal consolidations
- **Less Common**
  - mosaic patterns suggesting air trapping
  - cavitation
  - fibrosis
  - pleural thickening

Fig. 2. Radiographic findings on chest radiograph and chest CT in patients who have ABPA.

other conditions without ABPA, such as farmers' lung and hypersensitivity pneumonitis.[8,45,74,75,91] Some patients who may be sensitized to fungi other than *Aspergillus*, as is the case in ABPM, may have completely normal serology against *Aspergillus*.[13] Other diagnostic markers have been explored. Recently, Nguyen and colleagues[92] looked at the utility of measuring galactomannan in the bronchoalveolar lavage fluid (BALF) of nonimmunocompromised patients to differentiate colonization from infection. They found that there was a high rate of false-positive results, making this test a poor predictor of disease in this population.

Physicians must always consider the diagnosis of ABPA and be vigilant in the appropriate clinical setting, because some patients may have mild disease with only infiltrates on chest radiographs, and if unrecognized, these patients may progress to more advanced stages. Pulmonary infiltrates, eosinophilia, and precipitating antibodies may be apparent only during acute exacerbations. Likewise, IgE may fluctuate with flares and on steroid therapy; however, it usually remains abnormally elevated.[93]

Diagnosis In Patients Who Have Cystic Fibrosis

In CF, the diagnosis of ABPA can be especially difficult, because many of the laboratory, radiographic, and clinical manifestations of CF exacerbations can overlap. Patients who have CF can have pulmonary infiltrates, underlying bronchiectasis, and sensitization to *Aspergillus*, with elevated IgE levels at baseline.[6,94–96] One study found that the laboratory profile in patients who have CF can spontaneously change even without therapy.[96] In that study, the researchers followed 79 patients who had CF for 6 years. During that time, laboratory parameters, including skin prick test positivity, serum precipitins to *Aspergillus*, and *Aspergillus*-specific antibodies, spontaneously became positive or negative, with only 4 patients fulfilling criteria for APBA. The researchers concluded that patients who have CF can have variable immune responses to *Aspergillus* and that diagnosis should not be based on

Fig. 3. Chest radiograph of an asthmatic patient who has APBA demonstrates right middle lobe infiltrates and atelectasis secondary to mucous plugging. (*Courtesy of* J. Allen, MD, Columbus, OH.)

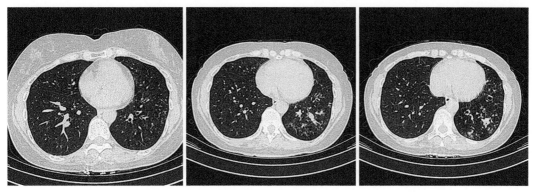

Fig. 4. Several CT sections of an asthmatic patient who has ABPA demonstrate CB with surrounding tree-in-bud opacities. (*Courtesy of* J. Allen, MD, Columbus, OH.)

laboratory results alone.[96] Cortese and colleagues[85] performed serial chest radiographs in 11 patients who had CF with ABPA at baseline, during an ABPA exacerbation, and after exacerbation. They found that radiographic findings overlapped in all stages of disease and were unreliable to diagnose exacerbations.

In 2003, the Cystic Fibrosis Foundation revised the guidelines for the diagnosis of ABPA in patients who have CF. They also made screening and management recommendations.[6] **Fig. 7** summarizes the diagnostic criteria in patients who have CF. The panel recommends that physicians should have a high level of suspicion for ABPA in patients who have CF and are older than 6 years of age and should check serum IgE levels yearly.[6]

DIAGNOSTIC CHALLENGES

Recognizing specific immunity toward *Aspergillus* antigens is key in making the diagnosis of ABPA. Unfortunately, there is a lack of antigen standardization, and different laboratories use different antigen preparations to establish the diagnosis.[97] Growth conditions, nutrients, culture media, and genetic variation may account for the expression of different proteins under different conditions, which results in variability among laboratories.[98] More than 20 recombinant purified allergens, designated as Asp *f* (1–22), have been produced.[97,99–102] Although some studies look-ing at recombinant allergens have proved promsing,[98–104] others have failed to show a difference.[97,98]

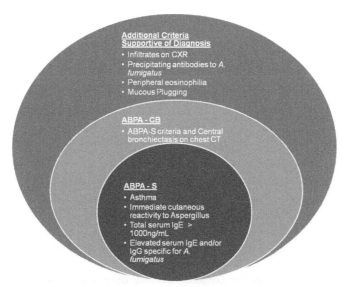

Fig. 5. Diagnostic criteria for ABPA in patients who have asthma (ABPA-S or ABPA-CB). CXR, chest radiograph.

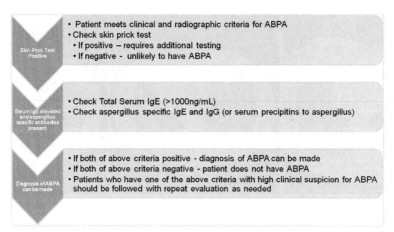

Fig. 6. Laboratory evaluation for patients suspected of having ABPA.

Staging

ABPA is divided into five stages, as described by Patterson and colleagues[88] in 1982. All stages except stage V (fibrosis) are reversible, and the stages do not always progress in order. Stages I, II, and III represent acute disease, remission, and exacerbation, respectively. Patients can present with stage III or IV disease as a result of missing the diagnosis at an earlier point in time.[88] In stage IV, patients usually require continuous oral corticosteroids to keep their symptoms controlled, and steroid-dependent asthmatics are often identified in this phase of the disease. These patients usually have elevated *Aspergillus*-specific IgE/IgG, positive serum precipitins to *Aspergillus*, and persistent pulmonary infiltrates. They may develop CB despite steroid therapy. The dose of steroids prescribed to control their asthma is often not enough to control ABPA, and distinguishing between asthma exacerbation and ABPA flare

can be difficult.[73,88,105] Patients who have prolonged or unrecognized disease may have irreversible damage, including fibrosis, severe bronchiectasis, and cavitation (stage V). These patients can present with clubbing and cyanosis from chronic hypoxia, and their pulmonary function tests may show restriction and irreversible obstructive defects. Steroids are usually not effective at this stage. These patients may also have complicating concomitant infections with *Staphylococcus*, *Pseudomonas*, and non-*Tuberculosis mycobacterium*.[88] Rarely, patients may present with stage V disease. The diagnosis should be considered in asthmatics who have a long history of poorly controlled asthma and are found to have end-stage fibrotic changes with CB.[106]

Treatment

Treatment is focused on limiting the inflammatory response and antigen availability. Treatment is

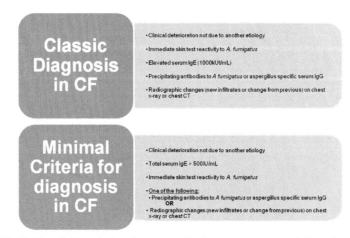

Fig. 7. Summary of Cystic Fibrosis Foundation Consensus Conference recommendations for diagnosis of ABPA in patients who have CF.

similar in asthma and CF, and optimal therapy for these underlying conditions is essential. The goal is to prevent the irreversible fibrotic stage of ABPA. Steroids and antifungals are the two main drug classes used to accomplish these goals, although antifungals serve as an adjuvant therapy. More recently, anti-IgE (omalizumab) has been used successfully in two separate case reports;[107,108] however, no controlled trials using this medication are available. Success of therapy is measured by improvement of symptoms, resolution or improvement of pulmonary infiltrates, disappearance of eosinophilia, a drop in total serum IgE to baseline, and improved lung function.[70,109]

Steroids

Although there are no long-term randomized controlled trials using corticosteroids in the treatment of ABPA, several studies have shown them to be effective in reducing the systemic inflammatory response and in improving bronchospasm in acute exacerbations.[70,109–112]

For patients with acute exacerbations, corticosteroids at a dosage equal to or greater than 0.5 mg/kg are started for a 2-week period. This dosage can be tapered over the next 6 to 8 weeks depending on the patient's response, and alternate-day dosing can be used. Patients receiving steroids should be monitored clinically by symptoms and pulmonary function tests, radiographically, and with serial laboratory assessment (**Fig. 8**). IgE levels and pulmonary infiltrates can take up to 6 to 8 weeks to improve.[6,73] Serum IgE is followed every 6 to 8 weeks for 1 year after the first exacerbation, and an increase in IgE level greater than 100% of the patient's baseline usually signifies exacerbation requiring treatment.[89] Even if successfully treated, IgE levels often remain elevated, and it is important to establish a baseline. It is not necessary to target steroid doses to normalize this value.[73] Some patients have recurrent infiltrates on chest radiographs with no symptoms and should be treated to prevent long-term complications.[70] If patients fail to improve with steroids, physicians should consider misdiagnosis,

suspect noncompliance, or consider using higher dose steroids.[113] Some patients who have steroid-dependent disease (stage IV) require continuous corticosteroid therapy and should be kept on the lowest dose possible to minimize side effects, such as opportunistic infections, osteoporosis, cataracts, hyperglycemia, and weight gain.[109,111,112] Even though steroids seem to mitigate symptoms in acute exacerbations, they have not been shown to prevent progression of disease and are not effective in all patients.[70,88,110] Exacerbations can occur during steroid therapy.[70,110,111,114] Therefore, chronic steroids are not recommended during periods of remission. Acute exacerbations should be treated, and steroids should be tapered off or to the lowest dose tolerated in a timely fashion.

Inhaled corticosteroids may be important as adjuvant therapy, especially in controlling underlying asthma. Some studies have shown inhaled corticosteroids to be effective in controlling symptoms and exacerbation frequency in ABPA; however, other studies have shown inhaled corticosteroids to be less effective.[114–116] Intravenous steroids have also been used in at least one small study to control patients' symptoms.[117]

Antifungals

Antifungal agents may reduce fungal burden in the airways and have been shown to improve symptoms and also to decrease necessary daily steroid doses in ABPA.[118–120] Several studies have been done looking at the efficacy of antifungals for treatment of APBA, including those with nystatin, amphotericin B, clotrimazole, miconazole, ketoconazole, itraconazole, and, more recently, voriconazole and posaconazole. Oral, intravenous, and inhaled preparations have been used. Currently, the most studied and most commonly used antifungal is itraconazole.[15,48,110,119–124]

Itraconazole has been shown to be effective at improving patient symptoms, clearing pulmonary infiltrates on chest radiographs, lowering the required dose of maintenance steroid therapy, and preventing exacerbations.[15,118–120,125] It has a broader spectrum than ketoconazole and has

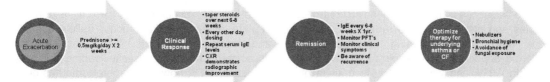

Fig. 8. Treatment of acute exacerbations and management of stable disease. CXR, chest radiograph; PFT, pulmonary function test.

also been shown to prevent progression in steroid-dependent patients, with the most notable side effect being gastrointestinal upset.[119,123]

Two placebo-controlled studies suggested that treatment with itraconazole for 16 weeks improves clinical outcomes and reduces inflammation, at least over the short period studied.[119,122] There was no evidence that itraconazole improved lung function, and longer treatment trials are needed.[124] There are no randomized trials with antifungals available in patients who have CF; however, antifungals have been used effectively to control symptoms in these patients in several studies.[125–127] Nepomuceno and colleagues[127] demonstrated that patients who had CF and were receiving itraconazole had a 47% dose reduction in the daily steroid required and a 55% reduction in acute exacerbations.

At this point, antifungal therapy is recommended as adjuvant therapy for ABPA, especially in those patients requiring high-dose steroids. These patients should be monitored with itraconazole levels and by sputum cultures to ensure that the organism is susceptible to the prescribed therapy, especially if the response is poor.[13] Itraconazole has poor absorption at high pH and may need to be taken with meals. It is important to avoid acid-suppressive therapy, such as a proton pump inhibitor, at the time of dosing.[123] Azole metabolism can interfere with CYP3A4, causing decreased cyclosporine metabolism, impaired glucocorticoid metabolism, and impaired mineralocorticoid synthesis.[128] This can lead to increased levels of exogenous steroid, decreased corticotropin secretion, and adrenal suppression.[128]

Voriconazole is typically used as the treatment of choice in severely immunocompromised patients, and because of a much safer side-effect profile, it has replaced amphotericin B for invasive infections.[129] It has also been demonstrated to be effective in pediatric patients who have CF with ABPA.[130] It is more expensive than amphotericin B and is also limited by its drug-drug interactions, pharmacokinetics, and side-effect profile. Posaconazole is the newest azole agent, with an even better safety profile than voriconazole.[129]

Other therapies

Recently, anti-IgE (omalizumab) has been used with some success. There have been no controlled studies and only a few case reports.[107,108] One case study reported using omalizumab in a steroid-dependent 12-year-old patient who had CF with ABPA and was able to discontinue her steroids.[107] A small case series of three children who had ABPA and CF, who were steroid dependent and all failing to improve with adjuvant itraconazole therapy, showed clinical improvement and tapering off steroids completely after initiation of omalizumab.[108]

Other treatment measures are important in ABPA, including controlling underlying conditions, such as asthma or CF, with optimal inhaler therapy and bronchial hygiene. Immunizations, including pneumococcal vaccine and yearly influenza vaccines, are helpful. Limiting exposure to *Aspergillus* by avoiding areas where the fungus might grow and the use of high-efficiency particulate air filtration units can also help to control disease.[57,131]

Prognosis

For patients who are diagnosed early and treated, the prognosis for ABPA is usually good. Exacerbations can be managed with steroid and antifungal therapy, and these patients do not usually have long-term or irreversible changes in lung function. Few patients progress to stage V, and in these cases, the prognosis is poor. Standard therapy may be of minimal benefit. Underlying lung damage causes irreversible respiratory impairment and can be complicated by chronic bacterial infections.[73,88,105,106] ABPA has also been shown to cause more underlying lung destruction or worse pulmonary function in patients who have concomitant CF.[132]

Future Directions

Thus far, attempts to develop an *Aspergillus* vaccine have been met with limited success.[133] There have been efforts to change the exaggerated Th2 response characterized by production of IgE and eosinophilia toward a Th1 response in an attempt to mitigate the disease process.[54] The presence of certain HLA phenotypes may help to identify patients at risk for ABPA, who should be closely monitored. In addition, understanding how certain HLA types tailor the immune response may help to develop immunotherapy in the future.[19]

ASPERGILLOMA

Aspergilloma is defined as the presence of a fungus ball inside a cavity or dilated airway. Histologically, aspergillomas are a mixture of septate hyphae, fibrin, mucus, cellular debris, and other blood products.[134] The most common associated underlying disease leading to cavity formation is TB; however, aspergilloma has been reported with sarcoidosis, emphysema, bronchiectasis, ankylosing spondylitis, and other prior infections.[135–138]

Initially, aspergillomas were classified as simple or complex;[139] however, more recent guidelines distinguish the two conditions as simple and chronic cavitary pulmonary aspergillosis (CCPA).[140] Simple aspergillomas are encased by thin-walled cysts with little surrounding parenchyma disease, whereas CCPA is associated with thick walls, multiple cavities, and surrounding parenchymal changes.

Clinical Features

Some aspergillomas are asymptomatic and seen as an incidental finding on radiographic studies. The most common symptom associated with simple aspergilloma is hemoptysis. Hemoptysis is reported in 69% to 83% of cases in two of the largest studies and ranges from extremely mild to life threatening.[141,142] Other associated symptoms are fever, weight loss, malaise, and clubbing.[138] These symptoms may be associated with the underlying lung disease itself, however.

Pathophysiology

In most cases, the hemoptysis associated with aspergillomas is believed to be from a bronchial arterial source. Speculation about the underlying mechanisms involved has included damage to arteries from the fungal ball rolling around in the cavity or localized invasion of surrounding blood vessels.[13,68] One recent pathologic review of 41 patients suggests that the source of bleeding may be the anastomotic plexus between pulmonary and bronchial arteries.[134]

Natural History

Aspergillus commonly seems to colonize old cavitary lung lesions. One large retrospective review of patients with preexisting cavitary disease from prior TB infection showed that 11% to 25% had evidence of *Aspergillus* colonization (25% with serum precipitins for *Aspergillus* and 11%–14% with radiographic evidence of aspergillomas.)[142] As the incidence of TB has declined, the occurrence of aspergilloma may also be declining.[143]

Some patients who have aspergilloma remain relatively asymptomatic. One analysis of 41 patients at a single institution over 26 years showed a favorable prognosis for those patients who had absence of symptoms or no superimposed bacterial infections or in those who received surgery. They reported 5 asymptomatic patients who demonstrated no progression in disease.[144] Other reviews have also reported patients without progression and those who had spontaneous resolution.[141,142]

Patients who have aspergillomas are more likely to have chronic cough and hemoptysis, which can be quite severe at times.[142] One study of 23 patients revealed chronic cough as the most common symptom, with hemoptysis also being frequent (12 of 23 patients).[138] The investigators reported 5 patients who progressed to invasive disease and five deaths directly attributed to aspergillomas (2 patients who had invasive disease, 2 who had massive hemoptysis, and 1 patient after surgery for massive hemoptysis).[138]

Mortality in patients who have aspergillomas has been reported to be 5% to 6% per year. Jewkes and colleagues[141] retrospectively reviewed 85 cases over 24 years and reported 56% overall mortality over 10 years, with 10 deaths directly attributable to aspergillomas (3 attributable to hemoptysis in medically treated patients and 7 after surgery). Another large study reported 18% mortality over 3 years. This rate closely mirrored that of patients with old tuberculous cavities without aspergillomas. The increased mortality in this population is likely attributable to the age of the patients and underlying comorbid lung disease.

Another outcome is progression of disease beyond a simple aspergilloma. It is likely that there is a spectrum of lung disease ranging from a simple fungal ball to invasive aspergillosis, with semi-invasive disease (CPA) in the middle. Progression of aspergilloma to a chronic necrotizing form or to invasive aspergillosis is a particular concern in neutropenic patients. Kibbler and colleagues[145] presented 4 cases and reviewed the literature (including another 34 cases) for aspergillomas in neutropenic patients. The most common underlying diagnosis was acute myelogenous leukemia. They report hemoptysis occurring in approximately 50% and approximately 25% mortality for neutropenic patients who develop aspergillomas. They suggest the term *mycotic lung sequestration*, because these lesions are not formed in a preexisting cavity but rather develop from necrotic lung tissue with fungal invasion.[145] Another study looked at aspergillomas in HIV-infected patients and found that hemoptysis was less common (although still present in 10% of patients). Disease progression was more likely in HIV, however, and specifically in the subset of patients with a CD4+ count less than 100 cells/mm^3 blood.[146] Two cases of aspergilloma have been reported after single lung transplantation, both of which had symptoms of hemoptysis.[147] Because of the concern for progression of disease, immunosuppressed patients who have aspergilloma should be monitored closely and may need to be treated as if they have chronic pulmonary or invasive aspergillosis with antifungal therapy or surgery.

Diagnosis

Diagnosis of aspergilloma is usually made by classic radiographic findings, but *Aspergillus* precipitins (IgG) are also usually detectable and BALF or sputum cultures are often positive. On a CT scan, an aspergilloma appears as a ball within a cavity. If the patient is rotated during the scan, the aspergilloma often moves because it can be mobile within the cavity.[148]

Treatment

Simple aspergilloma in a nonimmunocompromised patient with no symptoms does not usually require treatment. The most recent Infectious Diseases Society of America (IDSA) guidelines support this and recommend treatment if disease progresses or the patient develops hemoptysis. Itraconazole or voriconazole is recommended as the agent in this case. The guidelines also discuss surgical resection, bronchial artery embolization (BAE), or intracavitary therapies as options for patients who have hemoptysis.[140]

Medical

Itraconazole has been used for chronic forms of aspergillosis, including aspergillomas, with some success. In one study, encouraging results were noted in a small number of patients who received greater than 6 months of therapy, but no improvement was reported in those who discontinued treatment before 6 months.[149] Another study examined 14 patients on itraconazole therapy for greater than 6 months and demonstrated improvement in 8, with cure in 2.[150] Voriconazole may be preferred based on studies in CPA as discussed elsewhere in this article.

Several studies in neutropenic patients seem to support combined medical and surgical intervention, but this is based on a small and limited number of studies. Interestingly, one study compared surgery in 20 patients who had aspergilloma with previous TB infection versus that in 10 patients who had acute leukemia.[151] In the leukemia group, there was 0% morbidity or mortality, compared with one postoperative death and 25% morbidity in the post-TB group. Others studies support surgical intervention in localized aspergillosis for neutropenic patients, even in the case of invasive aspergillosis.[152,153]

Surgical

Many surgical procedures have been used to treat aspergillomas. These have included lobectomy, segmentectomy, pneumonectomy, and cavernostomy. Because the approach is difficult, surgery is not thought of first-line therapy, and the literature has reported high morbidity and mortality, although this seems to have improved over time.[139,143] **Table 2** summarizes nine studies published since 2000 regarding surgical treatment for aspergillomas.[154–162] Overall, there were 537 patients who underwent surgical resection of aspergillomas. The indication for surgery was hemoptysis in 73% of patients. The most common underlying lung disease was TB (57%). Most of the studies reported the number of complex or simple aspergillomas in their series. Of 456 cases for which this information was available (all but one study), there were 300 cases of complex and 156 cases of simple aspergillomas. Averaging the nine studies, mortality was 2.3%. Looking the 156 cases of simple aspergilloma alone, however, mortality was less than 1%. High complication rates remain problematic for surgical intervention. The overall morbidity in these nine studies was 30.3%. The most common complications were prolonged air leak, hemorrhage, empyema, incomplete lung reexpansion, wound infection, respiratory insufficiency, and chylothorax. Because of the high morbidity associated with surgery, this should be reserved for carefully selected patients with low surgical risk.

Embolization

Although BAE has been used successfully to stop bleeding in some conditions, the results have not been as promising for patients who have aspergilloma.[163] Kim and colleagues[164] reviewed 118 patients who were followed for 1 year after BAE for hemoptysis. The only significant factor associated with rebleeding (32 patients) was the presence of aspergilloma, leading them to favor surgical intervention over BAE for patients who have aspergilloma and massive hemoptysis. Others have reported success with BAE and acryl microspheres; however, researchers recommend this as a short-term treatment in preparation for (not replacement of) surgery.[165] IDSA guidelines recommend BAE as a short-term therapy to stabilize patients for more definitive treatment, including surgery.[140]

Interventional

Several researchers have reported on the use of intracavitary amphotericin B for aspergillomas,[166–169] with some success, whereas others have not had encouraging results.[137,170] One group reported good results using an amphotericin paste. Of 40 patients, 35 had clinical improvement and all had resolution of hemoptysis.[171]

Table 2
Recent surgical outcomes for aspergilloma

Year Published	Study Years	No. Patients/No. Operations	Simple Aspergilloma (SA)	Complex Aspergilloma (CA)	Morbidity % Total (SA/CA)	Mortality % Total (SA/CA)
2008	2001–2008	42	12	30	28.5 (25/30)	2.4 (0/3.3)
2006	1992–2006	24	8	16	41.6	4.2
2006	1976–2004	31	17	14	19	0
2006	1999–2004	11	0	11	18.2	0
2005	1981–1999	88	16	72	24	1.1
2005	1985–2003	60	14	46	20 (0/26.1)	3.3 (0/4.3)
2002	1987–2000	110	81	29	23.6	0
2000	1959–1988	84/90	NR	NR	64	4
2000	1977–1997	87/89	8	82	33.7	5.6

Abbreviation: NR, not reported.

CHRONIC PULMONARY ASPERGILLOSIS

Although invasive aspergillosis and ABPA are fairly well defined, chronic forms of *Aspergillus* infection span a wide range of clinical presentations and histopathologic findings. As mentioned previously, the surgical literature has broken aspergillomas into simple (thin-walled with fungus ball alone) and complex (CCPA; thick-walled with surrounding parenchymal infiltration). Chronic necrotizing aspergillosis (CNA), also known as semi-invasive aspergillosis, is thought to be a distinct form of disease. CNA has been defined as slowly progressive inflammation and destruction of lung tissue attributable to *Aspergillus* in patients who have underlying lung disease and mild degrees of immunosuppression. Distinguishing CCPA and CNA becomes difficult, however, because there is much overlap between these conditions.[148] Recent IDSA guidelines distinguish them based on chronicity and genetic differences leading to defects in the innate immune system in CCPA. For this review, the authors discuss CCPA and CNA together as CPA. This approach has been used by others as well.[172]

Clinical Features

The clinical course for CPA is less dramatic and more indolent than for invasive pulmonary aspergillosis (IPA). Patients often present with symptoms of fever, weight loss, cough, chronic sputum production, or hemoptysis.[173] Other less common symptoms include chest pain or dyspnea. Symptoms are usually present between 1 and 6 months before the diagnosis is made.[173,174] Symptoms of CPA differ from those of IPA because of the indolent nature of the disease. Clinical symptoms and lung destruction may progress over months to years.[174,175] CCPA has been reported to develop into pulmonary fibrosis in some patients.[176]

Pathophysiology

Defects in the innate immune system may predispose to CPA. Polymorphisms in mannose-binding lectin, SP-A, and toll-like receptors have been associated with CCPA.[177–179] Mild degrees of immunosuppression may also lead to chronic forms of pulmonary aspergillosis. Patients often have underlying lung disease or systemic conditions, such as COPD, diabetes mellitus, chronic steroid use, HIV, alcohol abuse, or advanced age.[174,180] CNA has also been reported complicating previous pulmonary *Mycobacterium avium* complex disease and cryptococcal infection.[181,182] A history of occupational lung disease may also contribute to risk.[175]

Diagnosis

Upper lobe infiltrates are the most common radiographic abnormalities; however, cavitation, nodular opacities, and pleural thickening may also be seen.[183,184] Gradually expanding cavities with surrounding pleural thickening and parenchymal inflammation have also been described.[185] As cavitation develops, there may be an associated "crescent sign," and, later, there is often mycetoma formation associated with CNA.[174,176,185]

Aspergillus precipitins are usually positive with disease but are not specific. Positive cultures are desired for the diagnosis. Sputum cultures, bronchoalveolar lavage cultures, and surgical biopsy specimens may reveal the organism. The diagnosis can be made in the appropriate clinical setting in patients with compatible radiographs and positive cultures for *Aspergillus*. A pathologic examination demonstrating tissue invasion with fungal hyphae is confirmatory, however. Surgical biopsy has been reported most often, but transbronchial biopsies may also be diagnostic.[180,186]

Yousem[187] described the pathologic manifestations in 10 patients who had chronic necrotizing forms of pulmonary aspergillosis. He classified the pathologic findings into three distinct entities: necrotizing granulomatous pneumonia, granulomatous bronchiectatic cavities, and bronchocentric granulomatosis. Others have described the histologic findings as active parenchymal inflammation, intra-alveolar hemorrhage, tissue necrosis, and *Aspergillus* organisms.[183]

Treatment

Current recommendations for treatment of CPA include oral therapy using one of the triazoles, with voriconazole being the drug of choice.[140] Several studies have examined the use of voriconazole in the treatment of chronic forms of aspergillosis.[188] Camuset and colleagues[188] looked at 24 patients who had chronic forms of aspergillosis (9 who had CCPA and 15 who had CNA). Voriconazole was given as first-line therapy (13 patients) or after a failure of another treatment (11 patients). They reported 67% clinical improvement, which compares favorably with historical controls treated with itraconazole. Two similar studies showed voriconazole to be effective in CCPA, with a partial response rate of 67% (10 of 15 patients)[189] and 64% (7 of 11 patients).[190]

The use of interferon-γ (IFNγ) for chronic aspergillosis has also been reported. One study reported three patients who had a clinical response with the addition of IFNγ to antifungal therapy.[176] Another two patients have been reported with defective IFNγ responses from peripheral blood mononuclear cells, who responded to the addition of subcutaneous IFNγ to systemic antifungals.[191]

Surgical intervention has been used in a limited number of studies. One study reported 0% mortality and 30% morbidity in 10 patients. The indication for resection was prolonged illness in 4 patients and hemoptysis in the other 6 patients. These results are similar to those for CCPA.[192] Similar to aspergilloma, the morbidity and mortality risks of the procedure should be carefully weighed with possible benefits and surgery should be reserved for those who develop severe hemoptysis.

SUMMARY

Pulmonary aspergillosis can cause a wide spectrum of disease depending on underlying host immune function. This includes allergic or hypersensitivity reactions (ABPA), saprophytic infections (aspergilloma), and chronic disease (CPA). ABPA is most commonly seen in patients who have asthma or CF and results from a combination of cellular, humoral, and cytokine interactions. Patients may have refractory respiratory symptoms, fleeting infiltrates, elevated IgE, and eosinophilia. Early diagnosis is essential to prevent advanced disease and is made by specific clinical, radiographic, and laboratory assessments. The mainstay of treatment is corticosteroids, and antifungal agents are used as adjuvant therapy. New medications like anti-IgE (omalizumab) and continued efforts in defining the immunopathogenesis should lead to new therapies down the road. Aspergillomas commonly occur in patients with a previous history of cavitary lung disease. The most serious complication can be life-threatening hemoptysis. Antifungals have been used with some success, but more serious cases may require interventional therapies, including bronchial arterial embolization or surgery. CPA bridges the gap between invasive and noninvasive disease. It is usually seen with mild degrees of immunosuppression, including COPD, diabetes mellitus, and chronic steroid use. The clinical course may be indolent, and successful therapy has been employed using triazole antifungal agents.

REFERENCES

1. Hohl TM, Feldmesser M. *Aspergillus fumigatus*: principles of pathogenesis and host defense. Eukaryot Cell 2007;6(11):1953–63.

2. Latge JP. *Aspergillus fumigatus* and aspergillosis. Clin Microbiol Rev 1999;12(2):310–50.

3. Soubani AO, Chandrasekar PH. The clinical spectrum of pulmonary aspergillosis. Chest 2002; 121(6):1988–99.

4. Hinson KF, Moon AJ, Plummer NS. Broncho-pulmonary aspergillosis; a review and a report of eight new cases. Thorax 1952;7(4):317–33.

5. Denning DW, O'Driscoll BR, Hogaboam CM, et al. The link between fungi and severe asthma: a summary of the evidence. Eur Respir J 2006; 27(3):615–26.

6. Stevens DA, Moss RB, Kurup VP, et al. Allergic bronchopulmonary aspergillosis in cystic fibrosis—state of the art: Cystic Fibrosis Foundation Consensus Conference. Clin Infect Dis 2003; 37(Suppl 3):S225–64.

7. Greenberger PA, Smith LJ, Hsu CC, et al. Analysis of bronchoalveolar lavage in allergic bronchopulmonary aspergillosis: divergent responses of antigen-specific antibodies and total IgE. J Allergy Clin Immunol 1988;82(2):164–70.

8. Eaton T, Garrett J, Milne D, et al. Allergic bronchopulmonary aspergillosis in the asthma clinic. A prospective evaluation of CT in the diagnostic algorithm. Chest 2000;118(1):66–72.

9. Schwartz HJ, Greenberger PA. The prevalence of allergic bronchopulmonary aspergillosis in patients with asthma, determined by serologic and radiologic criteria in patients at risk. J Lab Clin Med 1991;117(2):138–42.

10. Henderson AH. Allergic aspergillosis: review of 32 cases. Thorax 1968;23(5):501–12.

11. Moss RB. Allergic bronchopulmonary aspergillosis. Clin Rev Allergy Immunol 2002;23(1):87–104.

12. Glancy JJ, Elder JL, McAleer R. Allergic bronchopulmonary fungal disease without clinical asthma. Thorax 1981;36(5):345–9.

13. Judson MA. Noninvasive Aspergillus pulmonary disease. Semin Respir Crit Care Med 2004;25(2): 203–19.

14. Slavin RG, Bedrossian CW, Hutcheson PS, et al. A pathologic study of allergic bronchopulmonary aspergillosis. J Allergy Clin Immunol 1988;81(4): 718–25.

15. Tillie-Leblond I, Tonnel AB. Allergic bronchopulmonary aspergillosis. Allergy 2005;60(8): 1004–13.

16. Graves TS, Fink JN, Patterson R, et al. A familial occurrence of allergic bronchopulmonary aspergillosis. Ann Intern Med 1979;91(3):378–82.

17. Halwig JM, Kurup VP, Greenberger PA, et al. A familial occurrence of allergic bronchopulmonary aspergillosis: a probable environmental source. J Allergy Clin Immunol 1985;76(1):55–9.

18. Chauhan B, Santiago L, Kirschmann DA, et al. The association of HLA-DR alleles and T cell activation with allergic bronchopulmonary aspergillosis. J Immunol 1997;159(8):4072–6.

19. Chauhan B, Santiago L, Hutcheson PS, et al. Evidence for the involvement of two different MHC class II regions in susceptibility or protection in allergic bronchopulmonary aspergillosis. J Allergy Clin Immunol 2000;106(4):723–9.

20. Khan MA, Mathieu A, Sorrentino R, et al. The pathogenetic role of HLA-B27 and its subtypes. Autoimmun Rev 2007;6(3):183–9.

21. Wen L, Wong FS, Tang J, et al. In vivo evidence for the contribution of human histocompatibility leukocyte antigen (HLA)-DQ molecules to the development of diabetes. J Exp Med 2000; 191(1):97–104.

22. Raju R, Munn SR, David CS. T cell recognition of human pre-proinsulin peptides depends on the polymorphism at HLA DQ locus: a study using HLA DQ8 and DQ6 transgenic mice. Hum Immunol 1997;58(1):21–9.

23. Chauhan B, Hutcheson PS, Slavin RG, et al. MHC restriction in allergic bronchopulmonary aspergillosis. Front Biosci 2003;8:s140–8.

24. Miller PW, Hamosh A, Macek M Jr, et al. Cystic fibrosis transmembrane conductance regulator (CFTR) gene mutations in allergic bronchopulmonary aspergillosis. Am J Hum Genet 1996;59(1): 45–51.

25. Marchand E, Verellen-Dumoulin C, Mairesse M, et al. Frequency of cystic fibrosis transmembrane conductance regulator gene mutations and 5T allele in patients with allergic bronchopulmonary aspergillosis. Chest 2001;119(3):762–7.

26. Saxena S, Madan T, Shah A, et al. Association of polymorphisms in the collagen region of SP-A2 with increased levels of total IgE antibodies and eosinophilia in patients with allergic bronchopulmonary aspergillosis. J Allergy Clin Immunol 2003; 111(5):1001–7.

27. Chauhan B, Knutsen A, Hutcheson PS, et al. T cell subsets, epitope mapping, and HLA-restriction in patients with allergic bronchopulmonary aspergillosis. J Clin Invest 1996;97(10):2324–31.

28. Berkin KE, Vernon DR, Kerr JW. Lung collapse caused by allergic bronchopulmonary aspergillosis in non-asthmatic patients. Br Med J (Clin Res Ed) 1982;285(6341):552–3.

29. Schubert MS. Allergic fungal sinusitis. Clin Rev Allergy Immunol 2006;30(3):205–16.

30. Braun JJ, Pauli G, Schultz P, et al. Allergic fungal sinusitis associated with allergic bronchopulmonary aspergillosis: an uncommon sinobronchial allergic mycosis. Am J Rhinol 2007;21(4):412–6.

31. deShazo RD, Chapin K, Swain RE. Fungal sinusitis. N Engl J Med 1997;337(4):254–9.

32. Sher TH, Schwartz HJ. Allergic Aspergillus sinusitis with concurrent allergic bronchopulmonary

Aspergillus: report of a case. J Allergy Clin Immunol 1988;81(5 Pt 1):844–6.

33. Grammer LC, Greenberger PA, Patterson R. Allergic bronchopulmonary aspergillosis in asthmatic patients presenting with allergic rhinitis. Int Arch Allergy Appl Immunol 1986;79(3):246–8.

34. Knutsen AP, Bellone C, Kauffman H. Immunopathogenesis of allergic bronchopulmonary aspergillosis in cystic fibrosis. J Cyst Fibros 2002; 1(2):76–89.

35. Beaumont F, Kauffman HF, van der Mark TH, et al. Volumetric aerobiological survey of conidial fungi in the North-East Netherlands. I. Seasonal patterns and the influence of meteorological variables. Allergy 1985;40(3):173–80.

36. Robertson MD, Seaton A, Milne LJ, et al. Suppression of host defences by Aspergillus fumigatus. Thorax 1987;42(1):19–25.

37. Robertson MD, Seaton A, Milne LJ, et al. Resistance of spores of Aspergillus fumigatus to ingestion by phagocytic cells. Thorax 1987;42(6):466–72.

38. Roilides E, Uhlig K, Venzon D, et al. Prevention of corticosteroid-induced suppression of human polymorphonuclear leukocyte-induced damage of Aspergillus fumigatus hyphae by granulocyte colony-stimulating factor and gamma interferon. Infect Immun 1993;61(11):4870–7.

39. Fraser RS. Pulmonary aspergillosis: pathologic and pathogenetic features. Pathol Annu 1993;28(Pt 1): 231–77.

40. Kauffman HF, Tomee JF, van der Werf TS, et al. Review of fungus-induced asthmatic reactions. Am J Respir Crit Care Med 1995;151(6):2109–15 [discussion: 2116].

41. Kauffman HF. Immunopathogenesis of allergic bronchopulmonary aspergillosis and airway remodeling. Front Biosci 2003;8:e190–6.

42. Tomee JF, Wierenga AT, Hiemstra PS, et al. Proteases from Aspergillus fumigatus induce release of proinflammatory cytokines and cell detachment in airway epithelial cell lines. J Infect Dis 1997; 176(1):300–3.

43. Kauffman HF, Tomee JF, van de Riet MA, et al. Protease-dependent activation of epithelial cells by fungal allergens leads to morphologic changes and cytokine production. J Allergy Clin Immunol 2000;105(6 Pt 1):1185–93.

44. Malo JL, Inouye T, Hawkins R, et al. Studies in chronic allergic bronchopulmonary aspergillosis. 4. Comparison with a group of asthmatics. Thorax 1977;32(3):275–80.

45. McCarthy DS, Pepys J. Allergic broncho-pulmonary aspergillosis. Clinical immunology. 2. Skin, nasal and bronchial tests. Clin Allergy 1971;1(4): 415–32.

46. Gibson PG, Wark PA, Simpson JL, et al. Induced sputum IL-8 gene expression, neutrophil influx and MMP-9 in allergic bronchopulmonary aspergillosis. Eur Respir J 2003;21(4):582–8.

47. Malo JL, Hawkins R, Pepys J. Studies in chronic allergic bronchopulmonary aspergillosis. 1. Clinical and physiological findings. Thorax 1977;32(3): 254–61.

48. Vlahakis NE, Aksamit TR. Diagnosis and treatment of allergic bronchopulmonary aspergillosis. Mayo Clin Proc 2001;76(9):930–8.

49. Schuyler MR. Allergic bronchopulmonary aspergillosis. Clin Chest Med 1983;4(1):15–22.

50. Wark PA, Saltos N, Simpson J, et al. Induced sputum eosinophils and neutrophils and bronchiectasis severity in allergic bronchopulmonary aspergillosis. Eur Respir J 2000;16(6): 1095–101.

51. Chu HW, Wang JM, Boutet M, et al. Immunohistochemical detection of GM-CSF, IL-4 and IL-5 in a murine model of allergic bronchopulmonary aspergillosis. Clin Exp Allergy 1996;26(4):461–8.

52. Schuyler M. The Th1/Th2 paradigm in allergic bronchopulmonary aspergillosis. J Lab Clin Med 1998; 131(3):194–6.

53. Kurup VP, Grunig G, Knutsen AP, et al. Cytokines in allergic bronchopulmonary aspergillosis. Res Immunol 1998;149(4–5):466–77 [discussion: 515–466].

54. Berger A. Th1 and Th2 responses: what are they? BMJ 2000;321(7258):424.

55. Knutsen AP, Mueller KR, Levine AD, et al. Asp f I CD4 + TH2-like T-cell lines in allergic bronchopulmonary aspergillosis. J Allergy Clin Immunol 1994;94(2 Pt 1):215–21.

56. Khan S, McClellan JS, Knutsen AP. Increased sensitivity to IL-4 in patients with allergic bronchopulmonary aspergillosis. Int Arch Allergy Immunol 2000;123(4):319–26.

57. Moss RB. Pathophysiology and immunology of allergic bronchopulmonary aspergillosis. Med Mycol 2005;43(Suppl 1):S203–6.

58. Greenberger PA, Liotta JL, Roberts M. The effects of age on isotypic antibody responses to Aspergillus fumigatus: implications regarding in vitro measurements. J Lab Clin Med 1989;114(3):278–84.

59. Patterson R, Rosenberg M, Roberts M. Evidence that Aspergillus fumigatus growing in the airway of man can be a potent stimulus of specific and nonspecific IgE formation. Am J Med 1977;63(2):257–62.

60. Knutsen AP. Lymphocytes in allergic bronchopulmonary aspergillosis. Front Biosci 2003;8: d589–602.

61. Knutsen AP, Hutchinson PS, Albers GM, et al. Increased sensitivity to IL-4 in cystic fibrosis patients with allergic bronchopulmonary aspergillosis. Allergy 2004;59(1):81–7.

62. Schuh JM, Blease K, Kunkel SL, et al. Chemokines and cytokines: axis and allies in asthma and allergy. Cytokine Growth Factor Rev 2003;14(6):503–10.

63. Grunig G, Kurup VP. Animal models of allergic bronchopulmonary aspergillosis. Front Biosci 2003;8:e157–71.

64. Kradin RL, Mark EJ. The pathology of pulmonary disorders due to Aspergillus spp. Arch Pathol Lab Med 2008;132(4):606–14.

65. Jelihovsky T. The structure of bronchial plugs in mucoid impaction, bronchocentric granulomatosis and asthma. Histopathology 1983;7(2):153–67.

66. Bosken CH, Myers JL, Greenberger PA, et al. Pathologic features of allergic bronchopulmonary aspergillosis. Am J Surg Pathol 1988;12(3):216–22.

67. Zander DS. Allergic bronchopulmonary aspergillosis: an overview. Arch Pathol Lab Med 2005;129(7):924–8.

68. Zmeili OS, Soubani AO. Pulmonary aspergillosis: a clinical update. QJM 2007;100(6):317–34.

69. Rosenberg IL, Greenberger PA. Allergic bronchopulmonary aspergillosis and aspergilloma. Long-term follow-up without enlargement of a large multiloculated cavity. Chest 1984;85(1):123–5.

70. Safirstein BH, D'Souza MF, Simon G, et al. Five-year follow-up of allergic bronchopulmonary aspergillosis. Am Rev Respir Dis 1973;108(3):450–9.

71. Slavin RG, Hutcheson PS, Chauhan B, et al. An overview of allergic bronchopulmonary aspergillosis with some new insights. Allergy Asthma Proc 2004;25(6):395–9.

72. Malo JL, Longbottom J, Mitchell J, et al. Studies in chronic allergic bronchopulmonary aspergillosis. 3. Immunological findings. Thorax 1977;32(3):269–74.

73. Greenberger PA. Allergic bronchopulmonary aspergillosis. J Allergy Clin Immunol 2002;110(5):685–92.

74. Schwartz HJ, Citron KM, Chester EH, et al. A comparison of the prevalence of sensitization to Aspergillus antigens among asthmatics in Cleveland and London. J Allergy Clin Immunol 1978;62(1):9–14.

75. Bahous J, Malo JL, Paquin R, et al. Allergic bronchopulmonary aspergillosis and sensitization to *Aspergillus fumigatus* in chronic bronchiectasis in adults. Clin Allergy 1985;15(6):571–9.

76. McCarthy DS, Simon G, Hargreave FE. The radiological appearances in allergic broncho-pulmonary aspergillosis. Clin Radiol 1970;21(4):366–75.

77. Neeld DA, Goodman LR, Gurney JW, et al. Computerized tomography in the evaluation of allergic bronchopulmonary aspergillosis. Am Rev Respir Dis 1990;142(5):1200–5.

78. Malo JL, Pepys J, Simon G. Studies in chronic allergic bronchopulmonary aspergillosis. 2. Radiological findings. Thorax 1977;32(3):262–8.

79. Buckingham SJ, Hansell DM. Aspergillus in the lung: diverse and coincident forms. Eur Radiol 2003;13(8):1786–800.

80. Angus RM, Davies ML, Cowan MD, et al. Computed tomographic scanning of the lung in patients with allergic bronchopulmonary aspergillosis and in asthmatic patients with a positive skin test to *Aspergillus fumigatus*. Thorax 1994;49(6):586–9.

81. Ward S, Heyneman L, Lee MJ, et al. Accuracy of CT in the diagnosis of allergic bronchopulmonary aspergillosis in asthmatic patients. AJR Am J Roentgenol 1999;173(4):937–42.

82. Franquet T, Muller NL, Gimenez A, et al. Spectrum of pulmonary aspergillosis: histologic, clinical, and radiologic findings. Radiographics 2001;21(4):825–37.

83. Currie DC, Goldman JM, Cole PJ, et al. Comparison of narrow section computed tomography and plain chest radiography in chronic allergic bronchopulmonary aspergillosis. Clin Radiol 1987;38(6):593–6.

84. Sandhu M, Mukhopadhyay S, Sharma SK. Allergic bronchopulmonary aspergillosis: a comparative evaluation of computed tomography with plain chest radiography. Australas Radiol 1994;38(4):288–93.

85. Cortese G, Malfitana V, Placido R, et al. Role of chest radiography in the diagnosis of allergic bronchopulmonary aspergillosis in adult patients with cystic fibrosis. Radiol Med 2007;112(5):626–36.

86. Nichols D, Dopico GA, Braun S, et al. Acute and chronic pulmonary function changes in allergic bronchopulmonary aspergillosis. Am J Med 1979;67(4):631–7.

87. Kraemer R, Delosea N, Ballinari P, et al. Effect of allergic bronchopulmonary aspergillosis on lung function in children with cystic fibrosis. Am J Respir Crit Care Med 2006;174(11):1211–20.

88. Patterson R, Greenberger PA, Radin RC, et al. Allergic bronchopulmonary aspergillosis: staging as an aid to management. Ann Intern Med 1982;96(3):286–91.

89. Patterson R, Greenberger PA, Halwig JM, et al. Allergic bronchopulmonary aspergillosis. Natural history and classification of early disease by serologic and roentgenographic studies. Arch Intern Med 1986;146(5):916–8.

90. Greenberger PA, Miller TP, Roberts M, et al. Allergic bronchopulmonary aspergillosis in patients with and without evidence of bronchiectasis. Ann Allergy 1993;70(4):333–8.

91. Hoehne JH, Reed CE, Dickie HA. Allergic bronchopulmonary aspergillosis is not rare. With a note on preparation of antigen for immunologic tests. Chest 1973;63(2):177–81.

92. Nguyen MH, Jaber R, Leather HL, et al. Use of bronchoalveolar lavage to detect galactomannan for diagnosis of pulmonary aspergillosis among nonimmunocompromised hosts. J Clin Microbiol 2007;45(9):2787–92.

93. Wark P. Pathogenesis of allergic bronchopulmonary aspergillosis and an evidence-based review of azoles in treatment. Respir Med 2004;98(10):915–23.

94. Nikolaizik WH, Moser M, Crameri R, et al. Identification of allergic bronchopulmonary aspergillosis in cystic fibrosis patients by recombinant *Aspergillus fumigatus* I/a-specific serology. Am J Respir Crit Care Med 1995;152(2):634–9.

95. Zeaske R, Bruns WT, Fink JN, et al. Immune responses to Aspergillus in cystic fibrosis. J Allergy Clin Immunol 1988;82(1):73–7.

96. Hutcheson PS, Rejent AJ, Slavin RG. Variability in parameters of allergic bronchopulmonary aspergillosis in patients with cystic fibrosis. J Allergy Clin Immunol 1991;88(3 Pt 1):390–4.

97. de Oliveira E, Giavina-Bianchi P, Fonseca LA, et al. Allergic bronchopulmonary aspergillosis' diagnosis remains a challenge. Respir Med 2007;101(11):2352–7.

98. Kurup VP. Aspergillus antigens: which are important? Med Mycol 2005;43(Suppl 1):S189–96.

99. Banerjee B, Kurup VP, Greenberger PA, et al. Cloning and expression of *Aspergillus fumigatus* allergen Asp f 16 mediating both humoral and cell-mediated immunity in allergic bronchopulmonary aspergillosis (ABPA). Clin Exp Allergy 2001; 31(5):761–70.

100. Hemmann S, Menz G, Ismail C, et al. Skin test reactivity to 2 recombinant Aspergillus fumigatus allergens in A fumigatus-sensitized asthmatic subjects allows diagnostic separation of allergic bronchopulmonary aspergillosis from fungal sensitization. J Allergy Clin Immunol 1999;104(3 Pt 1):601–7.

101. Knutsen AP, Hutcheson PS, Slavin RG, et al. IgE antibody to *Aspergillus fumigatus* recombinant allergens in cystic fibrosis patients with allergic bronchopulmonary aspergillosis. Allergy 2004; 59(2):198–203.

102. Kurup VP, Banerjee B, Hemmann S, et al. Selected recombinant *Aspergillus fumigatus* allergens bind specifically to IgE in ABPA. Clin Exp Allergy 2000; 30(7):988–93.

103. Crameri R, Hemmann S, Ismail C, et al. Disease-specific recombinant allergens for the diagnosis of allergic bronchopulmonary aspergillosis. Int Immunol 1998;10(8):1211–6.

104. Kurup VP, Knutsen AP, Moss RB, et al. Specific antibodies to recombinant allergens of *Aspergillus fumigatus* in cystic fibrosis patients with ABPA. Clin Mol Allergy 2006;4:11.

105. Greenberger PA, Patterson R. Diagnosis and management of allergic bronchopulmonary aspergillosis. Ann Allergy 1986;56(6):444–8.

106. Lee TM, Greenberger PA, Patterson R, et al. Stage V (fibrotic) allergic bronchopulmonary aspergillosis. A review of 17 cases followed from diagnosis. Arch Intern Med 1987;147(2):319–23.

107. van der Ent CK, Hoekstra H, Rijkers GT. Successful treatment of allergic bronchopulmonary aspergillosis with recombinant anti-IgE antibody. Thorax 2007;62(3):276–7.

108. Zirbes JM, Milla CE. Steroid-sparing effect of omalizumab for allergic bronchopulmonary aspergillosis and cystic fibrosis. Pediatr Pulmonol 2008; 43(6):607–10.

109. Capewell S, Chapman BJ, Alexander F, et al. Corticosteroid treatment and prognosis in pulmonary eosinophilia. Thorax 1989;44(11):925–9.

110. Wark PA, Gibson PG. Allergic bronchopulmonary aspergillosis: new concepts of pathogenesis and treatment. Respirology 2001;6(1):1–7.

111. Wang JL, Patterson R, Roberts M, et al. The management of allergic bronchopulmonary aspergillosis. Am Rev Respir Dis 1979;120(1):87–92.

112. Rosenberg M, Patterson R, Roberts M, et al. The assessment of immunologic and clinical changes occurring during corticosteroid therapy for allergic bronchopulmonary aspergillosis. Am J Med 1978; 64(4):599–606.

113. Ricketti AJ, Greenberger PA, Patterson R. Serum IgE as an important aid in management of allergic bronchopulmonary aspergillosis. J Allergy Clin Immunol 1984;74(1):68–71.

114. Inhaled beclomethasone dipropionate in allergic bronchopulmonary aspergillosis. Report to the Research Committee of the British Thoracic Association. Br J Dis Chest 1979;73(4):349–56.

115. Hilton AM, Chatterjee SS. Bronchopulmonary aspergillosis—treatment with beclomethasone dipropionate. Postgrad Med J 1975;51(Suppl 4): 98–103.

116. Seaton A, Seaton RA, Wightman AJ. Management of allergic bronchopulmonary aspergillosis without maintenance oral corticosteroids: a fifteen-year follow-up. QJM 1994;87(9):529–37.

117. Thomson JM, Wesley A, Byrnes CA, et al. Pulse intravenous methylprednisolone for resistant allergic bronchopulmonary aspergillosis in cystic fibrosis. Pediatr Pulmonol 2006;41(2):164–70.

118. Salez F, Brichet A, Desurmont S, et al. Effects of itraconazole therapy in allergic bronchopulmonary aspergillosis. Chest 1999;116(6):1665–8.

119. Stevens DA, Schwartz HJ, Lee JY, et al. A randomized trial of itraconazole in allergic bronchopulmonary aspergillosis. N Engl J Med 2000;342(11): 756–62.

120. Leon EE, Craig TJ. Antifungals in the treatment of allergic bronchopulmonary aspergillosis. Ann Allergy Asthma Immunol 1999;82(6):511–6, quiz 516–9.

121. Shale DJ, Faux JA, Lane DJ. Trial of ketoconazole in non-invasive pulmonary aspergillosis. Thorax 1987;42(1):26–31.

122. Wark PA, Hensley MJ, Saltos N, et al. Anti-inflammatory effect of itraconazole in stable allergic

bronchopulmonary aspergillosis: a randomized controlled trial. J Allergy Clin Immunol 2003; 111(5):952–7.

123. Saag MS, Dismukes WE. Azole antifungal agents: emphasis on new triazoles. Antimicrobial Agents Chemother 1988;32(1):1–8.

124. Wark PA, Gibson PG, Wilson AJ. Azoles for allergic bronchopulmonary aspergillosis associated with asthma. Cochrane Database Syst Rev 2003;(3): CD001108.

125. Denning DW, Van Wye JE, Lewiston NJ, et al. Adjunctive therapy of allergic bronchopulmonary aspergillosis with itraconazole. Chest 1991; 100(3):813–9.

126. Mannes GP, van der Heide S, van Aalderen WM, et al. Itraconazole and allergic bronchopulmonary aspergillosis in twin brothers with cystic fibrosis. Lancet 1993;341(8843):492.

127. Nepomuceno IB, Esrig S, Moss RB. Allergic bronchopulmonary aspergillosis in cystic fibrosis: role of atopy and response to itraconazole. Chest 1999;115(2):364–70.

128. Skov M, Main KM, Sillesen IB, et al. Iatrogenic adrenal insufficiency as a side-effect of combined treatment of itraconazole and budesonide. Eur Respir J 2002;20(1):127–33.

129. Zonios DI, Bennett JE. Update on azole antifungals. Semin Respir Crit Care Med 2008;29(2): 198–210.

130. Hilliard T, Edwards S, Buchdahl R, et al. Voriconazole therapy in children with cystic fibrosis. J Cyst Fibros 2005;4(4):215–20.

131. Lazarus AA, Thilagar B, McKay SA. Allergic bronchopulmonary aspergillosis. Dis Mon 2008;54(8): 547–64.

132. Mastella G, Rainisio M, Harms HK, et al. Allergic bronchopulmonary aspergillosis in cystic fibrosis. A European epidemiological study. Epidemiologic Registry of Cystic Fibrosis. Eur Respir J 2000; 16(3):464–71.

133. Kurup VP, Grunig G. Animal models of allergic bronchopulmonary aspergillosis. Mycopathologia 2002;153(4):165–77.

134. Shah R, Vaideeswar P, Pandit SP. Pathology of pulmonary aspergillomas. Indian J Pathol Microbiol 2008;51(3):342–5.

135. Hours S, Nunes H, Kambouchner M, et al. Pulmonary cavitary sarcoidosis: clinico-radiologic characteristics and natural history of a rare form of sarcoidosis. Medicine (Baltimore) 2008;87(3): 142–51.

136. Sarosi GA, Silberfarb PM, Saliba NA, et al. Aspergillomas occurring in blastomycotic cavities. Am Rev Respir Dis 1971;104(4):581–4.

137. Kawamura S, Maesaki S, Tomono K, et al. Clinical evaluation of 61 patients with pulmonary aspergilloma. Intern Med 2000;39(3):209–12.

138. Rafferty P, Biggs BA, Crompton GK, et al. What happens to patients with pulmonary aspergilloma? Analysis of 23 cases. Thorax 1983;38(8):579–83.

139. Belcher JR, Plummer NS. Surgery in bronchopulmonary aspergillosis. Br J Dis Chest 1960;54: 335–41.

140. Walsh TJ, Anaissie EJ, Denning DW, et al. Treatment of aspergillosis: clinical practice guidelines of the Infectious Diseases Society of America. Clin Infect Dis 2008;46(3):327–60.

141. Jewkes J, Kay PH, Paneth M, et al. Pulmonary aspergilloma: analysis of prognosis in relation to haemoptysis and survey of treatment. Thorax 1983;38(8):572–8.

142. Aspergilloma and residual tuberculous cavities—the results of a resurvey. Tubercle 1970;51(3):227–45.

143. Chatzimichalis A, Massard G, Kessler R, et al. Bronchopulmonary aspergilloma: a reappraisal. Ann Thorac Surg 1998;65(4):927–9.

144. Ueda H, Okabayashi K, Ondo K, et al. Analysis of various treatments for pulmonary aspergillomas. Surg Today 2001;31(9):768–73.

145. Kibbler CC, Milkins SR, Bhamra A, et al. Apparent pulmonary mycetoma following invasive aspergillosis in neutropenic patients. Thorax 1988;43(2):108–12.

146. Addrizzo-Harris DJ, Harkin TJ, McGuinness G, et al. Pulmonary aspergilloma and AIDS. A comparison of HIV-infected and HIV-negative individuals. Chest 1997;111(3):612–8.

147. Westney GE, Kesten S, De Hoyos A, et al. Aspergillus infection in single and double lung transplant recipients. Transplantation 1996;61(6):915–9.

148. Denning DW. Chronic forms of pulmonary aspergillosis. Clin Microbiol Infect 2001;7(Suppl 2):25–31.

149. Campbell JH, Winter JH, Richardson MD, et al. Treatment of pulmonary aspergilloma with itraconazole. Thorax 1991;46(11):839–41.

150. Dupont B. Itraconazole therapy in aspergillosis: study in 49 patients. J Am Acad Dermatol 1990; 23(3 Pt 2):607–14.

151. Al-Kattan K, Ashour M, Hajjar W, et al. Surgery for pulmonary aspergilloma in post-tuberculous vs. immuno-compromised patients. Eur J Cardiothorac Surg 2001;20(4):728–33.

152. Baron O, Guillaume B, Moreau P, et al. Aggressive surgical management in localized pulmonary mycotic and nonmycotic infections for neutropenic patients with acute leukemia: report of eighteen cases. J Thorac Cardiovasc Surg 1998;115(1): 63–8 [discussion: 68–9].

153. Danner BC, Didilis V, Dorge H, et al. Surgical treatment of pulmonary aspergillosis/mycosis in immunocompromised patients. Interact Cardiovasc Thorac Surg 2008;7(5):771–6.

154. Brik A, Salem AM, Kamal AR, et al. Surgical outcome of pulmonary aspergilloma. Eur J Cardiothorac Surg 2008;34(4):882–5.

155. Okubo K, Kobayashi M, Morikawa H, et al. Favorable acute and long-term outcomes after the resection of pulmonary aspergillomas. Thorac Cardiovasc Surg 2007;55(2):108–11.

156. Endo S, Otani S, Tezuka Y, et al. Predictors of postoperative complications after radical resection for pulmonary aspergillosis. Surg Today 2006;36(6): 499–503.

157. Shiraishi Y, Katsuragi N, Nakajima Y, et al. Pneumonectomy for complex aspergilloma: is it still dangerous? Eur J Cardiothorac Surg 2006;29(1): 9–13.

158. Kim YT, Kang MC, Sung SW, et al. Good long-term outcomes after surgical treatment of simple and complex pulmonary aspergilloma. Ann Thorac Surg 2005;79(1):294–8.

159. Akbari JG, Varma PK, Neema PK, et al. Clinical profile and surgical outcome for pulmonary aspergilloma: a single center experience. Ann Thorac Surg 2005;80(3):1067–72.

160. Park CK, Jheon S. Results of surgical treatment for pulmonary aspergilloma. Eur J Cardiothorac Surg 2002;21(5):918–23.

161. Babatasi G, Massetti M, Chapelier A, et al. Surgical treatment of pulmonary aspergilloma: current outcome. J Thorac Cardiovasc Surg 2000;119(5): 906–12.

162. Regnard JF, Icard P, Nicolosi M, et al. Aspergilloma: a series of 89 surgical cases. Ann Thorac Surg 2000; 69(3):898–903.

163. Kato A, Kudo S, Matsumoto K, et al. Bronchial artery embolization for hemoptysis due to benign diseases: immediate and long-term results. Cardiovasc Intervent Radiol 2000;23(5):351–7.

164. Kim YG, Yoon HK, Ko GY, et al. Long-term effect of bronchial artery embolization in Korean patients with haemoptysis. Respirology 2006; 11(6):776–81.

165. Corr P. Management of severe hemoptysis from pulmonary aspergilloma using endovascular embolization. Cardiovasc Intervent Radiol 2006; 29(5):807–10.

166. Rumbak M, Kohler G, Eastrige C, et al. Topical treatment of life threatening haemoptysis from aspergillomas. Thorax 1996;51(3):253–5.

167. Munk PL, Vellet AD, Rankin RN, et al. Intracavitary aspergilloma: transthoracic percutaneous injection of amphotericin gelatin solution. Radiology 1993; 188(3):821–3.

168. Hargis JL, Bone RC, Stewart J, et al. Intracavitary amphotericin B in the treatment of symptomatic pulmonary aspergillomas. Am J Med 1980;68(3): 389–94.

169. Krakowka P, Traczyk K, Walczak J, et al. Local treatment of aspergilloma of the lung with a paste containing nystatin or amphotericin B. Tubercle 1970;51(2):184–91.

170. Jackson M, Flower CD, Shneerson JM. Treatment of symptomatic pulmonary aspergillomas with intracavitary instillation of amphotericin B through an indwelling catheter. Thorax 1993;48(9):928–30.

171. Giron J, Poey C, Fajadet P, et al. CT-guided percutaneous treatment of inoperable pulmonary aspergillomas: a study of 40 cases. Eur J Radiol 1998; 28(3):235–42.

172. Denning DW. Aspergillosis. In: Fauci AS, Kasper DL, Longo DL, et al, editors. Harrison's principles of internal medicine. 17th edition. USA: The McGraw-Hill Companies, Inc.; 2008. Available at. http://online.statref.com/document.aspx?fxid=55&docid=1616. November 11, 2008.

173. Binder RE, Faling LJ, Pugatch RD, et al. Chronic necrotizing pulmonary aspergillosis: a discrete clinical entity. Medicine (Baltimore) 1982;61(2):109–24.

174. Gefter WB, Weingrad TR, Epstein DM, et al. "Semiinvasive" pulmonary aspergillosis: a new look at the spectrum of aspergillus infections of the lung. Radiology 1981;140(2):313–21.

175. Kato T, Usami I, Morita H, et al. Chronic necrotizing pulmonary aspergillosis in pneumoconiosis: clinical and radiologic findings in 10 patients. Chest 2002;121(1):118–27.

176. Denning DW, Riniotis K, Dobrashian R, et al. Chronic cavitary and fibrosing pulmonary and pleural aspergillosis: case series, proposed nomenclature change, and review. Clin Infect Dis 2003;37(Suppl 3):S265–80.

177. Vaid M, Kaur S, Sambatakou H, et al. Distinct alleles of mannose-binding lectin (MBL) and surfactant proteins A (SP-A) in patients with chronic cavitary pulmonary aspergillosis and allergic bronchopulmonary aspergillosis. Clin Chem Lab Med 2007;45(2):183–6.

178. Carvalho A, Pasqualotto AC, Pitzurra L, et al. Polymorphisms in toll-like receptor genes and susceptibility to pulmonary aspergillosis. J Infect Dis 2008; 197(4):618–21.

179. Crosdale DJ, Poulton KV, Ollier WE, et al. Mannose-binding lectin gene polymorphisms as a susceptibility factor for chronic necrotizing pulmonary aspergillosis. J Infect Dis 2001;184(5):653–6.

180. Saraceno JL, Phelps DT, Ferro TJ, et al. Chronic necrotizing pulmonary aspergillosis: approach to management. Chest 1997;112(2):541–8.

181. Kobashi Y, Fukuda M, Yoshida K, et al. Chronic necrotizing pulmonary aspergillosis as a complication of pulmonary Mycobacterium avium complex disease. Respirology 2006;11(6):809–13.

182. Kitazaki T, Osumi M, Miyazaki Y, et al. Chronic necrotizing pulmonary aspergillosis following cryptococcal infection of the lung. Scand J Infect Dis 2005;37(5):393–5.

183. Franquet T, Muller NL, Gimenez A, et al. Semiinvasive pulmonary aspergillosis in chronic obstructive

pulmonary disease: radiologic and pathologic findings in nine patients. AJR Am J Roentgenol 2000; 174(1):51–6.

184. Kim SY, Lee KS, Han J, et al. Semiinvasive pulmonary aspergillosis: CT and pathologic findings in six patients. AJR Am J Roentgenol 2000;174(3):795–8.

185. Thompson BH, Stanford W, Galvin JR, et al. Varied radiologic appearances of pulmonary aspergillosis. Radiographics 1995;15(6):1273–84.

186. Caras WE. Chronic necrotizing pulmonary aspergillosis: approach to management. Chest 1998; 113(3):852–3.

187. Yousem SA. The histological spectrum of chronic necrotizing forms of pulmonary aspergillosis. Hum Pathol 1997;28(6):650–6.

188. Camuset J, Nunes H, Dombret MC, et al. Treatment of chronic pulmonary aspergillosis by voriconazole in nonimmunocompromised patients. Chest 2007; 131(5):1435–41.

189. Sambatakou H, Dupont B, Lode H, et al. Voriconazole treatment for subacute invasive and chronic pulmonary aspergillosis. Am J Med 2006;119(6):527, e517–24

190. Jain LR, Denning DW. The efficacy and tolerability of voriconazole in the treatment of chronic cavitary pulmonary aspergillosis. J Infect 2006;52(5): e133–7.

191. Kelleher P, Goodsall A, Mulgirigama A, et al. Interferon-gamma therapy in two patients with progressive chronic pulmonary aspergillosis. Eur Respir J 2006;27(6):1307–10.

192. Endo S, Sohara Y, Murayama F, et al. Surgical outcome of pulmonary resection in chronic necrotizing pulmonary aspergillosis. Ann Thorac Surg 2001;72(3):889–93 [discussion: 894].

Molds: Hyalohyphomycosis, Phaeohyphomycosis, and Zygomycosis

Susanna Naggie, MD*, John R. Perfect, MD

KEYWORDS

- Mold • Hyalohyphomycosis • Phaeohyphomycosis
- Zygomycosis • Invasive fungal infection
- Emerging fungal infection • Epidemiology • Transplant

We have witnessed a change in the epidemiology of invasive fungal infections (IFIs) over the past 2 decades. Emerging fungal organisms previously thought to be nonpathogenic or extremely rare pathogens are now recognized as playing a significant role in the increased incidence of invasive fungal disease. Before this shift, *Candida* spp (particularly *Candida albicans*) were the most common cause of fungal bloodstream infection and *Aspergillus* spp (particularly *Aspergillus fumigatus*) were the most common cause of invasive fungal pneumonia. Yet, there are increasing descriptions of severe invasive mycoses from emerging pathogens, including hyaline septated molds (*Fusarium* spp, *Scedosporium* spp, *Trichoderma* spp, and *Paecilomyces* spp), dematiaceous molds (*Dactylaria/Ochroconis* spp, *Wangiella/Exophilia* spp, and *Cladophialophora* spp), and Zygomycetes (*Rhizopus* spp, *Cunninghamella* spp, and *Mucor* spp).[1–7] The significant morbidity and mortality associated with these infections are not only related to the host populations and state of the underlying disease but to delayed recognition and diagnosis, coupled with high rates of clinical resistance in some of these emerging pathogens to standard antifungal therapies.

Several factors are contributing to this changing epidemiology: expanded at-risk patient populations, changes in medical treatments and interventions, and new diagnostic methods. The increase in the incidence of IFIs over the past 20 years has been in transplant recipients (solid organ transplant [SOT] and hematopoietic stem cell transplant [HSCT]), patients who have cancer, recipients of immunosuppressive and chemotherapeutic agents, patients who have HIV/AIDS, premature birth infants, the elderly, and those undergoing major surgery.[8] Aggressive new therapies for HSCT and for malignancies have led to profound immunosuppression of longer duration and have extended the survival of these critically ill patients. Specifically, increasing rates of IFIs in patients who have prolonged neutropenia or graft-versus-host disease (GVHD) and those on high-dose steroids or antithymocyte antibody have been described.[9] Antibiotic selection pressure from new antifungal agents and changes in the use of antifungals for prophylaxis, especially in the transplant and cancer populations, is also contributing to this shift in epidemiology.[10] Distinguishing colonization with an environmental mold from IFIs can be difficult at times; thus, emerging technologies in diagnostics do and are likely to continue to play a role in differentiating pathogens from "innocent bystanders."[11]

Advances in medical technology and medical therapies for many medical conditions, including malignancies and autoimmune diseases, in addition to changes in prophylaxis, therapies, and diagnostics for invasive mycoses have combined

Division of Infectious Diseases, Department of Internal Medicine, Duke University Medical Center, DUMC Box 3824, Durham, NC 27710, USA
* Corresponding author.
E-mail address: naggi001@mc.duke.edu (S. Naggie).

Clin Chest Med 30 (2009) 337–353
doi:10.1016/j.ccm.2009.02.009

to form the "perfect storm," with conditions that have forever altered the epidemiology of IFIs. It is now recognized that there is an enlarging menu of pathogenic fungi and that in the severely immunocompromised host, poorly virulent fungi must be considered possible pathogens. This review focuses on these emerging fungal pathogens: microbiology, pathogenesis, clinical presentations, diagnosis, treatment (**Table 1**), and outcomes.

HYALINE SEPTATE MOLDS: HYALOHYPHOMYCOSIS

Hyalohyphomycosis refers to infections caused by colorless septate fungal hyphae in affected tissue. Often misidentified as *Aspergillus* spp, these molds are differentiated by their conidia and phialide morphologies. Although *Aspergillus* spp are the most common filamentous fungi causing opportunistic infection in immunocompromised hosts, non-*Aspergillus* hyaline fungi, such as *Fusarium*, *Scedosporium*, *Trichoderma*, and *Paecilomyces*, are being increasingly described in cases of IFIs. Because of the ubiquitous nature of these fungi in the environment, exposure primarily by inhalation or cutaneous trauma is common. Nevertheless, it is because of frequent exposure that distinguishing colonization from true infection can be difficult. In one study of 85 cases of saprophytic molds isolated from the lower respiratory tract, 58% were consistent with colonization.[12] Host factors that were determined to be associated with true IFIs in these saprophytic mold isolates included allogeneic bone marrow

Table 1
Management of invasive fungal infections

Fungal Disease	First-Line Therapy	Other Considerations
Hyalohyphomycosis		
Fusarium infections		
F solani F oxysporon F moniliforme	AmB lipid (5 mg/kg/d)[a] D-AmB (1.0–1.5 mg/kg/d) or voriconazole or posaconazole	Combination therapy
Scedosporium apiospermum/ Pseudallescheria boydii	Voriconazole or posaconazole	Combination therapy
Trichoderma spp		
T longibrachiatum T viride	AmB lipid (5 mg/kg/d)[a] D-AmB (1.0–1.5 mg/kg/d)	Voriconazole or combination therapy
Paecilomyces spp		
P lilacinus P variotii	Posaconazole or voriconazole AmB lipid (5 mg/kg/d)[a] D-AmB (1.0–1.5 mg/kg/d)	Posaconazole or voriconazole or combination therapy
Zygomycosis		
Rhizopus spp *Absidia corymbifera* *Mucor spp* *Cunninghamella spp*	AmB lipid (5 mg/kg/d)[a] D-AmB (1.0–1.5 mg/kg/d)	Posaconazole or combination therapy (GCSF or GM-CSF, deferasirox, hyperbaric oxygen therapy)
Phaeohyphomycosis		
Bipolaris spp Cladophialophora spp Ochroconis spp Alternaria spp Wangiella spp Curvularia spp	Severe disease: AmB lipid (5 mg/kg/d)[a] D-AmB (1.0–1.5 mg/kg/d) + triazole ± 5-FC Non–life-threatening: voriconazole or posaconazoleor itraconazole	Combination therapy or systemic therapy with local antiseptic used to washout surgical bed to eliminate spores

Antifungal therapies recommended here should be combined with surgical debridement or intervention when available or appropriate.

Abbreviations: AmB, amphotericin B; D-AmB, deoxycholate amphotericin B; 5-FC, flucytosine; GCSF, granulocyte colony-stimulating factor; GMCSF, granulocyte-macrophage colony-stimulating factor.

[a] Lipid products of amphotericin B are favored over D-AmB.

transplantation, leukemia, and corticosteroid treatment. Among the molds identified, two had the greatest positive predictive value for IFIs in high-risk patients: *Scedosporium* spp and *Paecilomyces* spp. Similar conclusions were drawn from the same group in the evaluation of blood cultures positive for saprophytic molds, wherein 55% were consistent with contamination.[13] Again, high-risk hosts included those who had hematologic malignancies and HSCT, but no patient who had a solid organ malignancy had definite or probable fungemia. The most common mold causing true fungemia was *Scedosporium* spp. Thus, a positive culture from blood or other specimens alone does not always correlate with an IFI; attempts to elucidate the significance of a culture should include pursuit of histopathologic specimens or risk stratification by host factors and identification of organisms.

Fusarium

Fungi of the genus *Fusarium* are commonly found in soil, water, and decaying material and are well-recognized plant pathogens causing extensive crop destruction and contamination. The most common species are *Fusarium solani*, *Fusarium oxysporum*, and *Fusarium moniliforme*.[1] One of the most common airborne molds, *Fusarium*, has been identified as a colonizer of the throat in 17% of nonhospitalized healthy adults and of the conjunctival sac, especially in diseased eyes.[14,15] In immunocompetent hosts, *Fusarium* causes a more localized disease. For example, it is the most common cause of fungal keratitis worldwide. It can also produce onychomycosis with or without paronychia and cutaneous infection, especially in patients who have burn injuries. Increasingly, hospital centers are reporting *Fusarium* as the second most common filamentous mold (second to *Aspergillus*) causing respiratory and disseminated infection in severely immunocompromised patients.[16] Risk factors for invasive fusariosis include acute leukemia, HSCT, prolonged neutropenia, and GVHD.[1,17] Fusariosis has also been described in outbreaks related to contaminated environmental water supplies.[17]

Similar to *Aspergillus*, *Fusarium* can be angioinvasive and leads to tissue infarction in immunocompromised patients. Common clinical presentation includes fever and pulmonary infiltrates or sinusitis, because these are the initial routes of exposure with inhalation of spores. In contrast to *Aspergillus*, from infarcted tissue, *Fusarium* can undergo intravascular adventitious sporulation with continuous releases of spores into the bloodstream.[18] This morphologic mechanism of dissemination results in positive blood cultures in as many as 60% to 75% of disseminated cases.[8,19] The hallmark of disseminated fusariosis is positive blood cultures and characteristic "bull's eye" skin lesions.[19] The skin lesions are most commonly found on the extremities and are typically described as subcutaneous painful and often pruritic nodules that can ulcerate to ecthyma gangrenosum-like necrotic lesions.[1,17,19,20]

In a large cohort of HSCT recipients at a single center, *Fusarium* was the most common non-*Aspergillus* mold causing proved invasive infection, and there was an increase in the frequency of such infections over the study period.[16] Significant risk for developing *Fusarium* infection included multiple myeloma and receipt of a graft from a human leukocyte antigen-mismatched or unrelated donor. Clinically, 19% of cases were isolated sinusitis, but most (81%) had invasive fungal pneumonia and dissemination was common (74%). In another study, the same group provided a further description of the radiographic presentation of pulmonary fusariosis with nonspecific alveolar infiltrates (8 unilateral, 19 bilateral), nodules (3 unilateral, 6 bilateral), interstitial infiltrates (1 unilateral, 6 bilateral), and cavities in 84 patients.[17] Mortality in the first 1 to 2 months was approximately 80%, and the 1-year survival rate was 20%. In another multicenter cohort study in HSCT recipients, the overall incidence of fusariosis was 5.97 cases per 1000 transplants, with the highest rates of disease occurring in mismatched donors.[1] The median survival after diagnosis was 13 days, with an 87% 90-day mortality rate, and predictors of death included GVHD and persistent neutropenia.

Definitive diagnosis is by histopathologic examination and culture of the affected tissue or blood. Treatment depends on the site of infection. Localized infection should be treated with surgical resection when possible. Initial therapy is often chosen before minimum inhibitory concentration (MIC) data are available; thus, decisions must be based on preliminary histopathologic or culture data (see **Table 1**). As noted previously, response to treatment of disseminated fusariosis is poor, because some *Fusarium* spp may be resistant to amphotericin B, with breakthrough infection on therapy reported.[21] Some strains, such as *F solani* and *Fusarium verticillioides*, are usually resistant to azoles; thus, high-dose amphotericin B or lipid formations of amphotericin B are recommended.[22,23] For strains resistant to amphotericin B or in other difficult-to-treat patients, voriconazole has been associated with some success (45%–63% response rates) and lower rates of mortality than previously reported for disseminated fusariosis.[24,25] There are also reports of successful treatment of refractory fusariosis with posaconazole (26 patients) and combination therapy of amphotericin B and voriconazole.[26,27] Echinocandins and limited-spectrum azoles, such as fluconazole and ketoconazole, are not active against *Fusarium* spp, and thus are not recommended. As important as initiation of antifungal therapy is for success of treatment, attention to immune reconstitution with use of granulocyte colony-stimulating factor (GCSF) or granulocyte-macrophage colony-stimulating factor (GM-CSF) for neutropenia or reduction of immunosuppressive therapy, when possible, is also an essential part of successful management.

Scedosporium

Scedosporium spp are ubiquitous filamentous fungi present in soil, sewage, polluted water, and decaying vegetation. The most medically significant species are *S apiospermun* (and its teleomorph or sexual state, *Pseudallescheria boydii*) and *Scedosporium prolificans* (a dematiaceous mold). Of 370 isolates of *Scedosporium* spp submitted to the Fungus Testing Laboratory at the University of Texas Health Science Center at San Antonio, 222 (60%) were from the thorax or lung; 31 (8%) each were from the sinuses and bones or joints; and 11 to 13 (approximately 3%) each were from the central nervous system (CNS), blood, hands, and feet.[28] As with most saprophytic molds, exposure in the environment is primarily by inhalation or cutaneous inoculation attributable to trauma. *Scedosporium* spp can be transient colonizers of the airway in any person in an endemic area with high environmental contamination and can become persistent colonizers (saprobic involvement) of previously damaged bronchopulmonary trees (prior exposure to pulmonary tuberculosis, cystic fibrosis, or bronchiectasis).[28,29] As a colonizer, these molds can lead to a mycetoma in empty pulmonary cavities or at sites of percutaneous inoculation (primarily legs and hands), can produce allergic bronchopulmonary disease in hosts who have underlying lung disease, or can cause IFIs in immunocompromised hosts.[29] A chronic infection with draining sinus tracts is characteristic of a tissue mycetoma, which can cause destruction of the underlying muscle, tendon, and bones.

Scedosporium spp are being increasingly reported as significant pathogens, primarily in immunocompromised hosts, including patients who have HIV/AIDS, primary immunodeficiencies (mainly chronic granulomatous disease [CGD] and Job's syndrome), or hematologic malignancies; HSCT recipients; and others undergoing therapy with antineoplastic or immunosuppressive therapies. Similar to *Fusarium*, *Scedosporium* can be angioinvasive and undergo characteristic adventitious sporulation leading to increased rates of hematogenous dissemination in susceptible hosts (30%–35%).[30] In a recent report of disseminated phaeohyphomycosis, *S prolificans* was the most common fungus, accounting for 42% of cases, in which 80% had positive blood cultures.[31]

In immunocompromised hosts, the clinical presentation most commonly involves fever and disseminated disease (46%) with CNS, pulmonary (bilateral focal and diffuse infiltrates, single or multiple nodules, and pleural effusions), and cutaneous involvement (nonpruriginous erythematous and nodular lesions with a necrotic center) in 29%, 43%, and 31% of cases, respectively.[32] In this cohort study, a total of 80 cases of *Scedosporium* infection were identified: 57 in SOT recipients and 23 in HSCT recipients. Most of these patients were on immunosuppressive therapy, with 95.6% on corticosteroids, and most HSCT recipients (64%) were on antifungal prophylaxis at the time of their diagnosis. *Scedosporium apiospermum* was the most common species (76%) causing disease overall, although rates of infection from *S prolificans* were higher in the HSCT recipients. Disseminated scedosporiosis was most common in HSCT recipients, and fungemia was found to be more common with *S prolificans* (57%) than *S apiospermum* (8%) infections. Mortality for all transplant recipients with disseminated scedosporiosis was 58%, with the highest rates in HSCT recipients (68%) and *S prolificans* infection with the worse prognosis (77.8% death rate in both transplant groups).

A clinically distinct syndrome of sinopulmonary and CNS infection from *S apiosperumum* (*P boydii*) has been described in 23 cases of immunocompetent near-drowning victims over the past 2 decades. In a published review, all 23 cases had evidence of aspiration pneumonitis or pneumonia with mostly diffuse, and less often focal, pulmonary infiltrates or abscess.[33] Twenty-one (91%) cases also had CNS infection with multiple or solitary parenchymal brain abscess. Less frequently, CNS involvement included meningitis, encephalitis, ventriculitis, ependymitis, or cerebral vascular disease. Diagnosis was most commonly made from culture of cerebrospinal fluid (CSF) or CNS tissue, with a few of the cases (26%) having isolated positive respiratory cultures. Overall mortality of scedosporiosis from near-drowning was 70%.

Diagnosis is most commonly made from recovery of the organism from clinical sites of infection, preferably by culture and histopathologic means. As compared with other saprophytic molds, *Scedosporium* spp are less likely to be colonizers or contaminants of the airways in the appropriate high-risk population (although they can be in some groups, such as patients who have cystic fibrosis). Because of generally low susceptibility of all antifungal agents to *S prolificans*, appropriate therapy is not clear (see **Table 1**). Localized infection or abscess should be treated with surgical resection or drainage when possible. *S prolificans* has inherent resistance (MIC >8 μg/mL) for most antifungal drugs.[23] The best in vitro activity has been found with voriconazole and caspofungin.[23,29] *S apiospermum* has lower MICs for most azoles, except fluconazole and ketoconazole, with the most potent in vitro activity observed with voriconazole.[23,29] Echinocandins also showed antifungal activity against *S apiospermum*.[23] One report of voriconazole use in refractory scedosporiosis had a global response rate of 30%, and the Kaplan-Meier estimate for survival was similar to other reports (0.300, 95% CI: 0.016–0.584).[24] In the cohort discussed previously, receipt of voriconazole was associated with a strong trend toward better survival in a multivariable analysis.[32] In a multicenter study, posaconazole was evaluated as salvage therapy in patients who had refractory *S apiospermum* infection, with a successful outcome in 43% of treated patients.[34] Combinations of antifungals for the treatment of scedosporiosis have been studied. Reports include synergy with terbinafine plus an azole, amphotericin B plus pentamidine, and amphotericin B plus voriconazole or miconazole or fluconazole or itraconazole.[28] Again, attention to immune reconstitution is crucial for successful treatment outcomes in the immunocompromised population, and in difficult cases, combination therapies may need to be used.

Trichoderma

Previously regarded as a nonpathogenic saprophytic environmental mold, several centers have now reported emerging infections attributable principally to *Trichoderma longibrachiatum*, although a total of five species have been identified as causing approximately 27 cases of IFIs over the past 2 decades.[3,35–37] Reports of IFIs have been primarily in immunocompromised hosts and patients receiving peritoneal dialysis.[3,8,37,38] The first case of *Trichoderma* infection was caused by the species *Trichoderma viride*, which was isolated from a pulmonary mycetoma in a patient who had underlying lung disease.[39] Since that report, 8 cases of peritonitis in patients undergoing dialysis have been identified, with overall mortality of 63%.[3,37] Five cases of *Trichoderma* spp IFIs

have been reported in SOT: (1) brain abscess with pulmonary involvement, (2) invasive sinusitis, (3) superinfected perihepatic hematoma, (4) subcapsular hepatic abscess, and (5) pneumonia with empyema in a lung transplant recipient.[3,36] In this group, mortality was 60% and success was associated with surgical resection or debridement. Seven cases of IFIs from *T longibrachiatum* have been reported in patients who had an underlying hematologic malignancy: (1) disseminated disease (2 cases), (2) mycetoma, (3) central venous catheter (CVC) infection, (4) stomatitis, (5) invasive pulmonary disease, and (6) invasive sinusitis with brain abscess.[3,37,40] Mortality was 43% for all infections, but disseminated disease was associated with 100% mortality.

Trichoderma spp is the perfect example of the emerging opportunistic infection in the era of extreme immunosuppression and increasing organ and bone marrow transplantation, with 80% of these reported cases occurring in the past 10 years. Based on the description of the previously reported IFIs, the likely source of contamination is from aerosols or nonsterile water sources. Because of its ubiquitous nature, diagnosis can be difficult and, ideally, should be based on demonstration of hyphae in tissue in association with positive culture of that same tissue specimen. Most isolates of *Trichoderma* spp are susceptible in vitro to amphotericin B, itraconazole, ketoconazole, voriconazole, and miconazole (see **Table 1**).[3,23,37,40] A recent report showed lower MICs (0.5–1 mg/L) for voriconazole in 15 isolates of *T longibrachiatum* as compared with amphotericin B and fluconazole.[41] There are two case reports of successful therapy of *Trichoderma* spp IFI using combination therapy with voriconazole and caspofungin.[37,40]

Paecilomyces

Paecilomyces spp are common environmental hyaline molds found worldwide. The fungi can be recovered from soil and air and are relatively resistant to common methods of sterilization, resulting in frequent contamination of body creams and lotions and colonization of medical foreign bodies, such as CVCs and medical implants. The two most common species associated with human infections are *Paecilomyces lilacinus* and *Paecilomyces variotii*. To date, approximately 160 cases of invasive *Paecilomyces* spp infection have been reported in the medical literature, 17 in the past 4 years.[42] The most common clinical presentation is of keratitis and endophthalmitis, usually related to lens implantation, contact lenses, or corneal injury, which account for more than 50% of cases.[42] Cutaneous and subcutaneous infections are the second most common presentations, occurring most commonly in immunocompromised patients (SOT, 28%; HSCT, 12%; corticosteroid, 9%; malignancy, 21%).[42] Historically, ocular and cutaneous infections have accounted for approximately 82% of all cases of *Paecilomyces* infections; however, over the past 4 years, reported IFIs (nonocular, noncutaneous) attributed to *Paecilomyces* have increased.[42] Because of the ability of *Paecilomyces* to sporulate adventitiously during tissue invasion (similar to *Fusarium* and *Scedosporium*), positive blood cultures potentially can occur but are not as common as its previously described counterparts.

The authors reviewed 43 cases of *Paecilomyces* IFI reported in the literature. The most common underlying risk factors are leukemia and HSCT, although there are also reports of IFIs in patients who have diabetes, solid organ malignancies, HIV/AIDS, and CGD.[42–51] The most common presentation was pulmonary (9 cases), with lobar and diffuse interstitial pneumonia being the most common presentation, in addition to pleural effusions and mycetomas.[43] Other possible presentations include sinusitis (6 cases), fungemia (6 cases), disseminated disease (4 cases), and peritoneal dialysis-associated peritonitis (8 cases all described with *P variotii*).[52] Even less common presentations include infectious endocarditis in patients who have prosthetic valve(s), splenic and pelvic abscess, pyelonephritis, otitis media, meningitis, and osteomyelitis.[53–56]

Reported clinical outcomes of IFIs attributable to *Paecilomyces* range from 100% recovery to significant rates of morbidity and mortality.[42,51] For localized infections, especially cutaneous infections, surgical intervention plays a significant role in successful outcomes. For invasive or disseminated infections, the optimal antifungal agent has not been identified, although species-specific susceptibility data can help (see **Table 1**). *P variotii* has lower MICs for amphotericin B and should be susceptible, whereas *P lilacinus* is generally resistant to polyenes in vitro. Conversely, in vitro data for *P lilacinus* with triazoles are reassuring, with low MIC ranges of posaconazole (0.12–0.5 mg/L), voriconazole (0.12–4 mg/L), albaconazole (0.06–0.5 mg/L), and ravuconazole (0.2–2 mg/L).[42] In vitro data for *P variotii* show MICs of less than 2 mg/L for amphotericin B, itraconazole, posaconazole, terbinafine, and the echinocandins, whereas more than 80% had MICs greater than 2 mg/L for voriconazole and ravuconazole.[57] Clinical evidence to support the in vitro susceptibility data are lacking. In one study of voriconazole treatment in refractory emerging fungal infections, only

three cases were attributable to *Paecilomyces* and one patient had a successful treatment response.[24] Otherwise, there are few case reports of successful treatment of *Paecilomyces* IFI with triazole therapies.[58–60] In vitro data of combination therapy with amphotericin B and azoles found additive effects and synergy in some isolates.[42] One case report of cutaneous *P lilacinus* had a successful treatment response with the combination of caspofungin and itraconazole.[4]

ASEPTATE MOLDS: ZYGOMYCOSIS

Zygomycosis refers to infections caused by fungi from the class Zygomycetes, which is composed of two orders, both causing disease in humans: Mucorales and Entomophthorales. This class of fungi is ubiquitous in soil; is commonly found in decaying organic matter; and, like other environmental molds, is commonly transmitted by means of inhalation or from percutaneous inoculation. The Entomophthorales can cause cutaneous and mucocutaneous infections, largely in immunocompetent hosts and primarily in tropical and subtropical regions, although the geographic distribution is broadening. Mucorales causes mucormycosis, which can be acute in onset and more often rapidly produces progressive angio-IFIs in immunocompromised hosts. The most common species causing human disease are *Rhizopus* spp (*Rhizopus arrhizus*), accounting for approximately half of all zygomycosis cases, but *Absidia corymbifera* and *Mucor* spp may also cause infection.[7,61] Unlike other opportunistic molds, the most common population afflicted with zygomycosis remains those with diabetes mellitus; other populations include those receiving deferoxamine therapy, injection drug users, and those with no underlying condition (frequently traumatic).[62–65] It is not yet certain whether with better glycemic control and the increased use of statins (with antifungal activity) in diabetic patients, there is likely to be a decline of disease rates in this population. Conversely, over the past decade, zygomycoses have re-emerged as increasingly important and dangerous pathogens, primarily described in HSCT recipients and patients who have hematologic malignancies.[7–10,16,66,67] Increasingly aggressive immunosuppression; medical advances, including organ transplantations; and the use of broader antifungal agents for therapy and prophylaxis have been suggested as major contributors to this changing epidemiology.

Phagocytes (macrophages and neutrophils) are recognized as the major host defenses against mucormycosis, using the generation of oxidative metabolites and cationic peptides defensins to kill the fungus.[68,69] Hyperglycemia and acidosis are known to impair the chemotactic function of phagocytes and have oxidative and nonoxidative killing mechanisms.[70] This is suggestive of the underlying pathophysiology of mucormycosis in patients who have diabetes and ketoacidosis, which have also been identified as risk factors in immunocompromised hosts.[7] Furthermore, the lack of phagocytes in neutropenic patients and the abnormal neutrophil function in patients on steroids (GVHD) lend clinical evidence to the role of these cells in normal host defenses against this group of molds. Another well-elucidated mechanism of Zygomycetes survival in the host is the role of iron in the pathogenesis of disease. It has been well described that patients with high serum iron levels (frequently on the iron chelator deferoxamine) have a significantly increased risk for invasive mucormycosis.[63] It has been shown that Rhizopus spp use deferoxamine as a sidero-phore to bind iron and allow the fungus to uptake the mineral, which is crucial for the pathogenicity of the mold.[71] Furthermore, patients who have systemic acidosis have elevated levels of available serum iron thought to be attributable to the release of iron from binding proteins, such as transferrin, in a more acidic environment, which may also contribute to the pathophysiology of zygomycosis in diabetic patients.[72]

A comprehensive review of all 929 cases (1940–2003) of zygomycosis reported in the literature has been published.[7] Underlying primary conditions included diabetes, injection drug users, deferox-amine therapy, SOT, malignancy, HSCT, and no underlying condition (eg, penetrating trauma, surgery, burn, accident). Although diabetes remained the most common underlying condition overall and across the decades, the contribution of other conditions, specifically malignancy (95% hematologic), SOT, and HSCT, has dramatically increased. The most common clinical presenta-tions were sinus (39%), pulmonary (24%), and cutaneous (19%). Less common presentations included cerebral, gastrointestinal, disseminated (3%), kidney, and other solid organs. Primary site of infection at the time of presentation was a func-tion of the host population. In patients who had underlying conditions of malignancy, HSCT, and SOT, the most common presentation was pulmo-nary, with 60%, 52%, and 37% of cases, respec-tively. Diabetics presented primarily with sinus disease (66%); deferoxamine therapy with disseminated (23%), sinus (26%), and pulmonary (28%) disease; intravenous drug users with cere-bral (62%) disease; and those with no underlying condition with cutaneous (50%) involvement.

Independent risk factors for pulmonary zygomyco-sis were infection with Cunninghamella species, neutropenia, and SOT. Survival with zygomycosis over the period of the review has significantly improved from 16% in the 1950s to 53% in the 1990s. Risk factors for mortality included dissem-inated disease, renal failure, and infection with Cunninghamella species. Improved outcomes were associated with receipt of antifungals and surgery, and the best outcomes were noted in those patients who had diabetes or without any underlying condition.

As noted previously, the incidence of cases of zygomycosis seems to have significantly increased over the past 2 decades, specifically in the transplant and malignancy populations. Some centers have reported increases only recently and have found an association with local change in epidemiology attributable to the use of voriconazole.[10,66,67] In a case-control study of 27 cases, zygomycosis was the second most common IFI over a 2-year period (2002–2004), with an increase in incidence from 0.0079 per 1000 patient-days to 0.095 per 1000 patient-days.[10] Hematologic malignancy was the under-lying diagnosis in all but 1 of these cases, 48% were HSCTs, and the most common presentation was pulmonary (59%). Compared with matched controls with invasive aspergillosis (IA), only vori-conazole prophylaxis and sinusitis were specifi-cally associated with zygomycosis. Interestingly, compared with matched controls without IFIs, voriconazole prophylaxis, diabetes mellitus, and malnutrition were associated with zygomycosis. A retrospective cohort found that Zygomycetes were the most common cause of breakthrough infection (46%) in HSCT recipients on voriconazole for therapy or for prophylaxis of an IFI.[67]

Diagnosis of mucormycosis is primarily by culture or histopathologic examination of affected tissue. Zygomycetes growth in culture from a sterile body site should never be considered a contaminant or colonizer, especially in an immu-nocompromised population. Conversely, histo-pathologic results may be positive and culture of tissue negative for fungal growth. Because of the lack of a rapid diagnostic tool for zygomycosis, empiric therapy must often be initiated based on clinical suspicion until more definitive data have been returned, which usually include tissue-related data. In the transplant and hematologic malignancy population, the most common cause of mold infection is IA, which is difficult to differen-tiate clinically from Zygomycetes infection because both are angioinvasive molds. Optimal therapies for these two IFIs are different, however; thus, early differentiation is crucial for improved outcome. An observational study has attempted to addresses this critical issue in the clinical decision-making process by comparing two cohorts with pulmonary disease caused by Zygomycetes versus *Aspergillus*.[73] The most common CT findings in pulmonary zygomycosis included nodular disease (79%) with peripheral distribution (82%). Furthermore, multiple nodules (≥ 10 nodules, seen in 64% of cases) and micronodules (<1 cm, seen in 55% of cases) were more indicative of pulmonary zygomycosis. In contrast, mass lesions, air-space consolidation, cavitary lesions, and the halo sign were less frequently identified on CT imaging (31%, 38%, 25%, and 25%, respectively). In the multivariable analysis, multiple nodules and the presence of pleural effusions were independently associated with pulmonary zygomycosis compared with pulmonary aspergillosis. Also, in a multivariate analysis of clinical features, sinus involvement (seen only in those patients who had pulmonary zygomycosis) and receipt of voriconazole prophylaxis were independently associated with pulmonary zygomycosis.

The core management of zygomycosis involves treatment with an antifungal agent, surgical resection or debridement of necrotic tissue, and attempts at immune reconstitution. Amphotericin B preparations (as amphotericin B deoxycholate or lipid/liposomal formulations of amphotericin B) are the most active agents against Zygomycetes, followed by posaconazole (see **Table 1**). Because of toxicity issues of the high-dose polyenes, most clinicians now prefer to use lipid formations. Although amphotericin B formulations are the first-line antifungal therapy for zygomycosis, there are increasing data on successful salvage therapy with posaconazole. The largest study, a compassionate use indication, included 91 cases of zygomycosis, in which 60% of patients had a complete or partial response and 17% failed.[74] Other antifungals commonly used for IFIs, including fluconazole, voriconazole, flucytosine, and echinocandins, have little to no efficacy alone, and therefore should not be considered for primary therapy for zygomycosis, although there are some in vivo data supporting use of echinocandins in combination therapy. It should also be noted that use of posaconazole (in the authors' opinion, one of only two antifungal agents with acceptable activity against Zygomycetes) is likely to become more frequent, because two large randomized controlled trials have recently shown posaconazole to be an acceptable alternative for the prevention of IFIs in neutropenic patients undergoing chemotherapy and in HSCT recipients who have GVHD.[75,76] Posaconazole was found to have a significantly lower rate of IFIs versus comparator regimens, although, there are case reports of breakthrough infections on this newest prophylactic broad-spectrum antifungal.[77,78]

The past decade has seen new developments in additional therapeutic options for this invasive fungal disease, including the lipid formulation of amphotericin B, deferasirox, combination therapy with echinocandins, and granulocyte growth factors (GCSF, GM-CSF).[79–84] In a retrospective single-center study, combination polyene-caspofungin therapy (polyene was lipid or liposomal formulation) was found to have a 100% success rate versus 45% success rate among patients treated with polyene monotherapy.[82] This same group found that *Rhizopus oryzae* expresses the gene encoding for the proteins of 1,3-β-D-glucan synthase complex, which they showed is inhibited by low doses of caspofungin, and led to improved survival in a diabetic murine model.[85] To date, use of deferasirox, granulocyte growth factors, and hyperbaric oxygen therapy is experimental, with success only documented in case reports.[81,83,84,86,87]

DEMATIACEOUS SEPTATE MOLDS: PHAEOHYPHOMYCOSIS

Phaeohyphomycosis is the term used to describe infections caused by darkly pigmented molds (black molds), also known as dematiaceous molds. This term was first introduced in 1974. Meaning "condition of fungi with dark hyphae," it describes the brown to black color within the cell wall of the vegetative cells.[88] This characteristic color of the hyphae is related to the presence of melanin in the cell wall of the fungi. It is thought that melanin may play an important role in the pathogenesis of infection caused by dematiaceous molds. The role of melanin as a virulence factor has been studied in the dematiaceous mold *Wangiella dermatitidis*.[89] A ubiquitous environmental mold found in soil, air, plants, and organic debris, the most common route of exposure to humans is by means of inhalation or percutaneous inoculation. Phaeohyphomycosis should also be differentiated from two specific pathologic entities caused by dematiaceous molds that are not described further in this review: chromoblastomycosis (sclerotic bodies in tissue, usually seen in tropical areas) and mycetoma (deep-tissue infection, usually of lower extremities, characterized by presence of mycotic granules). Phaeohyphomycosis has been attributed to more than 100 species of fungi; among the most prevalent causes of human infections include *Bipolaris* spp, *Cladophialophora bantania* (previously *Xylohypha bantiana*), *Ochroconis gallopava* (previously *Dactylaria gallopava*), *Alternaria* spp, *W dermatitidis* (previously *Exophilia dermatitidis*), *Phialophora* spp, and *Curvularia* spp. Unlike the other molds discussed in this review, phaeohyphomycosis can occur in immunocompetent hosts, primarily presenting as localized skin lesions, deep-tissue infection after percutaneous inoculation (usually related to trauma), or severe CNS infection. Still considered opportunistic pathogens in immunocompromised hosts, in a recent multicenter study, phaeohyphomycosis accounted for 9.4% of IFIs in SOT, presenting as sinusitis, pneumonia, CNS infection, and disseminated infection.[90]

A life-threatening phaeohyphomycosis occurs with involvement of the CNS. In a review of 101 cases of CNS infections, *C bantiana* was the most common responsible species (48%), followed by *Ramichloridium mackenziei* (13%) and *O gallopavum* (5%).[91] Unlike other IFIs discussed in this review, more than half (52%) of the cases occurred in patients who had no underlying disease or risk factor. Only 10% of patients had a diagnosed malignancy, 4% had neutropenia, 15% were SOT recipients, and 3% were HSCT recipients. The most common presentation was brain abscess, with 71% of cases occurring as a single lesion. Overall mortality in this review was 73%, and there was no difference in outcomes between immunocompetent and immunocompromised hosts. Improved outcomes were noted for those patients who underwent surgical excision (as compared with aspiration) and those treated with combination therapy of amphotericin B, flucytosine, and itraconazole.

A review of the 72 cases of disseminated phaeohyphomycosis found that *S prolificans* was the most frequent isolated species (42%), followed by *Bipolaris spicifera* (8%) and *W dermatitidis* (7%).[31] Unlike CNS phaeohyphomycosis, in this review, some degree of immune dysfunction was identified in 76% of patients: 54% had a diagnosed malignancy, 51% had neutropenia, and 18% were SOT or HSCT recipients. Ninety percent of the cases attributable to *S prolificans* occurred in patients who had persistent neutropenia. Interestingly, 14% of cases occurred in patients who had undergone recent cardiac surgery. Overall mortality was 79%, with a trend toward worse outcome in immunocompromised patients. There are also reports of disseminated infections occurring in outbreaks related to contaminated hospital water and in patients undergoing hemodialysis receiving care in the same unit.[92,93] Risk factors associated with fungemia in the hospital outbreak included neutropenia, longer duration of hospitalization, and use of corticosteroids.[92]

Sinusitis and pneumonia are two other common clinical presentations of phaeohyphomycosis. Because of the ubiquitous nature of this class of fungi, it is crucial to obtain histopathologic tissue when possible to confirm true invasive infection as opposed to "innocent bystander." The most common species presenting with sinusitis include *Bipolaris* spp, *Curvularia* spp, and *Alternaria* spp. Presentation can include invasive sinus disease with extension into the bone or brain (often in immunocompromised hosts), allergic sinusitis, or fungal ball formation. *Bipolaris* spp and *Curvularia* spp have also been associated with allergic bronchopulmonary disease (similar to *Scedosporium* spp). There are few descriptions of primary pulmonary phaeohyphomycosis in the literature; in fact, the authors were able to identify only 16 such cases (**Table 2**).[5,6,93–107] The most common species producing pneumonia were *Ochroconis* spp (5 cases), followed by *Cladophialophora* spp (3 cases), *Wangiella* spp (2 cases), and *Curvularia* spp (2 cases). Approximately 70% of patients were immunocompromised or had underlying lung disease. Common presentations included cough, shortness of breath, and hemoptysis. Fifty percent of these cases were diagnosed with culture and histopathologic specimens consistent with IFI. Mortality was low at approximately 19%, and just less than half of the patients had surgical cure. Common radiologic findings included nodules and lobar and bilateral infiltrates.

Black molds, such as *Rhinocladiella* spp and *Cladosporium* spp, can be frequently isolated from airway specimens (sputum, bronchoalveolar lavage [BAL]), and even in immunosuppressed patients, they can represent contamination or colonization rather than invasive disease. Thus, diagnosis of phaeohyphomycosis is primarily based on histopathologic findings of affected tissue and corresponding culture, with attention to the proper identification of black molds that are isolated. There are no current rapid diagnostic methods available. The first-line therapy for severe phaeohyphomycosis has not changed significantly over time and is primarily based on clinical experience: antifungal therapies and surgical resection or debridement when possible, although, as noted from the review of CNS infections, early combination therapy with amphotericin B, extended-spectrum azole, and flucytosine has improved outcomes and should be considered in severe CNS cases.[91] For less severe infections and for long-term treatment, however, extended-spectrum azoles, such as voriconazole or posaconazole, are a reasonable treatment option, with low MICs for most species.[23] There are increasing reports of successful salvage therapy in

Table 2
Primary pulmonary phaeohyphomycosis

Case No.	Underlying Disease	Pathogen	Clinical Presentation	Radiologic Findings	Diagnosis	Treatment	Resp	Ref
1	Pulmonary echinococcus	Not speciated	Hemoptysis, fever	Ruptured cyst with pleural invasion	Histopath	Surgical resection	S	94
2	Cardiac transplant (landscaper)	Ochroconis constricta	Cough, fever	Lingular cavity	Culture	Ampho B	S	5
3	Crohn's disease	Cladophialophora bantiana	FUO	LML solitary nodule	Histopath Culture	Surgical resection	S	95
4	Healthy Thai farmer	Cladophialophora bantiana	Hemoptysis, cough	Hilar consolidation	Unknown	Surgical resection	S	96
5	Bronchopulmonary sequestration	Exophiala jeanselmei	Chest pain, SOB	Unresolving LLL infiltrate	Histopath Culture	Surgical resection	S	97
6	HIV/AIDS bullous lung	Cladophialophora bantiana	Cough, SOB	Bilateral patchy interstitial infiltrates	Culture	None	D	98
7	Healthy, 38 years old	Fonsecaea pedrosoi	Dysphagia, cough	Mediastinal mass	Histopath Culture	Ampho B + itraconazole	S	99
8	HIV	Ochroconis gallopavum	Cough, DOE, fever, NS, Wt. loss	RML opacity bilateral infiltrates	Histopath Culture	Voriconazole	D	100

9	Bronchiectasis	*Wangiella dermatitidis*	Hemoptysis, Wt. loss	LLL, lingular infiltrates	Culture	Ampho B+ 5-FC	S	101
10	IVDU	*Scopulariopsis brumpti*	Chest pain, DOE, cough	Diffuse nodules LLL SS mass	Histopath Culture	Surgical resection	S	102
11	Bronchiectasis	*Wangiella dermatitidis*	Hemoptysis	RLL opacity and solitary nodule	Histopath Culture	Itraconazole	S	6
12	Healthy, 79 years old	*Ochroconis gallopavum*	SOB, fever, cough, NS	Diffuse nodules GGO	Culture	Voriconazole	S	103
13	Mentally retarded	*Curvularia pallescans*	Unknown	Diffuse infiltrates	Culture	Miconazole	D	104
14	Healthy, 41 years old	*Curvularia lunata*	SOB, seizures	Diffuse infiltrates	Histopath Culture	Ampho B	S	105
15	Lung transplant	*Ochroconis gallopavum*	Asymp	LUL, lingular solitary nodule	Culture	↓ IS Ampho B → Itra	S	106
16	Healthy, 38 years old (papermill worker)	*Ochroconis gallopavim*	Cough, hemoptysis	RUL nodules	Histopath Culture	Surgical resection+ Itra	S	107

Abbreviations: Ampho B, amphotericin B; Asymp, asymptomatic; D, died; DOE, dyspnea on exertion; 5-FC, flucytosine; FUO, fever of unknown origin; GGO, ground-glass opacities; Histopath, histopathologic examination; Itra, itraconazole; IVDU, intravenous drug use; LLL, left lower lobe; LML, left middle lobe; LUL, left upper lobe; NS, night sweats; Ref, references; Resp, response to therapy; RLL, right lower lobe; RUL, right upper lobe; S, survived; SOB, shortness of breath; SS, superior segment; Wt., weight; ↓ IS, decreased immunosuppression; → Itra, transition to itraconazole.

phaeohyphomycosis using posaconazole or voriconazole, and these agents may need to be integrated with a surgical approach as an appropriate first-line treatment option.[24,34,108,109]

DIAGNOSTICS

As discussed previously, appropriate and rapid diagnosis of these IFIs is often crucial for survival. This is especially important in the fungi discussed here because they may be resistant to available antifungal agents. Decision making for empiric therapy must be guided with as much data as possible to improve chances of a successful management strategy. Currently, conventional methods, such as direct microscopy, histopathologic examination, and culture, remain the cornerstone of diagnosis because of the lack of broad new technologies that are applicable to all fungi. There are several new rapid, sensitive, and specific fungal diagnostic tests that are helpful, however, and provide insight into what the future may hold.

Direct microscopy and histopathologic methods remain crucial to help provide preliminary information, such as yeast versus mold. Furthermore, visualization of fungal elements in tissue allows for assessment of the microscopic appearance of the hyphal elements, which can help to differentiate hyalohyphomycosis from zygomycosis from phaeohyphomycosis. Although this is certainly crucial, there are also significant limitations of these methods: slow turn-around time, invasive procedure required for tissue, and difficulty in differentiating the fungi causing hyalohyphomycosis from Aspergillus spp. Although there are reports of clear morphologic means to differentiate some hyaline molds from Aspergillus spp, because of the diversity of the hyaline septate molds in resistance to antifungals, a more rapid way to differentiate these molds from Aspergillus spp could be lifesaving.[110]

Galactomannan (GM) is a cell-wall polysaccharide specific to Aspergillus spp, and it is detectable in serum and other body fluids during IA. It is currently approved by the US Food and Drug Administration (FDA) for use only in two populations: HSCT recipients and patients who have leukemia. The diagnostic parameters of this test are reported at a sensitivity of 80.7% and a specificity of 89.2%.[11] Limitations include the fact that use of mold-active antifungals can decrease the sensitivity of the test and false-positive test results have been reported in patients on piperacillin-tazobactam and amoxicillin-clavulanate.[111,112] Use of this Aspergillus-specific antigen test can be helpful in attempting to differentiate Aspergillus from other hyaline molds that cause hyalohyphomycosis, thus allowing more rapid decision making for empiric therapy. Although GM is currently only approved for measurement in the serum, it has been studied for use in other body fluids, including BAL, urine, and CSF.

1,3-β-D-glucan (BG) is a cell-wall constituent found in multiple fungi, including Aspergillus spp and Candida spp, and it is used for detection of fungal products in the serum of a patient with clinical suspicion for IFI. BG has also been detectable in patients who have IFIs attributable to Fusarium, Trichosporon, Saccharomyces, and Acremonium.[113] This test has lacked sensitivity to detect IFIs attributable to zygomycosis.[11,114] The diagnostic parameters of the test are reported at a negative predictive value of 100% and a specificity of 90%.[114,115] Furthermore, the combination of these two tests in selected patients seems to increase sensitivity and specificity to 100% for the diagnosis of IA.[11]

Thus, although direct microscopy, histopathologic evaluation, and culture with expert mycologic identification remain the cornerstone of diagnosis and should be attained in all patients with suspicion of an IFI whenever possible, the use of rapid antigen-specific assays should also be considered as an adjuvant diagnostic method to help guide medical decision making and choices of preemptive therapy. Furthermore, other technologies, such as peptide nucleic acid fluorescence in situ hybridization, nucleic acid probes, amplification-based molecular approaches, and polymerase chain reaction (PCR), are being investigated for more rapid diagnostics in fungal disease.[11] The use of PCR for detection of zygomycosis in plasma, BAL, and lung tissue has had promising results.[115] It is hopeful these techniques not only provide more rapid means of detection of IFIs but help to differentiate true infection from colonization or contamination and correctly identify the infecting fungus.

SUMMARY

Emerging fungi previously thought to be nonpathogenic are now recognized as playing a significant role in the increased incidence of invasive fungal disease. This change in epidemiology of IFIs has occurred in the era of aggressive new therapies for HSCT and other malignancies that lead to profound immunosuppression for longer durations and has extended the survival of these critically ill patients. Specifically, increasing rates of IFIs in patients who have prolonged neutropenia or GVHD and those on high-dose steroids or an antithymocyte antibody have been reported.

Also, antimicrobial selection pressure from new antifungal agents and changes in use of antifungals for prophylaxis, especially in the transplant and cancer populations, are contributing to this shift in epidemiology. The significant morbidity and mortality associated with these infections are not only related to the host populations but to delayed recognition and diagnosis and high rates of resistance in some of these emerging pathogens to standard antifungal therapies.

Early recognition of IFI is crucial for improved outcome, and there are tools available for clinicians to improve chances of survival. These include increased suspicion of IFIs in high-risk populations, especially those on broad-spectrum antifungal prophylaxis; recognition of radiologic signs and clinical presentations that are suggestive of a certain IFI; aggressive pursuit of culture and histopathologic diagnosis; use of adjuvant diagnostics, such as galactomannan and 1,3-b-D-glucan BD assays, to differentiate IA or candidiasis from other emerging IFIs; aggressive surgical management when appropriate; and early appropriate empiric antifungal therapy, in addition to any other efficacious adjuvant therapies available, including change in the management of the underlying disease.

REFERENCES

1. Nucci M, Marr KA, Queiroz-Telles F, et al. *Fusarium* infection in hematopoietic stem cell transplant recipients. Clin Infect Dis 2004;38:1237–42.
2. Lamaris GA, Chamilos G, Lewis RE, et al. *Scedosporium* infection in a tertiary care cancer center: a review of 25 cases from 1989–2006. Clin Infect Dis 2006;43:1580–4.
3. Chouaki T, Lavarde V, Lachaud L, et al. Invasive infections due to *Trichoderma* species: report of 2 cases, findings of in vitro susceptibility testing, and review of the literature. Clin Infect Dis 2002;35:1360–7.
4. Safdar A. Progressive cutaneous hyalohyphomycosis due to *Paecilomyces lilacinus*: rapid response to treatment with caspofungin and itraconazole. Clin Infect Dis 2002;34:1415–7.
5. Mancini MC, McGinnis MR. *Dactylaria* infection of a human being: pulmonary disease in a heart transplant recipient. J Heart Lung Transplant 1992;11:827–30.
6. Ozawa Y, Suda T, Kaida Y, et al. A case of bronchial infection of Wangiella dermatitidis. Nihon Kokyuki Gakkai Zasshi 2007;45(11):907–11.
7. Roden MM, Zaoutis TE, Buchanan WL, et al. Epidemiology and outcome of zygomycosis: a review of 929 cases. Clin Infect Dis 2005;41:634–53.
8. Walsh TJ, Groll A, Hiemenz J, et al. Infections due to emerging and uncommon medically important fungal pathogens. Clin Microbiol Infect 2004;10(S1):48–66.
9. Baddley JW, Stroud TP, Salzman D, et al. Invasive mold infections in allogeneic bone marrow transplant recipients. Clin Infect Dis 2001;32:1319–24.
10. Kontoyiannis DP, Lionakis MS, Lewis RE, et al. Zygomycosis in a tertiary-care cancer center in the era of Aspergillus-active antifungal therapy: a case-control observational study of 27 recent cases. J Infect Dis 2005;191:1350–60.
11. Alexander BD, Pfaller MA. Contemporary tools for the diagnosis and management of invasive mycoses. Clin Infect Dis 2006;43:S15–27.
12. Lionakis MS, Kontoyiannis DP. The significance of isolation of saprophytic molds from the lower respiratory tract in patients with cancer. Cancer 2004;100:165–72.
13. Lionakis MS, Bodey GP, Tarrand JJ, et al. The significance of blood cultures positive for emerging saprophytic molds in cancer patients. Clin Microbiol Infect 2004;10:922–5.
14. Cohen R, Roth FJ, Delgado E, et al. Fungal flora of the normal human small and large intestine. N Engl J Med 1969;280:638–41.
15. Ando J, Takatori K. Fungal flora of the conjunctival sac. Am J Ophthalmol 1982;94:67–74.
16. Marr KA, Carter RA, Crippa F, et al. Epidemiology and outcome of mould infections in hematopoietic stem cell transplant recipients. Clin Infect Dis 2002;34:909–17.
17. Nucci M, Anaissie EJ, Queiroz-Telles F, et al. Outcome predictors of 84 patients with hematologic malignancies and Fusarium infection. Cancer 2003;98:315–9.
18. Schell WA. New aspects of emerging fungal pathogens: a multifaceted challenge. Clin Lab Med 1995;15:365–87.
19. Boutati EI, Anaissie EJ. *Fusarium*, a significant emerging pathogen in patients with hematologic malignancy: ten years' experience at a cancer center and implications for management. Blood 1997;90:999–1008.
20. Sampathkumar P, Paya CV. *Fusarium* infection after solid-organ transplantation. Clin Infect Dis 2001;32:1237–40.
21. Reuben A, Anaissie E, Nelson PE, et al. Antifungal susceptibility of 44 clinical isolates of Fusarium species. Antimicrobial Agents Chemother 1989;33:1647–9.
22. Nucci M, Anaissie E. *Fusarium* infections in immunocompromised patients. Clin Microbiol Rev 2007;20(4):695–704.
23. Pfaller MA, Diekema DJ. Rare and emerging opportunistic fungal pathogens: concern for resistance beyond Candida albicans and Aspergillus fumigatus. J Clin Micrbiol 2004;42(10):4419–31.
24. Perfect JR, Marr KA, Walsh TJ, et al. Voriconazole treatment for less-common, emerging, or refractory fungal infections. Clin Infect Dis 2003;36:1122–31.

25. Stanzani M, Tumietto F, Vianelli N, et al. Update on the treatment of disseminated fusariosis; focus on voriconazole. Ther Clin Risk Manag 2007;3(6): 1165–73.

26. Raad I, Hachem RY, Herbrecht R, et al. Posaconazole as salvage treatment for invasive fusariosis in patients with underlying hematological malignancies and other conditions. Clin Infect Dis 2006;42: 1398–403.

27. Ho DY, Lee JD, Rosso R, et al. Treating disseminated fusariosis: amphotericin B, voriconazole, or both? Mycoses 2007;50:227–31.

28. Cortez KJ, Roilides E, Quiroz-Telles F, et al. Infections caused by Scedosporium spp. Clin Microbiol Rev 2008;21(1):157–97.

29. Cimon B, Carrere J, Vinatier JP, et al. Clinical significance of Scedosporium apiospermum in patients with cystic fibrosis. Eur J Clin Microbiol Infect Dis 2000;19:53–6.

30. Castiglion B, Sutton DA, Rinaldi MG, et al. *Pseudallescheria boydii* (anamorph *Scedosporium apiospermum*) infection in organ transplant recipients in a tertiary medical center and review of the literature. Medicine 2002;81:333–48.

31. Revankar SG, Patterson JE, Sutton DA, et al. Disseminated phaeohyphomycosis: review of an emerging mycosis. Clin Infect Dis 2002;34:467–76.

32. Husain S, Munoz P, Forrest G, et al. Infections due to Scedosporium apiospermum and *Scedosporium prolificans* in transplant recipients: clinical characteristics and impact on antifungal agent therapy on outcome. Clin Infect Dis 2005;40:89–99.

33. Katragkou A, Dotis J, Kotsiou M, et al. *Scedosporium apiospermum* infection after near-drowning. Mycoses 2007;50:412–21.

34. Torres HA, Hachem RY, Chemaly RF, et al. Posaconazole: a broad-spectrum triazole antifungal. Lancet Infect Dis 2005;5:775–85.

35. Kuhls K, Lieckfeldt E, Borner T, et al. Molecular reidentification of human pathogenic *Trichoderma* isolates as *Trichoderma longibrachiatum* and *Trichoderma citrinoviride*. Med Mycol 1999;37:25–33.

36. Walsh TJ, Hiemenz JW, Seibel NL, et al. Amphotericin B lipid complex for invasive fungal infections: analysis of safety and efficacy in 556 cases. Clin Infect Dis 1998;26:1383–96.

37. Miguel DD, Gomez P, Gonzalez R, et al. Nonfatal pulmonary Trichoderma viride infection in an adult patient with acute myeloid leukemia: report of one case and review of the literature. Diagn Microbiol Infect Dis 2005;53:33–7.

38. Fleming RV, Walsh TJ, Anaissie EJ. Emerging and less common fungal pathogens. Infect Dis Clin North Am 2002;16:915–33.

39. Escudero Gil MR, Pino Corral E, Munoz R. Pulmonary mycetoma caused by *Trichoderma viride*. Actas Dermosifiliogr 1976;67:673–80.

40. Alanio A, Brethon B, Feuilhade de Chauvin M, et al. Invasive pulmonary infection due to Trichoderma longibrachiatum mimicking invasive Aspergillosis in a neutropenic patient successfully treated with voriconazole combined with caspofungin. Clin Infect Dis 2008;46:e116–8.

41. Kratzer C, Tobudic S, Schmoll M, et al. In vitro activity and synergism of amphotericin B, azoles, and cationic antimicrobials against the emerging pathogen *Trichderma* spp. J Antimicrob Chemother 2006;58:1058–61.

42. Pastor FJ, Guarro J. Clinical manifestations, treatment, and outcome of *Paecilomyces lilacinus* infections. Clin Microbiol Infect 2006;12:948–60.

43. Gutierrez F, Masia M, Ramos J, et al. Pulmonary mycetoma caused by an atypical isolate of Paecilomyces species in an immunocompetent individual: case report and literature review of *Paecilomyces* lung infections. Eur J Clin Microbiol Infect Dis 2005;24:607–11.

44. Salle V, Lecuyer E, Chouaki T, et al. *Paecilomyces variotii* fungemia in a patient with multiple myeloma: case report and literature review. J Infect 2005;51: e93–5.

45. Chamilos G, Kontoyiannis DP. Voriconazole-resistant disseminated *Paecilomyces variotii* infection in a neutropenic patient with leukaemia on voriconazole prophylaxis. J Infect 2005;51: e225–8.

46. Wang SM, Shieh CC, Liu CC. Successful treatment of *Paecilomyces variotii* splenic abscesses: a rare complication in a previously unrecognized chronic granulomatous disease child. Diagn Microbiol Infect Dis 2005;53(2):149–52.

47. Bertaina C, Giacchino M, Bezzio S, et al. Sepsis due to *Paecilomyces* in familial hemo-phagocytic lymphohistiocytosis after allogeneic transplant of hemopoietic stem cells. Minerva Pediatr 2007; 59(4):415.

48. Sanchez Yepes M, Maiquez Richard J, San Juan Gadea MC. Lung infection by *Paecilomyces variotii* in a patient with breast cancer. Med Clin 2007; 129(11):438.

49. Alkorta Gurrutxaga M, Saiz Camin M, Rodriguez Anton L. Fungal endocarditis in a patient bearing a valve prosthesis. Enferm Infecc Microbiol Clin 2007;25(8):549–50.

50. Jackson ST, Smikle MF, Antoine MG, et al. *Paecilomyces lilacinus* fungemia in a Jamaican neonate. West Indian Med J 2006;55(5):361.

51. Castro LG, Salebian A, Sotto MN. Hyalohyphomycosis by Paecilomyces lilacinus in a renal transplant patient and review of human *Paceilomyces* species infections. J Med Vet Mycol 1990;28:15–26.

52. Wright K, Popli S, Gandhi VC, et al. *Paecilomyces* peritonitis: case report and review of the literature. Clin Nephrol 2003;59(4):305–10.

53. Fagerburg R, Suh B, Buckley HR, et al. Cerebrospinal fluid shunt colonization and obstruction by *Paecilomyces variotii*. Case report. J Neurosurg 1981;54(2):257–60.

54. Sherwood JA, Dansky AS. *Paecilomyces* pyelonephritis complicating nephrolithiasis and review of Paecilomyces infections. J Urol 1983;130(3): 526–8.

55. Dhindsa MK, Naidu J, Singh SM, et al. Chronic suppurative otitis media caused by *Paecilomyces variotii*. J Med Vet Mycol 1995;33(1):59–61.

56. Lee J, Yew WW, Chiu CS, et al. Delayed sternotomy wound infection due to Paecilomyces variotii in a lung transplant recipient. J Heart Lung Transplant 2002;21(10):1131–4.

57. Castelli MV, Alastruey-Izquierdo A, Cuesta I, et al. Susceptibility testing and molecular classification of Paecilomyces spp. Antimicrobial Agents Chemother 2008;52(8):2926–8.

58. Martin CA, Roberts S, Greenberg RN. Voriconazole treatment of disseminated *Paecilomyces* infection in a patient with acquired immunodeficiency syndrome. Clin Infect Dis 2002;35(7):e78–81.

59. Van Schooneveld T, Freifeld A, Lesiak B, et al. *Paecilomyces lilacinus* infection in a liver transplant patient: case report and review of the literature. Transpl Infect Dis 2008;10(2):117–22.

60. Mullane K, Toor AA, Kalnicky C, et al. Posaconazole salvage therapy allows successful allogeneic hematopoietic stem cell transplantation in patients with refractory invasive mold infections. Transpl Infect Dis 2007;9(2):89–96.

61. Chayakulkeeree M, Ghannoum MA, Perfect JR. Zygomycosis: the re-emerging fungal infection. Eur J Clin Microbiol Infect Dis 2006;25:215–29.

62. Vazquez JA, Sobel JD. Fungal infections in diabetes. Infect Dis Clin North Am 1995;9:97–116.

63. Boelaert JR, Fenves AZ, Coburn JW. Deferoxamine therapy and mucormycosis in dialysis patients: report of an international registry. Am J Kidney Dis 1991;18:660–7.

64. Boelaert FR, van Roost GF, Vergauwe PL, et al. The role of desferrioxamine in dialysis-associated mucormycosis: report of three cases and review of the literature. Clin Nephrol 1988;29:261–6.

65. Hopkins RJ, Rothman M, Fiore A, et al. Cerebral mucormycosis associated with intravenous drug use: three case reports and review. Clin Infect Dis 1994;19:1133–7.

66. Siwek GT, Kodgson KJ, Magalhaes-Silverman M, et al. Invasive zygomycosis in hematopoietic stem cell transplant recipients receiving voriconazole prophylaxis. Clin Infect Dis 2004;39:584–7.

67. Imhof A, Balajee SA, Fredricks DN, et al. Breakthrough fungal infections in stem cell transplant recipients receiving voriconazole. Clin Infect Dis 2004;39:743–6.

68. Diamond RD, Haudenschild CC, Erickson NF. Monocyte-mediated damage to *Rhizopus oryzae* hyphae in vitro. Infect Immun 1982;38:292–7.

69. Waldorf AR, Ruderman N, Diamond RD. Specific susceptibility to mucormycosis in murine diabetes and bronchoalveolar macrophage defense against Rhizopus. J Clin Invest 1984;74:150–60.

70. Chinn RY, Diamond RD. Generation of chemotactic factors by Rhizopus oryzae in the presence and absence of serum: relationship to hyphal damage mediated by human neutrophils and effects of hyperglycemia and ketoacidosis. Infect Immun 1982;38:1123–9.

71. Boelaert JR, de Locht M, Van Cutsem J, et al. Mucormycosis during deferoxamine therapy is a siderophore-mediated infection. In vitro and in vivo animal studies. J Clin Invest 1993;91:1979–86.

72. Artis WM, Fountain JA, Delcher HK, et al. A mechanism of susceptibility to mucormycosis in diabetic ketoacidosis: transferrin and iron availability. Diabetes 1982;31:1109–14.

73. Chamilos G, Marom EM, Lewis RE, et al. Predictors of pulmonary zygomycosis versus invasive pulmonary aspergillosis in patients with cancer. Clin Infect Dis 2005;41:60–6.

74. van Burik JH, Hare RS, Solomon HF, et al. Posaconazole is effective as salvage therapy in zygomycosis: a retrospective summary of 91 cases. Clin Infect Dis 2006;42:e61–5.

75. Cornely OA, Maertens J, Winston DJ, et al. Posaconazole vs. fluconazole or itraconazole prophylaxis in patients with neutropenia. N Engl J Med 2007; 356:348–59.

76. Ullmann AJ, Liptom JH, Vesole DH, et al. Posaconazole or fluconazole for prophylaxis in severe graft-versus-host disease. N Engl J Med 2007; 356:335–47.

77. Ustun C, DeRemer DL, Steele JCH, et al. Fatal Aspergillus fumigatus and Candida glabrata infections with posaconazole prophylaxis after stem cell transplantation. Int J Antimicrob Agents 2008;32: 363–71.

78. Schlemmer F, Lagrange-Xelot M, Lacroix C, et al. Breakthrough Rhizopus infection on posaconazole prophylaxis following allogeneic stem cell transplant. Bone Marrow Transplant 2008;42:551–2.

79. Larkin JA, Montero JA. Efficacy and safety of amphotericin B lipid complex for zygomycosis. Infect Med 2003;20:201–6.

80. Ibrahim AS, Gebermariam T, Fu Y, et al. The iron chelator deferasirox protects mice from mucormycosis through iron starvation. J Clin Invest 2002; 117(9):2649–57.

81. Reed C, Ibrahim A, Edwards JE, et al. Deferasirox, an iron-chelating agent, as salvage therapy for rhinocerebral mucormycosis. Antimicrobial Agents Chemother 2006;50:3968–9.

82. Reed C, Bryant R, Ibrahim AS, et al. Combination polyene-caspofungin treatment of rhino-orbital-cerebral mucormycosis. Clin Infect Dis 2008;47: 364–71.

83. Gonzalez CE, Couriel DR, Walsh TJ. Disseminated zygomycosis in a neutropenic patient: successful treatment with amphotericin B lipid complex and granulocyte colony-stimulating factor. Clin Infect Dis 1997;24:192–6.

84. Garcia-Diaz JB, Palau L, Pankey GA. Resolution of rhinocerebral zygomycosis associated with adjuvant administration of granulocyte-macrophage colony-stimulating factor. Clin Infect Dis 2001;32: e166–70.

85. Ibrahim AS, Bowman JC, Avanessian V, et al. Caspfungin inhibits Rhizopus oryzae 1,3-β-D-glucan synthase, lowers burden in brain measured by quantitative PCR, and improves survival at a low but not a high dose during murine disseminated zygomycosis. Antimicrobial Agents Chemother 2005;49:721–7.

86. Ferguson BJ, Mitchell TG, Moore R, et al. Adjunctive hyperbaric oxygen for treatment of rhinocerebral mucormycosis. Rev Infect Dis 1988;10: 551–9.

87. John BV, Chamilos G, Kontoyiannis DP. Hyperbaric oxygen as an adjunctive treatment for zygomycosis. Clin Microbiol Infect 2005;11:515–7.

88. Ajello L, Georg LK, Steigbigel RT. A case of phaeohyphomycosis caused by a new species of Phialophora. Mycologia 1974;66:490–8.

89. Dixon DM, Polak A, Szaniszlo PJ. Pathogenicity and virulence of wild-type and melanin-deficient Wangiella dermatitidis. J Med Vet Mycol 1987;25: 97–106.

90. Husain S, Alexander BD, Munoz P, et al. Opportunistic mycelial fungal infections in organ transplant recipients: emerging importance of non-aspergillus mycelial fungi. Clin Infect Dis 2003;37:221–9.

91. Revankar SG, Sutton DA, Rinaldi MG. Primary central nervous system phaeohyphomycosis: a review of 101 cases. Clin Infect Dis 2004;38: 206–16.

92. Nucci M, Akiti T, Barreiros G, et al. Nosocomial outbreak of Exophiala jeanselmei fungemia associated with contamination of hospital water. Clin Infect Dis 2002;34:1475–80.

93. Proia LA, Hayden MK, Kammeyer PL, et al. *Phialemonium*: an emerging mold pathogen that caused 4 cases of hemodialysis-associated endovascular infection. Clin Infect Dis 2004;39:373–9.

94. Date A, Mathews MS, Varma SK, et al. Echinococcus with concurrent phaeohyphomycosis. Mycoses 1998;41:429–30.

95. Borges MC, Warren S, White W, et al. Pulmonary phaeohyphomycosis due to Xylohypha bantiana. Arch Pathol Lab Med 1991;115:627–8.

96. Limsila T, Stiltnimankarn T, Thasnakom P. Pulmonary cladosporoma: report of a case. J Med Assoc Thai 1970;53:586–90.

97. Samuels T, Morava-Protzner I, Youngson B, et al. Calcification in bronchopulmonary sequestration. J Can Assoc Radiol 1989;40:106–7.

98. Brenner SA, Morgan J, Rickert PD, et al. *Cladophialophora bantiana* isolated from an AIDS patient with pulmonary infiltrates. J Med Vet Mycol 1996; 34:427–9.

99. Singh N, Agarwal R, Gupta D, et al. An unusual case of mediastinal mass due to *Fonsecaea pedrosoi*. Eur Respir J 2006;28:662–4.

100. Boggild AK, Poutanen SM, Mohan S, et al. Disseminated phaeohyphomycosis due to *Ochroconis gallopavum* in the setting of advanced HIV infection. Med Mycol 2006;44:777–82.

101. Barenfanger J, Ramirez F, Tewari RP, et al. Pulmonary phaeohyphomycosis in a patient with hemoptysis. Chest 1989;95:1158–60.

102. Grieble HG, Rippon JW, Maliwan N, et al. Scopariopsosis and hypersensitivity pneumonitis in an addict. Ann Intern Med 1975;83:326–9.

103. Hollingsworth JW, Shofer S, Zaas A. Successful treatment of Ochroconis gallopavum infection in an immunocompetent host. Infection 2007;35(5): 367–9.

104. Lampert RP, Hutto JH, Donnelly WH, et al. Pulmonary and cerebral mycetoma caused by Curvularia pallescens. J Pediatr 1977;91:603–5.

105. de la Monte SM, Hutchins GM. Disseminated curvularia infection. Arch Pathol Lab Med 1985;109: 872.

106. Burns KEA, Ohori NP, Iacono AT. *Dactylaria gallopava* infection presenting as a pulmonary nodule in a single-lung transplant recipient. J Heart Lung Transplant 2000;19:900–2.

107. Odell JA, Alvarez S, Cvitkovich DG, et al. Multiple lung abscesses due to *Ochroconis gallopavum*, a dematiaceous fungus, in a nonimmunocompromised wood pulp worker. Chest 2000;118: 1503–5.

108. Al-Abdely HM, Alkhunaizi AM, Al-Tawfiq JA, et al. Successful therapy of cerebral phaeohyphomycosis due to Ramichloridium mackenziei with the new triazole posaconazole. Med Mycol 2005;43:91–5.

109. Segal BH, Barnhart LA, Anderson VL, et al. Posaconazole as salvage therapy in patients with chronic granulomatous disease and invasive filamentous fungal infection. Clin Infect Dis 2005;40:1684–8.

110. Liu K, Howell DN, Perfect JR, et al. Morphologic criteria for the preliminary identification of *Fusarium*, *Paecilomyces*, and *Acremonium* species by histopathology. Am J Clin Pathol 1998;109:45–54.

111. Maertens J, Theunissen K, Verhoef G, et al. False-positive Aspergillus galactomannan antigen test results. Clin Infect Dis 2004;39:289–90.

112. Mattei D, Rapezzi D, Mordini N, et al. False-positive Aspergillus galactomannan enzyme-linked immunoabsorbent assay results in vivo during amoxicillin-clavulanic acid treatment. J Clin Microbiol 2004;42:5362–3.

113. Yoshida M, Obayashi T, Iwama A, et al. Detection of plasma 1,3-β-D-glucan in patients with *Fusarium*, *Trichosporon*, *Saccharomyces*, and *Acremonium* fungaemias. J Med Vet Mycol 1997;35:371–4.

114. Ostrosky-Zeichner L, Alexander B, Kett DH, et al. Multicenter clinical evaluation of the 1,3-β-D-glucan assay as an aid to diagnosis of fungal infections in humans. Clin Infect Dis 2005;41:654–9.

115. Odabasi Z, Mattiuzzi G, Estey E, et al. β-D-glucan as a diagnostic adjunct for invasive fungal infections: validation, cutoff development, and performance in patients with acute myelogenous leukemia and myelodysplastic syndrome. Clin Infect Dis 2004;39:199–205.

Role of Bronchoalveolar Lavage Diagnostics in Fungal Infections

Kenneth S. Knox, MD[a],*, Laura Meinke, MD[b]

KEYWORDS

- Lavage • Fungus • Cytology • Antigen testing
- Lung • Endemic • Immunosuppressed

Bronchoscopy with bronchoalveolar lavage (BAL) is an important tool for the diagnosis of pulmonary infections and malignancies. Flexible fiberoptic bronchoscopy is a relatively safe and minimally invasive means by which to obtain bronchoalveolar lavage fluid (BALF). It is usually well tolerated by patients and can be performed safely even on those patients who are quite ill or debilitated.

Fungal diseases are emerging as important sources of infection, especially among the immunocompromised. Mortality attributable to invasive aspergillosis ranges from 30% to 70%. Immunosuppressed patients who have candidemia have 40% mortality.[1–3]

In some processes, such as pneumocystis pneumonia (PCP), BAL approaches the diagnostic sensitivity and specificity of biopsy, the "gold standard" for staining and culture. In other fungal illnesses, BAL falls well short. Until quite recently, rapid diagnosis of fungal infections was limited to direct cytologic examination of BALF. In recent years, fungal antigen detection and molecular techniques have been applied and have emerged as important adjuncts to the rapid diagnosis of several fungal infections.

TECHNIQUES FOR DIAGNOSIS

Methods of collection, shipping, and cytologic preparation of BAL samples continue to vary considerably among institutions. When examining submitted BAL specimens, 7% to 30% have been characterized as unsatisfactory because of lack of alveolar macrophages.[4,5]

It should also be noted that flexible fiberoptic bronchoscopy with BAL is not a sterile procedure. Contaminating organisms from the upper airways may be detected in BALF. In addition, certain organisms are known to colonize the tracheobronchial tree and may be collected in BALF samples. The question of colonization versus infection is of critical importance when treating patients who have presumed hospital- or ventilator-acquired pneumonia, necessitating rigorous collection standards. There are, however, relatively few fungal organisms known to colonize the tracheobronchial tree or upper airway. *Aspergillus* and *Candida* species are the most prominent such organisms, although *Pneumocystis* and *Cryptococcus* have been identified as potential colonizers. Boersma and colleagues[6] looked at the newer bronchoscopic techniques of protected BAL and protected specimen brushing and did not find that they provided improved diagnostic results in granulocytopenic patients.

PNEUMOCYSTIS

The utility of BAL in the diagnosis of fungal disease is best demonstrated in patients who have AIDS with PCP. Although some advocate biopsy at the time of bronchoscopy, BAL alone has a sensitivity nearing 98% in these patients.[7]

Pneumocystis, unlike many other fungal pathogens, cannot be cultured in the laboratory. Therefore, cytologic examination remains the mainstay of diagnosis. Characteristic findings of PCP in BALF include *Pneumocystis* cysts and clusters,

[a] Southern Arizona VA Health Care System (SAVAHCS), 3601 S. 6th Avenue (1-11C), Tucson, AZ 85723, USA
[b] Arizona Health Sciences Center, Pulmonary Critical Care, 1501 N. Campbell Avenue, PO BOX 254030, Tucson, AZ 85724, USA
* Corresponding author.
E-mail address: kenneth.knox2@va.gov (K.S. Knox).

Clin Chest Med 30 (2009) 355–365
doi:10.1016/j.ccm.2009.02.010
0272-5231/09/$ – see front matter. Published by Elsevier Inc.

chestmed.theclinics.com

foamy alveolar macrophages, foamy alveolar casts, and activated T cells (**Fig. 1**).[8] Several studies have compared staining techniques for the diagnosis of PCP. Results of these studies vary, but it seems that a Papanicolaou (Pap) stain can, with reliable sensitivity and specificity, lead to the diagnosis.[9–11] Institutional policy and experience with individual stains play an important role when rapid diagnosis of PCP or another fungal infection is required, however. In many centers, a Pap stain may not be readily available for rapid interpretation. In others, Gomori methenamine silver nitrate (GMS) staining may be done just as rapidly as a Pap stain and also has excellent positive and negative predictive values, as does calcofluor white (CW) staining.[9]

There is a higher detection sensitivity when commercialized fluorescein- or enzyme-labeled monoclonal or polyclonal antibodies are used on BALF smears in addition to routine stains.[12] They are, however, more expensive and time-consuming. In addition, although immunofluorescent staining increases sensitivity, it is less specific than standard staining, resulting in a need to confirm the diagnosis with a second method.[9]

Because of our inability to culture PCP, numerous studies have been performed on a variety of antigen testing techniques and molecular assays. DNA-based polymerase chain reaction (PCR) assays may be more sensitive than conventional microscopic examination.[13] They can be performed on oropharyngeal wash

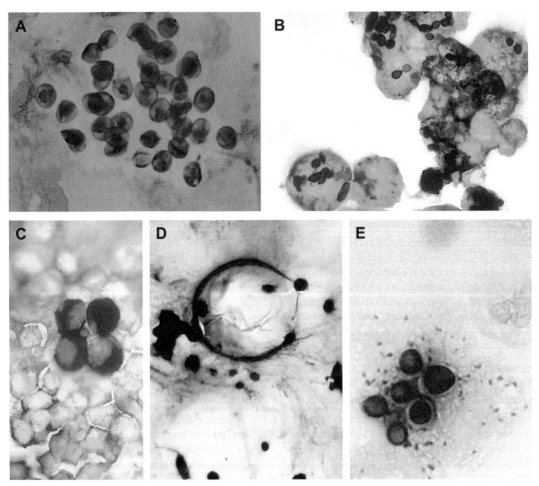

Fig. 1. Representative BAL stains of fungal pathogens. (*A*) Extracellularly located *Pneumocystis jirovecii* cysts (Gomori methenamine silver nitrate [GMS] stain, original magnification ×100). (*B*) Small budding *Histoplasma capsulatum* yeast in alveolar macrophages (GMS stain, original magnification ×400). (*C*) Large broad-based budding *Blastomyces dermatiditis* yeast (GMS stain, original magnification ×400). (*D*) Ruptured *Coccidioides immitis* spherule with release of small spores and a few spores located inside the spherule (Giemsa stain, original magnification ×500). (*E*) Small cluster of narrow budding *Cryptococcus neoformans* yeast extracellularly located (periodic acid–Schiff [PAS stain], original magnification ×400). Note that the sizes are not to scale, particularly because *Pneumocystis* (*A*) is magnified and is typically only 1 to 3 mm larger than *Histoplasma* (*B*).

specimens, sputum samples, or BALF. Several studies have shown sensitivities ranging from 50% to 94% and specificities ranging from 73% to 96%.[14–18] A prominent drawback of PCR testing is its ability to pick up minute amounts of *Pneumocystis* DNA. This results in a relatively high false-positive rate in patients without any laboratory or clinical evidence of disease.[19,20] In addition, it cannot distinguish between viable and nonviable organisms.[21] To overcome the difficulty in distinguishing viable from nonviable organisms, Maher and colleagues[22] and de Oliveira and colleagues[23] studied a reverse transcriptase (RT) PCR assay. Because the target is mRNA, and because mRNA rapidly degrades, it was thought that this type of assay would detect only viable organisms. When studied on BAL specimens, RT-PCR assays were shown to have a sensitivity of 67% to 100% and a specificity of 100%. It seems that RT-PCR assays are less sensitive and specific in induced sputum and oropharyngeal wash specimens and that results paralleled those obtained with simple staining methods.[23] This finding limits its clinical utility.

CRYPTOCOCCUS

Pulmonary infection by *Cryptococcus neoformans* has been reported in immunocompetent and immunocompromised patients. Colonization with *C neoformans* has also been reported.[24] Although the lungs are the portal of entry for *Cryptococcus*, pulmonary disease is relatively uncommon. Most patients, particularly those who are immunocompromised, present with meningoencephalitis. Local pulmonary infection may be seen in patients with higher CD4 cell counts[25] or in immunocompetent patients, who most often present with isolated pulmonary nodules.[26] Detection of cryptococcal antigen (CrAg) in serum or cerebrospinal fluid is the preferred method to establish the diagnosis of cryptococcosis. Bronchoscopic diagnosis may be valuable in cases of isolated lung infection, endobronchial cryptococcosis, and coinfection that would not otherwise be detected without sampling of respiratory secretions.[27] BAL has been reported as more sensitive than bronchial brushings in detection of pulmonary disease.[28]

Cryptococcus is an encapsulated yeast, 4 to 10 μm in diameter, with a clear halo and single narrow-based buds. It is easily visualized on routine fungal stains, such as Pap or GMS, but may be confused for *Candida* or *Histoplasma* species. A more definitive diagnosis may be confirmed by staining of capsular mucopolysaccharide with periodic acid–Schiff (PAS) or mucicarmine stain.[29,30] India ink stain, although useful

for diagnosis on samples of cerebrospinal fluid, is not practically performed on thick pulmonary secretions.

Measurement of CrAg can be done on samples from BAL. It can occasionally provide the diagnosis in patients with negative smears and negative serum antigen testing results.[31,32] A retrospective analysis indicated that the specificity and sensitivity of CrAg on BAL samples are 99% and 71%, respectively.[33] The false-positive rate, however, is quite high. Currently, CrAg testing on BAL fluid is recommended only in cases when direct examination of BAL or sputum samples suggests *Cryptococcus* and rapid confirmation is necessary.[32]

PCR has been studied mostly in tissue homogenates, and its usefulness in BAL diagnostics is unclear. In a study by Takahashi and colleagues,[34] detection of *C neoformans* in BAL fluid was possible through PCR but proved no better than staining, culture, or antigen testing.

CANDIDA

Candida is part of the normal flora of the oral cavity and gastrointestinal tract. Colonization of the tracheobronchial tree seems to be quite common, whereas invasive lung infection by *Candida* species is rare in immunocompetent patients. In a study by Wood and colleagues,[35] 62 critically ill mechanically ventilated trauma patients were noted to have BALF positive for *Candida* species. Most received no antifungal treatment. None developed systemic infection, and no excessive mortality was noted. The incidence of infection, especially among immunocompromised patients, seems to be increasing, as is the incidence of infection with resistant fungal organisms.[36–38]

Various studies show an incidence of candida pneumonia between 0.23% and 8%, with the highest incidence in immunocompromised patients who have disseminated candidiasis.[31,39] Isolation of *Candida* from sputum, tracheal aspirates, BALF, and even lung tissue may simply represent colonization rather than infection.[39] For this reason, clinical criteria for diagnosis of invasive infection caused by *Candida* species have been developed. The currently accepted criteria for diagnosis require a positive blood culture, a positive culture from a normally sterile site (other than urine, sinuses, or respiratory tract), or a histologically positive biopsy specimen.[40] Isolation of *Candida* from BAL samples alone does not indicate invasive infection, even in immunocompromised individuals.

There is a great deal of interest in identifying a means by which colonization can be differentiated from infection. In a prospective study on 25 patients performed by el-Ebiary and colleagues,[39] *Candida* was isolated from 40% of critically ill, mechanically ventilated, nonneutropenic, moribund patients. A definitive diagnosis of invasive infection was established in only 8% of the patients, however, based on histologically positive biopsy results obtained at autopsy. The use of quantitative respiratory samples did not seem to be helpful in determining whether patients were infected or colonized.[39]

Several studies involving PCR and DNA microarray-based detection of fungal pathogens have been performed. These studies show the ability to detect small amounts of candidal and other fungal DNA. The ability to do so does not seem to help in the distinction of colonization and invasive fungal infection, however.[41,42]

ASPERGILLUS

Invasive aspergillus is often difficult to diagnose in the early stages, when treatment is more likely to be of benefit. Among immunocompromised patients, mortality is as high as 92%.[43] The gold standard for diagnosis of infection with *Aspergillus* species is biopsy showing tissue invasion by the organism. Obtaining such samples in patients who have multiple comorbidities may be quite difficult. Further confounding our ability to diagnose invasive aspergillosis is the relative insensitivity of histologic examination and laboratory cultivation. Cytology or culture of BALF was positive in less than one quarter of cases in a study by Reichenberger and colleagues.[44] In high-risk patients, such as those with hematologic malignancies or with history of stem cell transplantation, the isolation of *Aspergillus* from the respiratory tract is predictive of pulmonary aspergillosis.[45,46] In patients with normal immune systems or who have underlying lung disease, however, colonization with *Aspergillus* is possible and differentiating infection from colonization may be difficult.

Galactomannan (GM) testing has been approved to monitor the serum of patients who have hematologic malignancies or hematopoietic stem cell transplants and to diagnose suspected cases of invasive aspergillosis in this patient population.[47] Maertens and colleagues[1] have reported a sensitivity of 100% and a specificity of 97.5% in this patient population, and a meta-analysis showed a sensitivity of 79% and a specificity of 86%.[2]

The *Aspergillus* enzyme immunoassay (EIA) may improve the diagnostic sensitivity of invasive pulmonary aspergillosis if used on BALF.[48–52] The utility of testing BAL specimens in patients who have received solid organ transplants is less clear, because there is a higher rate of false-positive results, especially in patients with colonization of the upper airways who have undergone lung transplantation.[53,54] There has been no proved benefit of BAL GM testing in immunocompetent hosts, and it should not be ordered in this patient population.[55] Meersseman and colleagues[56] examined the utility of BAL GM testing in critically ill patients. At an index cutoff of 0.5, the test had a sensitivity of 88% and a specificity of 87%, a significant improvement over serum GM or BAL with culture and direct staining examination. At present, the GM assay is not approved by the US Food and Drug Administration (FDA) for testing BALF, but it seems from the available data that such testing may significantly improve the diagnostic yield of bronchoscopy with BAL in immunocompromised patients.

As of this date, PCR testing for *Aspergillus* DNA has been performed on blood samples. It does not seem that this study is any more sensitive than antigenemia testing. Quantitative real-time PCR testing has been performed on BALF in a rabbit model of invasive pulmonary aspergillosis. Sensitivity was only 42%, and specificity was 100%.[57] Sensitivities dropped when the test animals were treated with antifungal medications.[57]

False-positive results in GM testing have been ascribed to the use of Plasmalyte (Plasmalyte, Baxter, Deerfield, Illinois) as the lavage solution.[31,58] It is also reported in patients treated with piperacillin-tazobactam, amoxicillin, amoxicillin-clavulanate, and other fungal infections.[59]

ENDEMIC FUNGAL DISEASES

It is important to consider endemic fungi in immunocompromised patients and in immunocompetent patients with nonresolving pulmonary infiltrates. Failure to include these organisms in the differential diagnosis often leads to a delayed diagnosis. Such delays add to the morbidity and mortality associated with infections by endemic fungi. Fungal culture remains the diagnostic gold standard. Fungal cultures may take weeks to yield results, however, and are therefore impractical in severely ill patients who have acute respiratory distress syndrome or progressive disseminated disease.

Rapid diagnosis can be achieved in many cases by cytopathologic examination of biologic samples such as BAL, peripheral blood smear, or biopsy material from infected organs. Testing for fungal antigens in serum and urine is a powerful diagnostic tool for the diagnosis of histoplasmosis. Antigen testing technology has improved over the years[60] and is now being applied to cerebrospinal fluid and BAL. The added benefit of antigen testing in BAL is, as of yet, poorly defined and is best demonstrated in the case of histoplasmosis (**Table 1**). At present, PCR, RT-PCR, and other molecular tests are available only as confirmatory tests once organisms have already grown in the laboratory, thus failing to aid in speedy diagnoses of these infections.

BLASTOMYCOSIS

Blastomyces dermatitidis is a systemic fungal pathogen that may affect immunocompetent or immunocompromised patients. Patients are often first diagnosed with and treated for bacterial pneumonia. This delay in diagnosis may result in progression of the infection, leading to respiratory failure and acute respiratory distress syndrome.[61,62] For this reason, it is desirable to have a rapid means of diagnosis.

Definitive diagnosis of blastomycosis requires isolation of the causative organism from culture. Cytologic examination of BALF or sputum may assist in more rapid diagnosis. The characteristic appearance of *B dermatitidis* is a large (10–15 μm), broad-based, budding yeast. The yeast may be detected using several staining techniques. If purulent sputum is expectorated, potassium hydroxide wet preparations can be an inexpensive way to make the diagnosis. The diagnostic yield on single specimens is quite low (36%), however, and improves only slightly when serial specimens are submitted (46%).[63–65] It is easier to recognize the yeast in specially stained specimens than in wet preparations.[64] Standard fungal stains, such as Giemsa and GMS, are quite useful.[5] PAS staining may also allow for identification of this organism. The diagnosis is best obtained using a Pap stain applied to a biopsy or BAL specimen, showing yeast with characteristic staining of internal structures.[5]

Cytologic examination alone may result in misdiagnosis, however. *C neoformans* and small immature spherules of *Coccidioides immitis* or *Coccidioides posadasii* can be mistaken for *Blastomyces*. This has led to interest in confirmatory testing for *Blastomyces*-specific antigens or *Blastomyces*-specific DNA. Commercially available DNA probes that recognize unique RNA sequences of *Blastomyces* may aid in more rapid diagnosis of blastomycosis from early cultures.[66] Testing for *Blastomyces* antigen is also available. It is detectable in at least one specimen (serum, urine, or BAL fluid) in more than 90% of patients who have disseminated or pulmonary blastomycosis.[67] The *Blastomyces* antigen test significantly cross-reacts with the *Histoplasma* antigen test.

PCR is not currently available for the diagnosis of blastomycosis on biologic samples. These techniques are labor-intensive and, as of yet, have not been prospectively tested on large numbers of patients.

COCCIDIOIDOMYCOSIS

Coccidioidomycosis is a major health problem in immunocompetent and immunocompromised individuals who live in the southwestern United States. In parts of Arizona, it has been estimated that *Coccidioides* causes 29% of community-acquired pneumonias.[68] Infections may be asymptomatic or present as a community-acquired pneumonia. In some patients, especially those who are immunocompromised, coccidioidomycosis may present as disseminated infection, rapidly progressive pulmonary infection, and respiratory failure.

Serology is the most widely used diagnostic test but is of little use in the rapid diagnosis of severely infected patients.[69] Blair and colleagues[70] found that the result of the immunodiffusion test was positive in 53% of immunosuppressed patients, compared with 73% of nonimmunosuppressed patients. The complement fixation test had similar results, with 67% positivity in immunosuppressed and 75% positivity in immunocompetent individuals.[70] Currently, rapid diagnosis can be achieved only by cytopathologic examination of biologic samples, such as BAL, sputum, or biopsy specimens. In some patients with negative cytopathologic findings by BAL, culture may result in diagnosis. The mean time for diagnosis by this means is nearly 1 week but may take as long as 3 weeks in some patients, again limiting its utility for rapid diagnosis. Bronchoscopy is particularly valuable in patients who have parenchymal lung infiltrates and cavitary disease.[71] Diagnosis can be rapidly established on BAL specimens in 30% to 70% of cases.[72,73] A Pap stain is superior to potassium hydroxide and CW stains.[74] Other stains, such as GMS, can also be used. The addition of a simultaneous transbronchial biopsy may increase the diagnostic yield of bronchoscopy.[73]

The diagnostic form of *Coccidioides* observed in biologic specimens is spherules that range in diameter from 20 to 200 μm and are filled with 2- to 4-μm diameter endospores. The mycelial form is uncommon but has been seen in fine needle aspiration and BAL specimens.[75]

Cross-reacting *Histoplasma* antigen has been detected in the BAL of patients who have pulmonary coccidiodomycosis.[76] Taking advantage of this cross-reactivity may prove helpful in the rapid diagnosis of isolated pulmonary infection in

Table 1
Usefulness of tests when applied specifically to bronchioalveolar lavage clinical samples.

	Pneumocystis	Histoplasma	Blastomyces	Coccidioides	Cryptococcus
BAL slide examination	Pap (++++) GMS (++++) CW (+++) Giemsa (++)	Pap (++) GMS (++++) Giemsa (+++) PAS (+)	Pap (++++) GMS (++++) PAS (+++) Giemsa (+++) KOH (sputum+++)	Pap (++++) GMS (++++) CW (+++) KOH (sputum++)	Pap (++++) GMS (++++) PAS (++++) Mucicarmine (capsular stain (+++))
BAL antigen	B-glucan insufficient evidence to recommend nonspecific test	Histoplasma antigen (+++) Well studied, limited experience with localized disease	Blastomyces antigen (++) Limited experience, cross-reactivity with Histoplasma antigen	None available Cross-reactivity with Histoplasma antigen assay	Cryptococcal antigen (+++) Limited experience with localized disease
BAL PCR	(++) Can detect colonization	Unclear role, under development	No data	Under development	Unclear role

Abbreviations: KOH, potassium hydroxide; ++++, most useful; +++, often useful; ++, limited utility; +, least helpful.

endemic areas. EIA testing for coccidioidomycosis has been performed on urine samples from patients with severe infection; however, this has not been adequately tested on BAL fluid.[72] There is enthusiasm for developing more specific antigen tests and using PCR technology for rapid identification of *Coccidioides* in clinical specimens, and a real-time PCR assay has shown some promise.[77]

HISTOPLASMOSIS

Histoplasmosis is the most common endemic mycosis in the United States. It causes various syndromes ranging from asymptomatic radiographic changes to fulminant respiratory failure. Rapid diagnosis is most important in immunocompromised patients and those who have severe pneumonia after large inocula, which are circumstances that may lead to respiratory failure. It is important to include histoplasmosis in the differential diagnosis, particularly when patients live in the endemic area or travel to such areas.

Testing urine and serum for *Histoplasma* antigen remains the preferred method for rapid diagnosis.[78] In fact, the antigen is detected in 92% of urine samples and 85% of blood samples in patients who have disseminated disease.[79] There are, however, plenty of patients who have histoplasmosis and are missed with urine or serum antigen testing. *Histoplasma* antigen can be detected in the urine in 80% of patients with acute diffuse pulmonary involvement, but it is seen in only 34% of patients with subacute pulmonary involvement and in 14% with chronic pulmonary involvement.[80] For this reason, BAL remains an important means of diagnosis.

BAL analysis should follow a protocol that includes several stains to detect *Histoplasma*. In contrast to *Pneumocystis*, GMS and Giemsa stains are superior to Pap and PAS stains for detecting yeast forms.[81,82] *Histoplasma* yeast is ovoid and small, measuring 2 to 5 μm in diameter with narrow-based budding. This morphology is not specific, and several other fungi, including *C neoformans*, *Candida glabrata*, *Pneumocystis*, and the spores released by a ruptured *Coccidioides* spherule, can be misidentified as *Histoplasma* yeast. Demonstration of the yeast inside of BAL phagocytes helps to differentiate it from *Pneumocystis* cysts and *Candida* species in some instances. Biopsy at the time of bronchoscopy likely improves the diagnostic yield of BAL.[83,84] Histopathologic examination of BAL specimens usually reveals the diagnosis in a few hours in those patients who have disseminated disease. Histopathologic findings may be falsely

negative, however, because of sampling error, low number of organisms, or inexperienced cytologists. As a result, the sensitivity of cytopathologic analysis of BAL varies among published studies, ranging from 40% to 85%.[78,85,86] In addition, culture may require several weeks to isolate and correctly identify the organism.[79]

Histoplasma antigen testing performed on BAL samples can improve the sensitivity of BAL analysis,[85,87] especially in concentrated specimens. Hage and colleagues[87] have reported false-positive results in 1.8% of BAL specimens from control patients, possibly attributable to cross-reaction with high levels of *Aspergillus* GM. One should note, however, that this test also reacts with *Blastomyces* species; therefore, in areas where both organisms are being considered, diagnosis must still be confirmed histologically. Sending BAL for antigen testing on nodules for chronic histoplasmosis is not recommended.

The Platelia (Bio-Rad Laboratories; Hercules, California) GM test is often positive in the BAL of patients who have disseminated histoplasmosis.[88,89] Thus, if GM is detected in BAL, confirmatory testing with *Histoplasma* antigen or cytologic examination is warranted.

Molecular diagnosis of histoplasmosis using PCR directly on BAL specimens is currently under development. In most studies, PCR is less sensitive than antigen testing and is not yet used in clinical practice.[90]

PARACOCCIDIOIDOMYCOSIS

Paracoccidioides brasiliensis is a dimorphic fungus endemic to Latin America. Cases are sporadically reported worldwide as a result of importation from endemic areas. The gold standard for diagnosis remains visualization of the yeast forms in clinical specimens. *P brasiliensis* is a 10- to 20-μm spherical thick-walled yeast with multiple daughter buds each attached by a narrow neck, a structure is often referred to as a "mariner's" or "pilot's wheel." The yeast may be detected by potassium hydroxide preparation and is easily seen with a Pap or GMS stain.[91] On occasion, the organism may not be readily visible by such methods. Additionally, growth of this fastidious organism is quite difficult, and culture results are often delayed. For this reason, there is significant interest in serologic, antigen detection, and PCR studies for diagnosis for paracoccidioidomycosis (PCM). *Paracoccidioides*-specific antibodies and antigens have been detected in BALF, perhaps improving the diagnostic yield of bronchoscopy in pulmonary PCM.[92–94] These tests remain cumbersome, however, and have been performed in relatively small numbers of patients. Their utility in the diagnosis of PCM remains unclear. PCR testing is also under development. San-Blas and his colleagues[93,94] have reported that primers designed on the 0.72-kb fragment are capable of identifying *P brasiliensis* DNA from sputum and cerebrospinal fluid of patients who have PCM. This test was able to detect as little as 10 pg of fungal DNA, preceding the ability to diagnose PCM by clinical, serologic, or mycologic tests. There are no published data regarding its efficacy on BAL samples, nor is this test currently approved for use in diagnostic testing of patients suspected of having PCM.

SUMMARY

Although a biopsy may need to be performed in complicated patients, BAL is an important adjunct to the diagnosis of pulmonary and disseminated fungal infections. Culture is the gold standard for diagnosis in many instances, but cytologic and morphologic analysis is often diagnostic. Although newer molecular and antigen techniques may be applied to BAL samples, the role of such tests is yet to be defined for many pathogens.

REFERENCES

1. Maertens J, Theunissen K, Lodewyck T, et al. Advances in the serological diagnosis of invasive aspergillus infections in patients with haematological disorders. Mycoses 2007;50(Suppl 1):2–17 [erratum in mycoses 2008; 51:179].
2. Pfeiffer CD, Fine JP, Safdar N. Diagnosis of invasive aspergillosis using a galactomannan assay: a meta-analysis. Clin Infect Dis 2006;42(10):1417–27.
3. Pfaller MA, Diekema DJ. Epidemiology of invasive candidiasis: a persistent public health problem. Clin Microbiol Rev 2007;20(1):133–63.
4. Chamberlain DW, Braude AC, Rebuck AS. A critical evaluation of bronchoalveolar lavage. Criteria for identifying unsatisfactory specimens. Acta Cytol 1987;31(5):599–605.
5. Lemos LB, Baliga M, Taylor BD, et al. Bronchoalveolar lavage for diagnosis of fungal disease. Five years' experience in a southern United States rural area with many blastomycosis cases. Acta Cytol 1995;39(6):1101–11.
6. Boersma WG, Erjavec Z, van der Werf TS, et al. Bronchoscopic diagnosis of pulmonary infiltrates in granulocytopenic patients with hematologic malignancies: BAL versus PSB and PBAL. Respir Med 2007;101(2):317–25.
7. Huang L, Morris A, Limper AH, et al. ATS Pneumocystis Workshop P. An official ATS workshop summary: recent advances and future directions in pneumocystis pneumonia (PCP). Proc Am Thorac Soc 2006;3(8):655–64.
8. Jacobs JA, Dieleman MM, Cornelissen EI, et al. Bronchoalveolar lavage fluid cytology in patients with pneumocystis carinii pneumonia. Acta Cytol 2001;45(3):317–26.
9. Procop GW, Haddad S, Quinn J. Detection of Pneumocystis jirovecii in respiratory specimens by four staining methods. J Clin Microbiol 2004;42:3333 3333–5.
10. Schumann GB, SJJ. Comparison of Papanicolaou's stain with the Gomori methenamine silver (GMS) stain for the cytodiagnosis of pneumocystis carinii in bronchoalveolar lavage (BAL) fluid. Am J Clin Pathol 1991;95(583):583–6.
11. Nassar A, Zapata M, Little JV, et al. Utility of reflex Gomori methenamine silver staining for Pneumocystis jirovecii on bronchoalveolar lavage cytologic specimens: a review. Diagn Cytopathol 2006; 34(719):719–23.
12. Lautenschlager I, Lyytikainen O, Jokipii L, et al. Immunodetection of pneumocystis carinii in bronchoalveolar lavage specimens compared with methenamine silver stain. J Clin Microbiol 1996; 34(3):728–30.
13. Arcenas RC, Uhl JR, Buckwalter SP, et al. A real-time polymerase chain reaction assay for detection of pneumocystis from bronchoalveolar lavage fluid. Diagn Microbiol Infect Dis 2006;54(3):169–75.
14. Atzori C, Agostoni F, Angeli E, et al. Combined use of blood and oropharyngeal samples for noninvasive diagnosis of pneumocystis carinii pneumonia using the polymerase chain reaction. Eur J Clin Microbiol Infect Dis 1998;17(4):241–6.
15. Fischer S, Gill VJ, Kovacs J, et al. The use of oral washes to diagnose pneumocystis carinii pneumonia: a blinded prospective study using a polymerase chain reaction-based detection system. J Infect Dis 2001;184(11):1485–8.
16. Helweg-Larsen J, Jensen JS, Benfield T, et al. Diagnostic use of PCR for detection of Pneumocystis carinii in oral wash samples. J Clin Microbiol 1998; 36(7):2068–72.
17. Larsen HH, Huang L, Kovacs JA, et al. A prospective, blinded study of quantitative touch-down polymerase chain reaction using oral-wash samples for diagnosis of pneumocystis pneumonia in HIV-infected patients. J Infect Dis 2004;189(9): 1679–83.
18. Matos O, Costa MC, Lundgren B, et al. Effect of oral washes on the diagnosis of pneumocystis carinii pneumonia with a low parasite burden and on detection of organisms in subclinical infections. Eur J Clin Microbiol Infect Dis 2001;20(8):573–5.
19. Durand-Joly I, Chabe M, Soula F, et al. Molecular diagnosis of pneumocystis pneumonia. FEMS Immunol Med Microbiol 2005;45(3):405–10.

20. Davis JL, Welsh DA, Beard CB, et al. Pneumocystis colonisation is common among hospitalised HIV infected patients with non-pneumocystis pneumonia. Thorax 2008;63(4):329–34.

21. Josephson KL, Gerba CP, Pepper IL. Polymerase chain reaction detection of nonviable bacterial pathogens. Appl Environ Microbiol 1993;59(10): 3513–5.

22. Maher NH, Vermund SH, Welsh DA, et al. Development and characterization of a molecular viability assay for pneumocystis carinii f sp hominis. J Infect Dis 2001;183(12):1825–7.

23. de Oliveira A, Unnasch TR, Crothers K, et al. Performance of a molecular viability assay for the diagnosis of pneumocystis pneumonia in HIV-infected patients. Diagn Microbiol Infect Dis 2007;57(2): 169–76.

24. Jarvis JN, Harrison TS. Pulmonary cryptococcosis. Semin Respir Crit Care Med 2008;29(2):141–50.

25. Meyohas MC, Roux P, Bollens D, et al. Pulmonary cryptococcosis: localized and disseminated infections in 27 patients with AIDS. Clin Infect Dis 1995; 21(3):628–33.

26. Pappas PG, Perfect JR, Cloud GA, et al. Cryptococcosis in human immunodeficiency virus-negative patients in the era of effective azole therapy. Clin Infect Dis 2001;33(5):690–9.

27. Chechani VKS. Pulmonary manifestations of disseminated cryptococcosis in patients with AIDS. Chest 1990;98:1060–6.

28. Gal AA, Koss MN, Hawkins J, et al. The pathology of pulmonary cryptococcal infections in the acquired immunodeficiency syndrome. Arch Pathol Lab Med 1986;110(6):502–7.

29. Kanjanavirojkul N, Sripa C, Puapairoj A. Cytologic diagnosis of Cryptococcus neoformans in HIV-positive patients. Acta Cytol 1997;41(2):493–6.

30. Rosen SE, Koprowska I. Cytologic diagnosis of a case of pulmonary cryptococcosis. Acta Cytol 1982;26(4):499–502.

31. Haron E, Vartivarian S, Anaissie E, et al. Primary candida pneumonia. Medicine (Baltimore) 1993;72: 137–42.

32. Bottone EJ, Sindone M, Caraballo V. Value of assessing cryptococcal antigen in bronchoalveolar lavage and sputum specimens from patients with AIDS. Mt Sinai J Med 1998;65(5–6):422–5.

33. Kralovic SM, Rhodes JC. Utility of routine testing of bronchoalveolar lavage fluid for cryptococcal antigen. J Clin Microbiol 1998;36(10):3088–9.

34. Takahashi T, Goto M, Kanda T, et al. Utility of testing bronchoalveolar lavage fluid for cryptococcal ribosomal DNA. J Int Med Res 2003;31(4):324–9.

35. Wood GC, Mueller EW, Croce MA, et al. Candida sp. isolated from bronchoalveolar lavage: clinical significance in critically ill trauma patients. Intensive Care Med 2006;32(4):599–603.

36. Bille J, Marchetti O, Calandra T. Changing face of health-care associated fungal infections. Curr Opin Infect Dis 2005;18(4):314–9.

37. Marchetti O, Bille J, Fluckiger U, et al. Epidemiology of candidemia in swiss tertiary care hospitals: secular trends, 1991-2000. Clin Infect Dis 2004;38(3): 311–20.

38. Maschmeyer G. The changing epidemiology of invasive fungal infections: new threats. Int J Antimicrob Agents 2006;27(Suppl 1):3–6.

39. el-Ebiary M, Torres A, Fabregas N, et al. Significance of the isolation of Candida species from respiratory samples in critically ill, non-neutropenic patients. An immediate postmortem histologic study. Am J Respir Crit Care Med 1997;156(2 Pt 1):583–90.

40. Ascioglu S, Rex JH, de Pauw B, et al. Defining opportunistic invasive fungal infections in immunocompromised patients with cancer and hematopoietic stem cell transplants: an international consensus. Clin Infect Dis 2002;34(1):7–14.

41. Spiess B, Seifarth W, Hummel M, et al. DNA microarray-based detection and identification of fungal pathogens in clinical samples from neutropenic patients. J Clin Microbiol 2007;45(11):3743–53.

42. Klingspor L, Jalal S. Molecular detection and identification of Candida and Aspergillus spp. from clinical samples using real-time PCR. Clin Microbiol Infect 2006;12(8):745–53.

43. Verdaguer V, Walsh TJ, Hope W, et al. Galactomannan antigen detection in the diagnosis of invasive aspergillosis. Expert Rev Mol Diagn 2007;7(1): 21–32.

44. Reichenberger F, Habicht J, Matt P, et al. Diagnostic yield of bronchoscopy in histologically proven invasive pulmonary aspergillosis. Bone Marrow Transplant 1999;24(11):1195–9.

45. Horvath JA, Dummer S. The use of respiratory-tract cultures in the diagnosis of invasive pulmonary aspergillosis. Am J Med 1996;100(2):171–8.

46. Yu VL, Muder RR, Poorsattar A. Significance of isolation of aspergillus from the respiratory tract in diagnosis of invasive pulmonary aspergillosis. Results from a three-year prospective study. Am J Med 1986;81(2):249–54.

47. Wheat LJ, Walsh TJ. Diagnosis of invasive aspergillosis by galactomannan antigenemia detection using an enzyme immunoassay. Eur J Clin Microbiol Infect Dis 2008;27(4):245–51.

48. Musher B, Fredricks D, Leisenring W, et al. Aspergillus galactomannan enzyme immunoassay and quantitative PCR for diagnosis of invasive aspergillosis with bronchoalveolar lavage fluid. J Clin Microbiol 2004;42(12):5517–22.

49. Salonen J, Lehtonen OP, Terasjarvi MR, et al. Aspergillus antigen in serum, urine and bronchoalveolar lavage specimens of neutropenic patients in relation

to clinical outcome. Scand J Infect Dis 2000;32(5): 485–90.

50. Sanguinetti M, Posteraro B, Pagano L, et al. Comparison of real-time PCR, conventional PCR, and galactomannan antigen detection by enzyme-linked immunosorbent assay using bronchoalveolar lavage fluid samples from hematology patients for diagnosis of invasive pulmonary aspergillosis. J Clin Microbiol 2003;41(8):3922–5.

51. Siemann M, Koch-Dorfler M. The Platelia aspergillus ELISA in diagnosis of invasive pulmonary aspergillosis (IPA). Mycoses 2001;44(7–8):266–72.

52. Becker MJ, Lugtenburg EJ, Cornelissen JJ, et al. Galactomannan detection in computerized tomography-based broncho-alveolar lavage fluid and serum in haematological patients at risk for invasive pulmonary aspergillosis. Br J Haematol 2003;121(3): 448–57.

53. Clancy CJ, Jaber RA, Leather HL, et al. Bronchoalveolar lavage galactomannan in diagnosis of invasive pulmonary aspergillosis among solid-organ transplant recipients. J Clin Microbiol 2007;45(6):1759–65.

54. Husain S, Paterson DL, Studer SM, et al. Aspergillus galactomannan antigen in the bronchoalveolar lavage fluid for the diagnosis of invasive aspergillosis in lung transplant recipients. Transplantation 2007;83(10):1330–6.

55. Nguyen MH, Jaber R, Leather HL, et al. Use of bronchoalveolar lavage to detect galactomannan for diagnosis of pulmonary aspergillosis among nonimmunocompromised hosts. J Clin Microbiol 2007; 45(9):2787–92.

56. Meersseman W, Lagrou K, Maertens J, et al. Galactomannan in bronchoalveolar lavage fluid: a tool for diagnosing aspergillosis in intensive care unit patients. Am J Respir Crit Care Med 2008;177(1):27–34.

57. Francesconi A, Kasai M, Petraitiene R, et al. Characterization and comparison of galactomannan enzyme immunoassay and quantitative real-time PCR assay for detection of aspergillus fumigatus in bronchoalveolar lavage fluid from experimental invasive pulmonary aspergillosis. J Clin Microbiol 2006; 44(7):2475–80.

58. Hage CA, Reynolds JM, Durkin M, et al. Plasmalyte as a cause of false-positive results for aspergillus galactomannan in bronchoalveolar lavage fluid. J Clin Microbiol 2007;45(2):676–7.

59. Aubry A, Porcher R, Bottero J, et al. Occurrence and kinetics of false-positive aspergillus galactomannan test results following treatment with beta-lactam antibiotics in patients with hematological disorders. J Clin Microbiol 2006;44(2):389–94.

60. Wheat LJ, Connolly P, Durkin M, et al. Elimination of false-positive histoplasma antigenemia caused by human anti-rabbit antibodies in the second-generation histoplasma antigen assay. Transpl Infect Dis 2006;8(4):219–21.

61. Sriram PS, Knox KS, Busk MF, et al. A 19-year-old man with nonresolving pneumonia. Chest 2004; 125(1):330–3.

62. Lemos LB, Baliga M, Guo M. Acute respiratory distress syndrome and blastomycosis: presentation of nine cases and review of the literature. Ann Diagn Pathol 2001;5(1):1–9.

63. Sarosi GA, Davies SF. Blastomycosis. Am Rev Respir Dis 1979;120(4):911–38.

64. Trumbull ML, Chesney TM. The cytological diagnosis of pulmonary blastomycosis. JAMA 1981; 245(8):836–8.

65. Martynowicz MA, Prakash UB. Pulmonary blastomycosis: an appraisal of diagnostic techniques. Chest 2002;121(3):768–73.

66. Stockman L, Clark KA, Hunt JM, et al. Evaluation of commercially available acridinium ester-labeled chemiluminescent DNA probes for culture identification of Blastomyces dermatitidis, Coccidioides immitis, Cryptococcus neoformans, and Histoplasma capsulatum. J Clin Microbiol 1993;31(4):845–50.

67. Durkin M, Witt J, Lemonte A, et al. Antigen assay with the potential to aid in diagnosis of blastomycosis. J Clin Microbiol 2004;42(10):4873–5.

68. Valdivia L, Nix D, Wright M, et al. Coccidioidomycosis as a common cause of community-acquired pneumonia. Emerg Infect Dis 2006;12(6):958–62.

69. Stevens DA. Coccidioidomycosis. N Engl J Med 1995;332(16):1077–82.

70. Blair JE, Coakley B, Santelli AC, et al. Serologic testing for symptomatic coccidioidomycosis in immunocompetent and immunosuppressed hosts. Mycopathologia 2006;162(5):317–24.

71. Wallace JM, Catanzaro A, Moser KM, et al. Flexible fiberoptic bronchoscopy for diagnosing pulmonary coccidioidomycosis. Am Rev Respir Dis 1981; 123(3):286–90.

72. Durkin M, Connolly P, Kuberski T, et al. Diagnosis of coccidioidomycosis with use of the coccidioides antigen enzyme immunoassay. Clin Infect Dis 2008;47(8):e69–73.

73. DiTomasso JP, Ampel NM, Sobonya RE, et al. Bronchoscopic diagnosis of pulmonary coccidioidomycosis. Comparison of cytology, culture, and transbronchial biopsy. Diagn Microbiol Infect Dis 1994;18(2):83–7.

74. Sarosi GA, Lawrence JP, Smith DK, et al. Rapid diagnostic evaluation of bronchial washings in patients with suspected coccidioidomycosis. Semin Respir Infect 2001;16(4):238–41.

75. Helig D, Giampoli EJ. Mycelial form of Coccidioides immitis diagnosed in bronchoalveolar lavage. Diagn Cytopathol 2007;35(8):535–6.

76. Kuberski T, Myers R, Wheat LJ, et al. Diagnosis of coccidioidomycosis by antigen detection using cross-reaction with a histoplasma antigen. Clin Infect Dis 2007;44(5):e50–4.

77. Binnicker MJ, Buckwalter SP, Eisberner JJ, et al. Detection of Coccidioides species in clinical specimens by real-time PCR. J Clin Microbiol 2007; 45(1):173–8.

78. Wheat LJ. Improvements in diagnosis of histoplasmosis. Expert Opin Biol Ther 2006;6(11):1207–21.

79. Williams B, Fojtasek M, Connolly-Stringfield P, et al. Diagnosis of histoplasmosis by antigen detection during an outbreak in Indianapolis, Ind. Arch Pathol Lab Med 1994;118(12):1205–8.

80. Wheat LJ, Conces D, Allen SD, et al. Pulmonary histoplasmosis syndromes: recognition, diagnosis and management. Semin Respir Crit Care Med 2004;25(2):129–44.

81. Valente PT, Calafati SA. Diagnosis of disseminated histoplasmosis by fine needle aspiration of the adrenal gland. Acta Cytol 1989;33(3):341–3.

82. Deodhare S, Sapp M. Adrenal histoplasmosis: diagnosis by fine-needle aspiration biopsy. Diagn Cytopathol 1997;17(1):42–4.

83. Salzman SH, Smith RL, Aranda CP. Histoplasmosis in patients at risk for the acquired immunodeficiency syndrome in a nonendemic setting. Chest 1988; 93(5):916–21.

84. Baughman RP, Kim CK, Bullock WE. Comparative diagnostic efficacy of bronchoalveolar lavage, transbronchial biopsy, and open-lung biopsy in experimental pulmonary histoplasmosis. J Infect Dis 1986;153(2):376–7.

85. Wheat LJ, Connolly-Stringfield P, Williams B, et al. Diagnosis of histoplasmosis in patients with the acquired immunodeficiency syndrome by detection of Histoplasma capsulatum polysaccharide antigen in bronchoalveolar lavage fluid. Am Rev Respir Dis 1992;145(6):1421–4.

86. Gutierrez ME, Canton A, Connolly P, et al. Detection of Histoplasma capsulatum antigen in Panamanian patients with disseminated histoplasmosis and AIDS. Clin Vaccine Immunol 2008;15(4):681–3.

87. Hage CA, Davis TE, Egan L, et al. Diagnosis of pulmonary histoplasmosis and blastomycosis by detection of antigen in bronchoalveolar lavage fluid using an improved second-generation enzyme-linked immunoassay. Respir Med 2007;101(1):43–7.

88. Wheat LJ. Evaluation of reagents for detection of Histoplasma capsulatum antigenuria. [author reply 1388]. Clin Vaccine Immunol 2007;14(10):1387–8.

89. Wheat LJ, Hackett E, Durkin M, et al. Histoplasmosis-associated cross-reactivity in the BioRad Platelia aspergillus enzyme immunoassay. Clin Vaccine Immunol 2007;14(5):638–40.

90. Tang YW, Li H, Durkin MM, et al. Urine polymerase chain reaction is not as sensitive as urine antigen for the diagnosis of disseminated histoplasmosis. Diagn Microbiol Infect Dis 2006;54(4):283–7.

91. de Mattos MC, Mendes RP, Marcondes-Machado J, et al. Sputum cytology in the diagnosis of pulmonary paracoccidioidomycosis. Mycopathologia 1991; 114(3):187–91.

92. Marques-da-Silva SH, Colombo AL, Blotta MH, et al. Diagnosis of paracoccidioidomycosis by detection of antigen and antibody in bronchoalveolar lavage fluids. Clin Vaccine Immunol 2006;13(12):1363–6.

93. San-Blas G, Nino-Vega G. Paracoccidioides brasiliensis: chemical and molecular tools for research on cell walls, antifungals, diagnosis, taxonomy. Mycopathologia 2008;165(4–5):183–95.

94. San-Blas G, Nino-Vega G, Barreto L, et al. Primers for clinical detection of Paracoccidioides brasiliensis. J Clin Microbiol 2005;43(8):4255–7.

Approach to the Diagnosis of Invasive Aspergillosis and Candidiasis

L. Joseph Wheat, MD

KEYWORDS

- Aspergillosis • Candidiasis
- Zygomycosis • Mucormycosis • Antigen detection
- Serology • Diagnosis • Mycosis

ASPERGILLOSIS

Invasive aspergillosis is a major cause for morbidity and mortality in immunocompromised patients,[1,2] especially those who are neutropenic or who have undergone bone marrow transplantation or solid-organ transplantation. In these settings the most common manifestations are pneumonia and sinusitis, but widespread disseminated disease may occur also. A favorable outcome depends on early initiation of treatment and improvement in the underlying immunosuppressive condition.

The diagnosis of invasive aspergillosis may be difficult. One obstacle is obtaining an adequate specimen for direct examination and culture. Because these patients may be severely ill and often are thrombocytopenic, biopsy may not be possible. Although bronchoscopy with bronchoalveolar lavage may be performed despite coagulation defects, direct examination and culture may be falsely negative, and several days may be required to isolate the organism when the culture is positive. Also, in some cases a positive culture may represent airway colonization rather than invasive aspergillosis. Furthermore, visualization of hyphae by direct examination is not specific for aspergillosis, because similar findings may be seen with other molds.

For these reasons methods other than direct examination of the tissue and culture have been developed, including galactomannan and β-glucan detection in serum or other body fluids.

Antigen Detection

Antigen detection is used increasingly for rapid diagnosis of aspergillosis, using the Platella (Bio-Rad Laboratories, Redmond, WA) *Aspergillus* enzyme immunoassay (EIA).[3–5] Evaluation of diagnostic tests in aspergillosis has been difficult because of the insensitivity and nonspecificity of direct examination and culture of respiratory specimens. In the absence of autopsy findings, proof of the diagnosis by tissue biopsy is extremely uncommon. The most accurate data are those of Maertens and colleagues,[6–8] made possible by the high autopsy rate at their institution, without which many of the positive results might have been regarded as false positive. Other studies, reviewed by meta-analysis,[9] are more difficult to evaluate because of differences in study design in the frequency of testing, in variable cut-offs used for the classification of results, in the level of laboratory experience performing the assay, and in other criteria.[10]

ANTIGENEMIA MONITORING

When testing is performed twice weekly and positive results in consecutive samples are required as a basis for diagnosis, sensitivity and specificity have been excellent in patients who have neutropenia or other hematologic conditions (**Table 1**).[9,12,13] In most studies, antigenemia precedes the diagnosis of aspergillosis and

---

The author is the president of MiraBella Technologies and MiraVista Diagnostics.

MiraVista Diagnostics and MiraBella Technologies, 4444 Decatur Boulevard, Indianapolis, IN 46241, USA

E-mail address: jwheat@miravistalabs.com

Clin Chest Med 30 (2009) 367–377
doi:10.1016/j.ccm.2009.02.012

Table 1
Monitoring for invasive aspergillosis in hematologic patients using the Platelia *Aspergillus* enzyme immunoassay

Sensitivity (%)	Specificity (%)	Reference
96 (N = 29)[a]	99 (N = 74)	Maertens (2004)[11]
92 (N = 38)	98 (N = 196)	Maertens (2007)[12]
88 (N = 24)	74 (N = 43)	Marr (2004)[13]
79 (N = 407)	86 (N = 3060)	Pfeiffer (2006)[9,a]

Abbreviation: N, number of cases.
[a] Results of meta-analysis.

initiation of therapy,[11,14] allowing a reduction in the use of empiric antifungal therapy.[15]

FALSE-POSITIVE AND FALSE-NEGATIVE RESULTS

The Platelia *Aspergillus* EIA is a high-complexity test, in which accuracy requires skilled technicians and a laboratory commitment to performance of complex, low-volume procedures; otherwise, false positivity and false negativity can be expected.[10] In skilled laboratories committed to high-complexity procedures, false results can be seen in a few well-recognized situations. False-positive results may occur in patients receiving the antibiotics piperacillin, amoxicillin, or ticarcillin, alone or combined with a beta-lactamase inhibitor. These antibiotics are fermentation products of *Penicillium* spp., a mold that produces a cross-reactive galactomannan (GM).[16,17] Furthermore, intratracheal or intravenous administration of Plasmalyte (Baxter Healthcare Corporation), a commercially available electrolyte replacement solution, also may cause false-positive results in serum[18] or bronchoalveolar lavage (BAL) fluid.[19] Plasmalyte contains sodium gluconate, a fermentation product of *Aspergillus flavus*. GM monitoring may not be appropriate in patients receiving these medications or fluids, unless their production processes are changed to exclude GM.

False-positive results also occur in patients who have infections caused by mold containing a cross-reactive GM, including *Penicillium, Paecilomyces, Alternaria, Geotrichum*, and a few others.[20–23] False positivity has been observed in histoplasmosis[24] and may occur in other endemic mycoses.[25] In patients from areas where endemic mycoses are common, antigen tests for these organisms should be performed to exclude false-positive results in the Platelia assay. False-positive results have been reported in cryptococcosis,[26] an observation that the authors could not substantiate.[27]

In some cases the cause for false positivity is uncertain. In a recent report, about half of the positive results were judged to be false positive, unrelated to known causes.[28] False-positive results were more common in patients who had chronic graft-versus-host disease of the gastrointestinal tract, suggesting that translocation of dietary GM was the cause for false positivity. False positivity once was thought to be more common in pediatric patients, a concern that was disproved recently.[29] As noted previously, without an autopsy excluding the diagnosis, some "false-positive" results may in fact represent undiagnosed aspergillosis.

False-negative results occur in 5% to 15% of patients who have invasive aspergillosis[4,10] but may be more common in several situations. False-negative results seem to be more common in patients receiving antifungal agents that are active against *Aspergillus*.[30] Antigen levels decline with effective therapy, explaining the negative results in these subjects. Results in serum also may be falsely negative in patients who have localized lesions. In such cases antigen may be detected in the infected fluid or tissue.

BRONCHOALVEOLAR LAVAGE FLUID

The Platelia *Aspergillus* EIA also may be used for detection of GM in BAL. In patients who have hematologic malignancy or who have received bone marrow transplantation, the sensitivity has been between 88% and 100%, and the specificity has been between 87% and 100% (**Table 2**).[8,31,32] In a report restricted to patients who had hematologic disorders, the specificity in BAL was 100% using a cut-off of 1.0.[31] The sensitivity for detection of GM in serum was only 47% in that study. In a subsequent study restricted to ICU patients, about one third of whom had hematologic disorders or graft-versus-host disease, sensitivity was 88% using a cut-off of 0.5,[8] and the sensitivity for detection of GM in serum was 44%. Four of the six false-positive results occurred in patients receiving piperacillin-tazobactam, in whom antigenemia also was detected.[8]

Table 2
Detection of galactomannan in bronchoalveolar lavage using the Platelia *Aspergillus* enzyme immunoassay

Group	Sensitivity (%)	Specificity (%)	Reference
Hematologic patients (CO 1.0)	100 (N = 17)	100 (N = 18)	Becker (2003)[31]
Hematopoietic stem cell transplantation (CO 0.5)	76 (N = 49)	94 (N = 50)	Musher(2004)[32]
Lung transplantation (CO 0.5)	67 (N = 6)	91 (N = 110)	Husain (2007)[33]
Solid organ transplantation (CO 0.5)	100 (N = 5)	84 (N = 76)	Clancy (2007)[34]
Nonimmunosuppressed (CO 0.5)	100 (N = 6)	78 (N = 67)	Nguyen (2007)[36]
Immunosuppressed ICU patients (CO 0.5)	88 (N = 26)	87 (N = 46)	Meerseman (2008)[8]

Abbreviations: CO, cut-off; N, number of patients.

In a third study, conducted at the Fred Hutchinson Cancer Research Center, sensitivity was 76% and specificity 94%.[32] Results in serum were not reported. Sensitivity was higher in the cases in which the BAL culture was positive (89%) than in those with negative cultures (59%). Of note is that more than three quarters of patients were receiving antifungal therapy and the specimens were obtained up to 30 days before or after the diagnosis was made, potentially reducing the sensitivity. This study was retrospective, so the results were not available for use in patient management. Nonetheless, the authors estimated that availability of this information might have eliminated the need for a second BAL or open lung biopsy in 90% of patients.

Testing for two studies in solid-organ transplant recipients was performed at MiraVista Diagnostics.[33,34] One study was conducted in lung transplant recipients who underwent BAL for diagnosis of suspected infection or routine monitoring following lung transplantation.[33] The second study included patients who had different types of organ transplantation who underwent diagnostic BAL for evaluation of pulmonary infiltrates.[34] With the 0.5 cut-off, sensitivity was 81.8% and specificity was 95.8% in lung transplant recipients who underwent surveillance BAL.[35] Sensitivity was unchanged, but specificity increased to 96.6% when the cut-off of 1.0 was used. The two false-negative results occurred in patients who were receiving mold-active antifungal agents. The test was positive in serum from one of the four (25%) aspergillosis cases for whom a matching serum specimen was tested. Among lung transplant controls with positive cultures for *Aspergillus* or other mold, 22.2% were positive when a 0.5 cut-off was used, compared with 16.7% when a cut-off of 1.0 was used.

A third study in non-immunosuppressed patients, for which the testing also was done at MiraVista Diagnostics, showed similar findings but concluded that the test may not be as useful in this patient group.[36] Sensitivity was 100% in BAL versus 60% in serum. Specificity was 78% when the 0.5 cut-off was used and 88% when the 1.0 cut-off was used. Two of the false-positive results were in specimens from which *Aspergillus* was isolated, and a third was in a patient who was receiving ticarcillin-clavulanate, an antibiotic that can cause false-positive results. Of the nine controls with false-positive results, two had chronic obstructive lung disease, and three had cavitary lung disease, conditions known to be associated with *Aspergillus* colonization or chronic invasive aspergillosis. Furthermore, histoplasmosis, a known cause for false-positive results in the Platelia *Aspergillus* EIA,[24] was not excluded in these controls, three of whom had radiographic findings consistent with that condition.

Colonization with *Aspergillus* is a strong risk factor for aspergillosis in lung transplant recipients.[37] Acknowledging the difficulty in diagnosis, positive results in some of these controls may have been caused by undiagnosed infection. The significance of positive results in lung transplant recipients who are colonized with *Aspergillus* or other cross-reactive mold merits further investigation to determine if these findings pose a risk for subsequent invasive disease and thus justify interventions to reduce that risk.

GM also has been detected in homogenized lung tissue specimens, positive in 86% of cases.[38] GM may be detected in other body fluids,[39] including cerebrospinal fluid, pleural fluid, and ocular fluid (L.J. Wheat, unpublished observations).

ANTIGEN CLEARANCE FOR MONITORING THERAPY

Several studies demonstrate reduction in antigenemia during therapy.[40–43] In a recent report GM antigenemia was monitored daily and outcome was evaluated in patients who had persistent antigenemia compared with those in whom antigenemia had cleared.[44] Death was significantly more common in patients who had persistent antigenemia. The same authors described an immune reconstitution inflammatory syndrome (IRIS), in which the clinical findings were caused by the immune response, not by progressive aspergillosis. In such cases clinical findings worsened despite clearance of antigenemia, suggesting IRIS as the cause for worsening.[45] Studies comparing antigen clearance in patients who responded versus those who did not respond to treatment have not been conducted, however.

(1→3)-β-D-Glucan Detection

(1→3)-β-D-Glucan (BG) is a cell wall component of Aspergillus and most other fungi. BG activates factor G of the horseshoe crab coagulation cascade, leading to production of a chromogenic substance.[46] The Fungitell BG assay (Associates of Cape Cod) was approved for use in the United States in 2005 and recommends a cut-off of 80 pg/mL for classification as positive. Some investigators recommend requirement of consecutive positive results to improve specificity, at the expense of sensitivity.[47]

The sensitivity for diagnosis of aspergillosis has ranged from 50% to 100%, and specificity ranges from 44% to 98% (Table 3).[48–51,53] A few studies have compared the BG and GM test and have shown similar[50] or reduced sensitivity[48] for the BG assay. The BG assay is not specific for aspergillosis. Positive results also occur in patients who have candidiasis,[49,51,53–56] gastrointestinal colonization with Candida spp.,[47] endemic mycoses,[54,57] cryptococcosis,[51,53,58] and Pneumocystis jiroveci pneumonia.[51,52,59]

False positivity in critically ill patients limits the usefulness of the BG test. High rates of false positivity have been reported in patients who have bacterial infections (54%[54] and 68%[55]). Persat[53] recently reported false-positive results in 44% of patients from hematology wards or ICUs who were at risk for invasive fungal infection. Ellis[56] reported false-positive results in 26% of patients who had neutropenic fever in whom an invasive fungal infection was not observed. Egan and colleagues[57] reported positive results in 44% of hospital controls without an identifiable mycosis. Others reported that 15% of immunocompetent noninfected children had positive BG tests,[60] compared with the reported rates of 7% in healthy adults[49] and 8% in adults without fungal infections.[51]

In addition to positivity in patients who have other mycoses or bacterial infection, false-positive results occur following hemodialysis, exposure to gauze, ingestion of certain foods or medications, use of filters in intravenous tubing, and administration of albumin or immunoglobulin. The assay should not be used in the presence of hemolysis, turbidity, lipemia, or bilirubinemia.

Serology

Serologic tests are not considered useful for the diagnosis of invasive or disseminated aspergillosis but are used for the diagnosis of aspergilloma and allergic bronchopulmonary aspergillosis, as reviewed elsewhere.[61,62]

Guidelines for Diagnosis and Monitoring Therapy

The Platelia Aspergillus EIA has emerged as a helpful method for diagnosing aspergillosis and seems to be more useful for this purpose than the BG assay. Twice weekly monitoring is recommended in hematology patients at risk for invasive aspergillosis, in the absence of mold-active antifungal prophylaxis or use of antibiotics or intravenous fluids that cause false-positive results. Monitoring for antigenemia is not recommended in solid-organ transplant recipients, except perhaps those who have undergone lung transplantation.[33] In such patients a positive result would suggest invasive infection with Aspergillus or another mold or airway colonization and would indicate the need for further evaluation and/or treatment. In patients undergoing bronchoscopy for evaluation of opportunistic infection, BAL fluid also should be tested for Aspergillus GM, improving the sensitivity for diagnosis of aspergillosis. Further studies are needed to establish the role of monitoring GM clearance as a surrogate marker for response to therapy and testing of tissues.

CANDIDIASIS

Candida spp. are common causes of nosocomial infections in patients in ICUs and are a cause for excess mortality.[63] Candida also may cause a variety of other invasive infections and colonization of mucosal surfaces. Blood cultures are positive in no more than half of patients who have invasive candidiasis, making diagnosis more difficult. Treatment of candidemia must be initiated within 12 to 24 hours of drawing the blood culture to improve the outcome of candidemia,[64,65] posing a challenge for diagnostic tests. To identify patients who require treatment this quickly, a test must be performed as soon as possible after the

Table 3
Detection of (1 → 3)-β-D-glucan in patients who have invasive aspergillosis

Design	Sensitivity (%)	Specificity (%)	Reference
Once-weekly monitoring, hematology patients, CO 11 pg/mL (BG Wako test)	55 (N = 11)	98 (N = 125)	Kawazu (2004)[48]
Twice-weekly monitoring, neutropenia, CO 60 ng/mL (Fungitell®)	100 (N = 4)	90 (N = 230)	Odabasi (2004)[48]
Twice-weekly monitoring, neutropenia, CO 120 pg/mL (Fungitell)	100 (N = 8)	90 (N = 29)	Pazos (2005)[50]
Single specimen, CO 80 (Fungitell®)	100 (N = 10)	92 (N = 170) healthy subjects: outpatients and inpatients without IFI	Ostrosky-Zeichner (2005)[51]
Liver transplantation, once-weekly monitoring, CO 40 pg/mL (Fungitec G test)	40 (N = 5)	83 (N = unknown)	Akamatsu (2007)[52]
Hematology or ICU, single test, CO 80 pg/mL (Fungitell)	68 (N = 70)	56 (N = 100)	Persat (2008)[53]

Abbreviations: CO, cut-off; IFI, invasive fungal infection; N, number of patients.

Table 4
Detection of (1 → 3)-β-D-glucan in patients who have candidiasis

Design	Sensitivity (%)	Specificity (%)	Reference
Candidemia, single specimen, CO 60 pg/mL	84 (N = 39)	88 (N = 40)	Mitsutake (1996)[66]
ICU patients, single specimen CO 100 pg/mL (Fungitell®)	57 (N = 7) candidemia	75 (N = 16) bacteremia	Digby (2003)[54]
Fungemia, single specimen, CO 60 pg/mL (Fungitell)	97 (N = 30) candidemia	93 (N = 30) healthy adults	Odabasi (2004)[48]
Fungemia, single specimen CO 80 pg/mL (Fungitell®)	87 (N = 15) candidemia	44 (N = 25) bacteremia	Pickering (2005)[55]
Fungemia, single specimen, CO 80 pg/mL (Fungitell)	78 (N = 92)	92 (N = 170) healthy subjects: outpatients, inpatients without IFI	Ostrosky-Zeichner (2005)[51]
Liver transplantation, once-weekly monitoring, CO 40 pg/mL (Fungitec G test)	57 (N = 14)	83 (N = unknown)	Akamatsu (2007)[52]
Hematology or ICU, single test, CO 80 pg/mL (Fungitell)	85 (N = 27)	56% (N = 100)	Persat (2008)[53]

Abbreviations: CO, cut-off; N, number of patients.

Table 5
Monitoring for (1→3)-β-D-glucan in patients at risk for invasive fungal infection

Design	Sensitivity (%)	Specificity (%)	Reference
Febrile patients, multiple specimens/patient, CO 20 pg/mL (G test-Seikagaku)	76 (N = 37)	84 (N = 161)	Obayaski (1995)[46]
Single specimen after diagnosis IFI, CO 80 pg/mL (Fungitell)	64 (N = 163)	92 (N = 170) healthy subjects, outpatients, inpatients without IFI	Ostrosky-Zeichner (2005)[51]
Neutropenia, twice-weekly monitoring, CO 7 pg/mL (Wako), single positive	67 (N = 30)	75 (N = 113)	Senn (2008)[47]
Neutropenia, twice-weekly monitoring, CO 7 pg/mL (Wako), consecutive positive	63 (N = 30)	96 (N = 113)	Senn (2008)[47]
Liver transplantation, once-weekly monitoring, CO 40 pg/ml (Fungitec G test)	58 (N = 24)	83 (N = unknown)	Akamatsu (2007)[52]
Neutropenia, alternate-day monitoring, CO 80 pg/mL (Fungitell), consecutive positive	87 (N = 38)	76 (N = 42)	Ellis (2008)[56]

Abbreviations: CO, cut-off; IFI, invasive fungal infection; N, number of patients.

specimen is obtained. Several studies address the role of BG testing for the diagnosis of candidiasis, but expert opinion concluded that "available evidence does not support the use of these tests as a reliable guide for clinicians."[63]

β-D-Glucan Detection

In an early report, the BG test was positive in 84% of patients who had candidemia (**Table 4**).[66] In other studies the sensitivity ranged from 57% to 100%, and specificity ranged from 44% to 92%.[49,50,52–54] If consecutive positive results were required for designation as positive, sensitivity fell from 100% to 75%, but specificity increased from 90% to 96%.[49] Based on a mean sensitivity of 89% and a specificity of 86%, derived from the studies in **Table 4**, and assuming a prevalence of 10% for candidemia or invasive candidiasis, the positive predictive value is 0.413, and the negative predictive value is 0.986. Based on these rates, treatment would be administered to patients without candidiasis more often than to those who have candidiasis.

As an alternative to testing at the time of suspected candidiasis, regular monitoring could identify cases in time to affect outcome. Several studies describe the use of BG to monitor patients at risk for invasive fungal infection, including candidiasis (**Table 5**). Sensitivity ranges from 58% to 87%, and specificity ranges from 75% to 92% in these studies.[46,47,51,52,56] Requiring consecutive positive results improved the specificity from 75% to 96%, with only a 4% reduction in sensitivity.[47]

Mohr and colleagues[67] reported a pilot study monitoring patients admitted to an ICU. A prospective pilot survey of β-glucan (BG) seropositivity and its relationship to invasive candidiasis in the surgical ICU). The BG test was performed three times weekly. Seventy-six percent of patients had a positive BG result at admission to the ICU, without evidence for candidiasis; this result reverted to negative in a few days. Although 100% of patients who had candidiasis had a positive result, the test was falsely positive in 20% of controls. Because the risk for a false-positive result would be 20% each time the test was performed, most patients would experience a false-positive result within the first week of testing.

Antigen Detection and Serology

Detection of *Candida* mannan antigenemia and anti-*Candida* antibodies has been described,[66–69] but studies to support their use are not convincing. Persat[53] reported detection of mannan antigenemia in only 42% of patients who had candidemia, compared with BG positivity in 77%.

Guidelines for Diagnosis and Monitoring Therapy

Accurate and convenient rapid methods for diagnosing candidemia or invasive candidiasis are not available. Problems include the logistics of performing the test rapidly enough to guide therapy and false-positive results in patients without fungal infections.

SUMMARY

With certain limitations, GM detection in BAL and serum is useful for the diagnosis of invasive aspergillosis in immunocompromised patients. The role of BG testing in the diagnosis of candidiasis is uncertain. Increasingly non-*Aspergillus* molds are causes for invasive mycoses in immunocompromised patients, but rapid tests for these organisms have not yet been developed. Additional research is needed to develop methods for rapid diagnosis of non-*Aspergillus* molds and to determine how best to use GM and BG detection assays.

REFERENCES

1. Meersseman W, Lagrou K, Maertens J, et al. Invasive aspergillosis in the intensive care unit. Clin Infect Dis 2007;45(2):205–16.
2. Maschmeyer G, Haas A, Cornely OA. Invasive aspergillosis: epidemiology, diagnosis and management in immunocompromised patients. Drugs 2007; 67(11):1567–601.
3. Maertens J, Theunissen K, Lodewyck T, et al. Advances in the serological diagnosis of invasive Aspergillus infections in patients with haematological disorders. Mycoses 2007;50(Suppl 1):2–17.
4. Wheat LJ, Walsh TJ. Diagnosis of invasive aspergillosis by galactomannan antigenemia detection using an enzyme immunoassay. Eur J Clin Microbiol Infect Dis 2008;27(4):245–51.
5. Mennink-Kersten MA, Donnelly JP, Verweij PE. Detection of circulating galactomannan for the diagnosis and management of invasive aspergillosis. Lancet Infect Dis 2004;4(6):349–57.
6. Maertens J, Van Eldere J, Verhaegen J, et al. Use of circulating galactomannan screening for early diagnosis of invasive aspergillosis in allogeneic stem cell transplant recipients. J Infect Dis 2002;186(9): 1297–306.
7. Maertens J, Verhaegen J, Demuynck H, et al. Autopsy-controlled prospective evaluation of serial screening for circulating galactomannan by a sandwich enzyme-linked immunosorbent assay for

hematological patients at risk for invasive Aspergillosis. J Clin Microbiol 1999;37(10):3223–8.

8. Meersseman W, Lagrou K, Maertens J, et al. Galactomannan in bronchoalveolar lavage fluid: a tool for diagnosing aspergillosis in intensive care unit patients. Am J Respir Crit Care Med 2008;177(1): 27–34.

9. Pfeiffer CD, Fine JP, Safdar N. Diagnosis of invasive aspergillosis using a galactomannan assay: a meta-analysis. Clin Infect Dis 2006;42(10):1417–27.

10. Wheat L. Rapid diagnosis of invasive aspergillosis by antigen detection. Transpl Infect Dis 2003;5(4): 158–66.

11. Maertens J, Theunissen K, Verbeken E, et al. Prospective clinical evaluation of lower cut-offs for galactomannan detection in adult neutropenic cancer patients and haematological stem cell transplant recipients. Br J Haematol 2004;126(6):852–60.

12. Maertens JA, Klont R, Masson C, et al. Optimization of the cutoff value for the Aspergillus double-sandwich enzyme immunoassay. Clin Infect Dis 2007; 44(10):1329–36.

13. Marr KA, Balajee SA, McLaughlin L, et al. Detection of galactomannan antigenemia by enzyme immunoassay for the diagnosis of invasive aspergillosis: variables that affect performance. J Infect Dis 2004;190(3):641–9.

14. Busca A, Locatelli F, Barbui A, et al. Usefulness of sequential Aspergillus galactomannan antigen detection combined with early radiologic evaluation for diagnosis of invasive pulmonary aspergillosis in patients undergoing allogeneic stem cell transplantation. Transplant Proc 2006;38(5):1610–3.

15. Maertens J, Theunissen K, Verhoef G, et al. Galactomannan and computed tomography-based preemptive antifungal therapy in neutropenic patients at high risk for invasive fungal infection: a prospective feasibility study. Clin Infect Dis 2005;41(9):1242–50.

16. Sulahian A, Touratier S, Ribaud P. False positive test for aspergillus antigenemia related to concomitant administration of piperacillin and tazobactam. N Engl J Med 2003;349(24):2366–7.

17. Walsh TJ, Shoham S, Petraitiene R, et al. Detection of galactomannan antigenemia in patients receiving piperacillin-tazobactam and correlations between in vitro, in vivo, and clinical properties of the drug-antigen interaction. J Clin Microbiol 2004;42(10): 4744–8.

18. Racil Z, Kocmanova I, Lengerova M, et al. Intravenous PLASMA-LYTE as a major cause of false-positive results of Platelia Aspergillus test for galactomannan detection in serum. J Clin Microbiol 2007;45(9):3141–2.

19. Hage CA, Reynolds JM, Durkin M, et al. Plasmalyte as a cause of false-positive results for Aspergillus galactomannan in bronchoalveolar lavage fluid. J Clin Microbiol 2007;45(2):676–7.

20. Stynen D, Sarfati J, Goris A, et al. Rat monoclonal antibodies against Aspergillus galactomannan. Infect Immun 1992;60(6):2237–45.

21. Swanink CMA, Meis JFGM, Rijs AJMM, et al. Specificity of a sandwich enzyme-linked immunosorbent assay for detecting Aspergillus galactomannan. J Clin Microbiol 1997;35(1):257–60.

22. Giacchino M, Chiapello N, Bezzio S, et al. Aspergillus galactomannan enzyme-linked immunosorbent assay cross-reactivity caused by invasive Geotrichum capitatum. J Clin Microbiol 2006;44(9):3432–4.

23. Huang YT, Hung CC, Liao CH, et al. Detection of circulating galactomannan in Penicillium marneffei infection and cryptococcosis among patients infected with human immunodeficiency virus. J Clin Microbiol 2007;45:2858–62.

24. Wheat LJ, Hackett E, Durkin M, et al. Histoplasmosis-associated cross-reactivity in the BioRad Platelia Aspergillus enzyme immunoassay. Clin Vaccine Immunol 2007;14(5):638–40.

25. Cummings JR, Jamison GR, Boudreaux JW, et al. Cross-reactivity of non-Aspergillus fungal species in the Aspergillus galactomannan enzyme immunoassay. Diagn Microbiol Infect Dis 2007;59(1):113–5.

26. Dalle F, Charles PE, Blanc K, et al. Cryptococcus neoformans galactoxylomannan contains an epitope(s) that is cross-reactive with Aspergillus galactomannan. J Clin Microbiol 2005;43(6):2929–31.

27. De Jesus M, Hackett E, Durkin M, et al. Galactoxylomannan does not exhibit cross-reactivity in the Platelia Aspergillus enzyme immunoassay. Clin Vaccine Immunol 2007;14(5):624–7.

28. Asano-Mori Y, Kanda Y, Oshima K, et al. False-positive Aspergillus galactomannan antigenaemia after haematopoietic stem cell transplantation. J Antimicrob Chemother 2008;61(2):411–6.

29. Hayden R, Pounds S, Knapp K, et al. Galactomannan antigenemia in pediatric oncology patients with invasive aspergillosis. Pediatr Infect Dis J 2008;27(9):815–9.

30. Marr KA, Laverdiere M, Gugel A, et al. Antifungal therapy decreases sensitivity of the Aspergillus galactomannan enzyme immunoassay. Clin Infect Dis 2005;40(12):1762–9.

31. Becker MJ, Lugtenburg EJ, Cornelissen JJ, et al. Galactomannan detection in computerized tomography-based broncho-alveolar lavage fluid and serum in haematological patients at risk for invasive pulmonary aspergillosis. Br J Haematol 2003;121(3): 448–57.

32. Musher B, Fredricks D, Leisenring W, et al. Aspergillus galactomannan enzyme immunoassay and quantitative PCR for diagnosis of invasive aspergillosis with bronchoalveolar lavage fluid. J Clin Microbiol 2004;42(12):5517–22.

33. Husain S, Paterson DL, Studer SM, et al. Aspergillus galactomannan antigen in the bronchoalveolar

lavage fluid for the diagnosis of invasive aspergillosis in lung transplant recipients. Transplantation
2007;83(10):1330–6.

34. Clancy CJ, Jaber RA, Leather HL, et al. Bronchoalveolar lavage galactomannan in diagnosis of invasive
pulmonary aspergillosis among solid-organ transplant recipients. J Clin Microbiol 2007;45(6):1759–65.

35. Husain S, Clancy CJ, Nguyen MH, et al. Performance characteristics of the platelia *aspergillus*
enzyme immunoassay for detection of *aspergillus*
galactomannan antigen in bronchoalveolar lavage
fluid. Clin Vaccine Immunol 2008;15(12):1760–3.

36. Nguyen MH, Jaber R, Leather HL, et al. Use of bronchoalveolar lavage to detect galactomannan for
diagnosis of pulmonary aspergillosis among nonimmunocompromised hosts. J Clin Microbiol 2007;
45(9):2787–92.

37. Husain S, Paterson DL, Studer S, et al. Voriconazole
prophylaxis in lung transplant recipients. Am J
Transplant 2006;12:3008–16.

38. Lass-Florl C, Resch G, Nachbaur D, et al. The value
of computed tomography-guided percutaneous
lung biopsy for diagnosis of invasive fungal infection
in immunocompromised patients. Clin Infect Dis
2007;45(7):e101–4.

39. Klont RR, Mennink-Kersten MA, Verweij PE. Utility of
Aspergillus antigen detection in specimens other
than serum specimens. Clin Infect Dis 2004;39(10):
1467–74.

40. Rohrlich P, Sarfati J, Mariani P, et al. Prospective
sandwich enzyme-linked immunosorbent assay for
serum galactomannan: early predictive value and
clinical use in invasive aspergillosis. Pediatr Infect
Dis J 1996;15(2):232–7.

41. Bretagne S, Marmorat-Khuong A, Kuentz M, et al.
Serum Aspergillus galactomannan antigen testing
by sandwich ELISA: practical use in neutropenic
patients. J Infect 1997;35(1):7–15.

42. Maertens J, Verhaegen J, Lagrou K, et al. Screening
for circulating galactomannan as a noninvasive
diagnostic tool for invasive aspergillosis in prolonged neutropenic patients and stem cell transplantation recipients: a prospective validation.
Blood 2001;97(6):1604–10.

43. Boutboul F, Alberti C, Leblanc T, et al. Invasive aspergillosis in allogeneic stem cell transplant recipients:
increasing antigenemia is associated with progressive disease. Clin Infect Dis 2002;34(7):939–43.

44. Miceli MH, Grazziutti ML, Woods G, et al. Strong
correlation between serum Aspergillus galactomannan index and outcome of aspergillosis in
patients with hematological cancer: clinical and
research implications. Clin Infect Dis 2008;46(9):
1412–22.

45. Miceli MH, Maertens J, Buve K, et al. Immune reconstitution inflammatory syndrome in cancer patients
with pulmonary aspergillosis recovering from

neutropenia: proof of principle, description, and clinical and research implications. Cancer 2007;110(1):
112–20.

46. Obayashi T, Yoshida M, Mori T, et al. Plasma (1–>3)-
beta-D-glucan measurement in diagnosis of invasive deep mycosis and fungal febrile episodes.
Lancet 1995;345(8941):17–20.

47. Senn L, Robinson JO, Schmidt S, et al. 1,3-Beta-D-
glucan antigenemia for early diagnosis of invasive
fungal infections in neutropenic patients with acute
leukemia. Clin Infect Dis 2008;46(6):878–85.

48. Kawazu M, Kanda Y, Nannya Y, et al. Prospective
comparison of the diagnostic potential of real-time
PCR, double-sandwich enzyme-linked immunosorbent assay for galactomannan, and a (1–>3)-
{beta}-D-glucan test in weekly screening for invasive
aspergillosis in patients with hematological disorders. J Clin Microbiol 2004;42(6):2733–41.

49. Odabasi Z, Mattiuzzi G, Estey E, et al. Beta-D-
Glucan as a diagnostic adjunct for invasive fungal
infections: validation, cutoff development, and
performance in patients with acute myelogenous
leukemia and myelodysplastic syndrome. Clin Infect
Dis 2004;39(2):199–205.

50. Pazos C, Ponton J, Palacio AD. Contribution of
(1–>3)-{beta}-D-glucan chromogenic assay to diagnosis and therapeutic monitoring of invasive aspergillosis in neutropenic adult patients: a comparison
with serial screening for circulating galactomannan.
J Clin Microbiol 2005;43(1):299–305.

51. Ostrosky-Zeichner L, Kontoyiannis D, Raffalli J, et al.
International, open-label, noncomparative, clinical
trial of micafungin alone and in combination for treatment of newly diagnosed and refractory candidemia. Eur J Clin Microbiol Infect Dis 2005;24(10):
654–61.

52. Akamatsu N, Sugawara Y, Kaneko J, et al. Preemptive treatment of fungal infection based on plasma
(1 –> 3)beta-D: -glucan levels after liver transplantation. Infection 2007;35(5):346–51.

53. Persat F, Ranque S, Derouin F, et al. Contribution of
the (1–>3)-beta-D-glucan assay for diagnosis of
invasive fungal infections. J Clin Microbiol 2008;
46(3):1009–13.

54. Digby J, Kalbfleisch J, Glenn A, et al. Serum glucan
levels are not specific for presence of fungal infections in intensive care unit patients. Clin Diagn Lab
Immunol 2003;10(5):882–5.

55. Pickering JW, Sant HW, Bowles CAP, et al. Evaluation of a (1–>3)-{beta}-D-glucan assay for diagnosis
of invasive fungal infections. J Clin Microbiol 2005;
43(12):5957–62.

56. Ellis M, Al Ramadi B, Finkelman M, et al. Assessment of the clinical utility of serial {beta}-D-glucan
concentrations in patients with persistent neutropenic fever. J Med Microbiol 2008;57(Pt 3):
287–95.

57. Egan L, Connolly P, Wheat LJ, et al. Histoplasmosis as a cause for a positive Fungitell (1->3)-beta-D-glucan test. Med Mycol 2008;46(1):93–5.

58. Tasaka S, Hasegawa N, Kobayashi S, et al. Serum indicators for the diagnosis of Pneumocystis pneumonia. Chest 2007;131(4):1173–80.

59. Smith PB, Benjamin DK Jr, Alexander BD, et al. Quantification of 1,3-beta-D-glucan levels in children: preliminary data for diagnostic use of the beta-glucan assay in a pediatric setting. Clin Vaccine Immunol 2007;14(7):924–5.

60. Stevens DA, Moss RB, Kurup VP, et al. Allergic bronchopulmonary aspergillosis in cystic fibrosis—state of the art: Cystic Fibrosis Foundation Consensus Conference. Clin Infect Dis 2003;37:S225–64.

61. Soubani AO, Chandrasekar PH. The clinical spectrum of pulmonary aspergillosis. Chest 2002; 121(6):1988–99.

62. Cruciani M, Serpelloni G. Management of Candida infections in the adult intensive care unit. Expert Opin Pharmacother 2008;9(2):175–91.

63. Morrell M, Fraser VJ, Kollef MH. Delaying the empiric treatment of Candida bloodstream infection until positive blood culture results are obtained: a potential risk factor for hospital mortality. Antimicrobial Agents Chemother 2005;49(9):3640–5.

64. Garey KW, Rege M, Pai MP, et al. Time to initiation of fluconazole therapy impacts mortality in patients with candidemia: a multi-institutional study. Clin Infect Dis 2006;43(1):25–31.

65. Mitsutake K, Miyazaki T, Tashiro T, et al. Enolase antigen, mannan antigen, Cand-Tec antigen, and beta-glucan in patients with candidemia. J Clin Microbiol 1996;34(8):1918–21.

66. Mohr JF, Paetznick V, Rodriguez J, et al. A Prospective pilot survey of B-glucan seropositivity and its relationship to invasive candidiasis in the surgical ICU [Abstract M-168]. 45th Interscience Conference on Antimicrobial Agents and Chemotherapy. Washington DC, 2005.

67. Alam FF, Mustafa AS, Khan ZU. Comparative evaluation of (1,3)-beta-D-glucan, mannan and anti-mannan antibodies, and Candida species-specific snPCR in patients with candidemia. BMC Infect Dis 2007;7(1):103.

68. Rimek D, Redetzke K, Steiner B, et al. [Experience with the Platelia Candida ELISA for the diagnostics of invasive candidosis in neutropenic patients]. Mycoses 2004;47(Suppl 1):27–31 [in German].

69. Sharafkhaneh A, Baaklini W, Gorin AB, et al. Yield of transbronchial needle aspiration in diagnosis of mediastinal lesions. Chest 2003;124(6):2131–5.

Approach to the Diagnosis of the Endemic Mycoses

L. Joseph Wheat, MD

KEYWORDS

- Histoplasmosis • Blastomycosis • Coccidioidomycosis
- Antigen detection • Serology • Diagnosis
- Mycosis

Endemic mycoses are frequently overlooked in the evaluation of pulmonary disease. They often are causes for community-acquired pneumonia in endemic areas and require specific testing for diagnosis. The role of and approach to diagnosis of endemic mycoses as causes for community-acquired pneumonia are superficially mentioned in the Infectious Diseases Society of America and American Thoracic Society guideline for management of community-acquired pneumonia.[1] Failure to consider the endemic mycoses may result in a fatal outcome, because progression may occur rapidly.[2–5] Now, histoplasmosis is three times more common than tuberculosis in patients receiving tumor necrosis factor blockers,[6] and it usually presents as a community-acquired pneumonia,[7] which often is overlooked (US Food and Drug Administration [FDA] alert link). Furthermore, exclusion of histoplasmosis often is not done in diagnosis of sarcoidosis,[8] leading to corticosteroid treatment and death as a result of progressive histoplasmosis in some cases.

Although there may be epidemiologic findings suggesting the endemic mycoses in these situations (**Table 1**), their absence does not exclude them as a cause for pulmonary disease in patients from endemic areas. Once considered, the diagnosis usually can be established within 3 to 7 days using a panel of tests (**Table 2**).

HISTOPLASMOSIS

Most infections caused by *Histoplasma capsulatum* are asymptomatic.[8,9] Symptomatic patients usually present with a mild pulmonary illness, at times complicated by pericarditis or rheumatologic complaints.[8,10] Histoplasmosis usually presents as a community-acquired pneumonia.[2,11] Radiographic or chest CT findings include hilar or mediastinal lymphadenopathy with localized or patchy infiltrates. Such cases are referred to as subacute pulmonary histoplasmosis (SPH)[8,10,12] and usually resolve without treatment. Treatment is reserved for those who do not show prompt improvement.[13]

After heavy exposure, patients may present acutely with pulmonary complaints that often include dyspnea.[8,10] Chest radiography or a CT scan typically shows diffuse reticulonodular or miliary infiltrates, referred to as the "epidemic type"[14] of acute pulmonary histoplasmosis (APH). This manifestation may be severe, requiring hospitalization for management of respiratory insufficiency. The published experience with APH is largely derived from case reports and small series of epidemic cases.[14–40] Although APH usually resolves without treatment,[14] recovery may be slow,[41] and, at times, prolonged hospitalization is required for management of respiratory failure.[27,32,38] APH can be fatal, however, as reported in a young woman who died as a result of respiratory failure after 14 days of hospitalization.[27] In approximately 40% of cases, nonprogressive extrapulmonary dissemination can be identified.[20,30,31,34,36,42,43] Rapid diagnosis is important, because early treatment may shorten the course and severity of APH,[17,18,44,45] and treatment is recommended for most cases.[13]

Dr. Wheat is the President of MiraBella Technologies and MiraVista Diagnostics.
MiraVista Diagnostics and MiraBella Technologies, 4444 Decatur Boulevard, Indianapolis, IN 46241, USA
E-mail address: jwheat@miravistalabs.com

Clin Chest Med 30 (2009) 379–389
doi:10.1016/j.ccm.2009.02.011

Table 1
Features suggesting the common endemic mycoses of North America

Features	Histoplasmosis	Coccidioidomycosis	Blastomycosis
Endemic areas in the United States[a]	Midwest but wider range distribution than other endemic mycoses	Southwest but spotty distribution	Midwest and southeast but spotty distribution
Exposure locations[a]	Old buildings containing bird or bat droppings, chicken coops, bird roosts, wood piles, caves	Deserts, archaeologic sites, prairie dog and armadillo habitats	Rivers and other wetlands, construction sites, wooded areas, prairie dog habitats, buildings with bat droppings
Radiographic[b] features	Mediastinal or hilar lymphadenopathy, diffuse or focal infiltrates	Diffuse or focal infiltrates	Diffuse or focal infiltrates
Extrapulmonary sites[c]	Liver, spleen, bone marrow, lymph nodes, CNS (meningitis or parenchymal lesions)	Skin, bone, joints, CNS (usually meningitis)	Skin, bone, genitourinary tract, CNS (usually parenchymal lesions)

Although these features may be clues to the diagnosis, they should not be expected in all cases and may only be detected by specific inquiry or evaluation.

Abbreviation: CNS, central nervous system.

[a] Of note is that exposure may occur miles away from the environmental site as a result wind-borne spread of the spores.

[b] In most cases, the radiographic features are not sufficiently distinct to suggest the diagnosis of an endemic mycosis. The exception might be acute histoplasmosis after heavy exposure causing diffuse reticulonodular, miliary, or nodular infiltrates and more focal infiltrates with hilar or mediastinal lymphadenopathy. These features are not specific for histoplasmosis, however, and should not be used as a basis for the diagnosis without supporting laboratory evidence.

[c] Any tissue may be involved in disseminated cases. Other uncommon sites for dissemination include the skin, gastrointestinal tract, and adrenal gland.

Data from Mandell LA, Wunderink RG, Anzueto A, et al. Infectious Diseases Society of America/American Thoracic Society consensus guidelines on the management of community-acquired pneumonia in adults. *Clin Infect Dis* 2007; 44(Suppl 2):S27–72.

Patients who have underlying obstructive lung disease typically exhibit progressive chronic pulmonary histoplasmosis (CPH).[8] Symptoms have usually been present for months to years before the diagnosis is established. Radiographs and CT scans show upper lobe infiltrates with cavity formation and parenchymal scarring. The urgency for diagnosis is usually low, because progression is slow; however, in some cases, the illness may be severe at the time the diagnosis is suspected or extrapulmonary dissemination may be present, heightening the importance of rapid diagnosis. The course is progressive without treatment, and treatment is indicated in all cases.[13]

Hematogenous dissemination is thought to occur in most patients after the initial infection with *H capsulatum*, but it is nonprogressive, clearing spontaneously within 1 or 2 months, with the development of cellular immunity. Findings supporting the occurrence of nonprogressive dissemination include occasional isolation of the fungus from the blood or bone marrow,[20,30,31,34,36,42,43] enlargement of the liver or spleen, demonstration of bone marrow suppression (anemia, leukopenia, or thrombocytopenia) or hepatic enzyme elevation,[12] and the presence of hepatic or splenic calcifications as incidental findings on radiographs or CT scans.[46] Immunosuppressed patients and those at the extremes of age experience progressive disseminated histoplasmosis (PDH),[47] however, which is ultimately fatal if not diagnosed and treated. PDH also may occur in patients who have other immunodeficiencies[48,49] or no underlying disease.[47] All patients who have PDH require treatment.[13]

Using a battery of tests, once suspected, the diagnosis of histoplasmosis can be made in most patients without difficulty. In patients who have

Table 2
Role of diagnostic tests for evaluation of endemic or invasive mycoses

	Histopathology/Cytology	Antigen Testing	Serology	Culture
Histoplasmosis	+	+	+	+
PDH	+	+	+	+
APH	+	+	+	+
SPH	±[a]	+	+	−
CPH	±[a]	+	+	+
Blastomycosis	+	+	−	+
Coccidioidomycosis	+	+	+	+

Abbreviations: APH, acute pulmonary histoplasmosis; CPH, chronic pulmonary histoplasmosis; PDH, progressive disseminated histoplasmosis; SPH, subacute pulmonary histoplasmosis.
[a] The diagnosis can usually be made based on serology (SPH) or serology and culture of sputum (CPH). Bronchoscopy may be needed in cases in which the diagnosis cannot be established noninvasively.

APH or PDH, or in any patient who has illness sufficiently severe to cause hospitalization, rapid diagnosis is imperative. In such cases, direct examination and antigen detection usually serve as the basis for rapid diagnosis. In asymptomatic cases and in those who have SPH and CPH, serologic tests are especially useful.

Direct Examination

H capsulatum yeast may be visualized by a variety of staining techniques, most commonly using the Gomori methenamine silver and Giemsa methods. Other yeast may be difficult to distinguish from *H capsulatum*, however, including *Blastomyces dermatitidis*, *Candida glabrata*, *Cryptococcus neoformans*, *Pneumocystis jirovecii*, *Leishmania*, and *Toxoplasma*. More common, however, is mistaking artifacts as yeast. The clinician should review the cytology or histopathology slides with the pathologist, and if uncertainty exists, evaluation by an expert should be sought. Also, other tests should be performed to strengthen the diagnosis. These include culture, antigen detection, and serology.

Direct examination is most useful for diagnosis of PDH. In PDH, fungal stains of bone marrow may be positive in approximately half of patients, with hematologic findings suggesting bone marrow involvement.[50] The results of histopathology were positive in bronchoalveolar lavage (BAL) specimens in 70% of patients who had AIDS with diffuse pulmonary infiltrates.[51] In pulmonary histoplasmosis without concurrent disseminated disease, examination of respiratory secretions is positive in less than one quarter of cases (**Table 3**).[52–54]

The histopathologic finding of tissue showing yeast does not distinguish active infection from past infection, however, because nonviable organisms persist in tissues.[46] Yeast may be seen by histopathology in a high proportion of pulmonary nodules biopsied to exclude malignancy, in which cultures are negative.[8] The results of histopathology also may be positive in biopsy specimens of extrapulmonary tissue, most often liver, resulting from past histoplasmosis. All body fluids and tissues submitted for cytology or histopathology for fungal stains also should be cultured for fungus.

Table 3
Sensitivity of diagnostic tests in histoplasmosis

Test	APH	SPH	CPH	PDH
Antigen	77 (N = 85)[a]	34 (N = 70)	21 (N = 14)	92 (N = 108)
Histopathology	35 (N = 26)	9 (N = 11)	17 (N = 6)	43 (N = 51)
Culture	41 (N = 44)	15 (N = 34)	85 (N = 13)	85 (N = 106)
Serology	70 (N = 43)	98 (N = 68)	100 (N = 14)	71 (N = 80)
Reference	Literature cases[b]	Williams et al[53]	Williams et al[53]	Williams et al[53]

Abbreviation: N, number of cases.
[a] Antigen results based on 85 cases tested by the author and 48 literature cases.
[b] Literature cases of APH.[14–40]

Antigen Detection

Antigen detection also is useful for rapid diagnosis of histoplasmosis.[52] This review is based on results using the MVista *Histoplasma* antigen enzyme immunoassay (EIA) (MiraVista Diagnostics, Indianapolis, Indiana)[55,56] and should not be applied to other methods, whose performance differs significantly.[57,58] Antigen is found in the urine of more than 95% of patients who have AIDS and PDH and in the serum of approximately 90%.[56,59] The sensitivity is lower (90%–95%) in patients who have PDH but do not have AIDS (L.J. Wheat, unpublished observation, 2009). Antigen can be detected in the urine in approximately 80% of patients who have APH, and in a lower proportion of those who have SPH (see **Table 3**). In some cases, antigenemia may be present in the absence of antigenuria (L.J. Wheat, unpublished observation, 2009), and both specimens should be tested. Antigen also can be detected in BAL, including cases in which the results of direct examination of the specimen are negative.[60]

Cross-reactivity occurs in patients who have penicilliosis marneffei, paracoccidioidomycosis, and blastomycosis,[56,61] and less so in patients who have coccidioidomycosis.[62] Cross-reactions are rare in patients who have aspergillosis[63] and do not occur with candidiasis or cryptococcosis.[56,64] Except for cross-reactions in patients who have endemic mycoses, false-positive results are uncommon, occurring in approximately 2% of healthy subjects or those with nonfungal infections.[55,56] Of note is that histoplasmosis may be a cause for false-positive results in the Platelia (Bio-Rad Laboratories; Hercules, California) *Aspergillus* antigen assay.[63]

The test also has been used to monitor therapy for PDH. Antigen concentration declines during treatment and increases with relapse.[52]

Serology

Serologic tests are useful for diagnosis of histoplasmosis, especially SPH and CPH.[52] In PDH, however, serology is less sensitive, probably because of underlying immunosuppression. In APH, serology may be negative during the first 2 months of infection.[65,66] Serology also may be negative in asymptomatic patients or in those with mild symptoms.[67]

Positive serology results can be misleading in some patients. Serologic tests may remain positive for several years,[29,68,69] incorrectly suggesting active histoplasmosis in patients who have other diseases. Furthermore, *Histoplasma* serology may be positive in patients who have other endemic mycoses because of the presence of cross-reactive antigens.

The complement fixation (CF) test using yeast and mycelial antigens is more sensitive than the immunodiffusion (ID) test. In SPH, the CF test is positive at titers of at least 1:8 in 90% of patients, M bands are present by ID in three quarters of patients, and H bands are present by ID in one quarter of patients.[54] CF titers of 1:8 or 1:16 are less helpful in differentiating active from past infection, but such low titers occur in one third of active cases and should not be disregarded. Antibodies also can be measured by EIA, but the available EIA methods are not as accurate as ID and CF.[52] Antibodies usually take a few years to decline after recovery from histoplasmosis,[29,68,69] but there are no data correlating antibody clearance with development of complications, treatment failure, or relapse. Thus, monitoring antibody titers is not recommended.

Guideline for Diagnosis and Monitoring Therapy

The highest sensitivity for diagnosis of histoplasmosis is made possible by use of a battery of tests (see **Table 2**). The need for rapid diagnosis is most important in patients who have APH or PDH, in whom the prompt initiation of therapy may be life-saving. In such cases, all the diagnostic modalities should be used. In patients who have severe manifestations (respiratory failure, hypotension, coagulopathy, or multiorgan failure), examination of a peripheral blood smear for intracellular yeast is appropriate. In all cases, serum and urine should be tested for antigen. If bronchoscopy is performed, BAL should be submitted for antigen testing. Cerebrospinal fluid (CSF) antigen testing is appropriate if central nervous system involvement is suspected. Fungal culture should also be obtained if tissues or body fluids are submitted for cytology, histopathology, or antigen testing. Despite its limitations, serology, including ID and CF, is recommended.

In patients who have SPH, CPH, or mediastinal manifestations of histoplasmosis, serology is most useful. The sensitivity of the antigen test is lower, but testing should be considered in the more severe cases. In cases in which the clinical findings are atypical and the serologic findings are negative or weak (ID negative, CF titer of 1:8 or 1:16), histopathology and culture of tissue may be required to establish the diagnosis.

To use the antigen test to monitor therapy for PDH, testing should be performed before starting treatment; at weeks 1, 2, 4, 8, and 12; at approximately 3-month intervals during therapy; and for 6 to 12 months after treatment is stopped. Guidelines for interpretation of changes in concentration are summarized in **Table 4**. Failure of antigen to decline or a sustained increase in antigen would raise concern about treatment failure.

BLASTOMYCOSIS

Patients who have blastomycosis exhibit a spectrum of pulmonary manifestations,[70,71] ranging from mild self-limited pneumonia[72] to diffuse pneumonia accompanied by acute respiratory distress syndrome (ARDS).[73–75] Patients often are initially suspected of having community-acquired pneumonia caused by bacterial or atypical pathogens.[3,73] Findings of extrapulmonary dissemination also are common.[70,76] Although some patients may recover spontaneously,[72] the risk for a severe and even fatal outcome is high enough to justify a recommendation to treat all patients who have not shown complete recovery clinically and radiographically at the time the diagnosis is established.[77]

ARDS occurs in approximately 10% of cases, of which nearly three quarters are fatal.[73–75] In two thirds of the fatal cases, the diagnosis was not suspected before death or was considered only after the patient became moribund.[75] Survival was more likely if amphotericin B was initiated within 24 hours of the development of ARDS.[75] These findings highlight the importance of a high index of suspicion for blastomycosis in patients who have community-acquired pneumonia, especially those who have ARDS. Once suspected, the diagnosis may be established rapidly by direct examination of respiratory secretions or tissues or by antigen detection.

Direct Examination

Rapid diagnosis may be accomplished by potassium hydroxide (KOH) wet mount or cytology of respiratory secretions or by histopathology of tissue specimens. Typical broad-based budding

yeast could be seen in approximately 90% of cases (**Table 5**).[76] Cultures were positive in two thirds of cases but were rarely the basis for diagnosis because of the delay needed to identify the organism. The diagnostic yield may be improved by testing bronchoscopy specimens. The sensitivity for culture was higher in BAL than in sputum in one study, and KOH wet mount was positive in half of BAL specimens.[78]

Antigen Detection

Antigen can be detected in the urine and serum of patients who have blastomycosis using the MVista *Blastomyces* antigen EIA.[79] The sensitivity was 93% and the specificity was 98% in healthy subjects or patients who had candidiasis, aspergillosis, or cryptococcosis. Cross-reactions were common in histoplasmosis. Antigen also may be detected in BAL.[60] Antigen clears with treatment, providing a method to monitor the success of therapy and diagnose relapse.[80]

Serology

Most experts do not recommend using the currently available serologic tests for diagnosis of blastomycosis.[70,71] In pulmonary blastomycosis, the results of ID were positive in 40% of cases and the results of CF were positive in 16% of cases.[78] In cases identified during an outbreak, the sensitivity was 28% for ID and 9% for CF (**Table 6**).[81] In another review comprised mostly (~80%) of patients who had proved blastomycosis, the results of ID were positive in 29% and the results of CF were positive in 25%.[75] Cross-reactivity was noted in approximately half of patients who had histoplasmosis[82] but may be reduced using a 120-kD protein antigen.[83]

Table 4
Interpretation of changes in *Histoplasma* antigen concentration

Change	Interpretation
Low to moderate positive results (<0.6–19.9 ng/mL)	
>3 ng/mL increase	Probable treatment failure/relapse
≤3 ng/mL decrease	Possible treatment failure
>3 ng/mL decrease	Probable treatment response
High positive results (≥20 ng/mL)	
>15% increase	Probable treatment failure/relapse
≤15% decrease	Possible treatment failure
>15% decrease	Probable treatment response

Table 5
Sensitivity of diagnostic tests in blastomycosis

Test	Pulmonary	Extrapulmonary	Reference
Antigen (N = 42)	100	89	Durkin et al[79]
Histopathology (N = 127)	79	87	Lemos et al[76]
Culture (N = 127)	62	77	Lemos et al[76]

Abbreviation: N, population size.

Guideline for Diagnosis and Monitoring Therapy

Sputum should be evaluated by fungal stain and culture, and antigen testing should be performed on urine and serum. If the results of these tests are negative, or the patient is unable to produce sputum, bronchoscopy should be performed and respiratory secretions should be examined microscopically, cultured for fungus, and tested for antigen. Skin lesions should be aspirated or biopsied and evaluated by direct examination and culture. The currently available serologic tests are not recommended but, in rare cases, may provide the only laboratory basis for the diagnosis. Antigen testing may be used to monitor therapy, as described in histoplasmosis.

COCCIDIOIDOMYCOSIS

Coccidioidomycosis is a common cause of pneumonia in patients from endemic areas.[5] In a survey of cases of community-acquired pneumonia in Arizona, coccidioidomycosis accounted for 29% of cases.[84] Risk factors for severe illness include immunosuppression, pregnancy, old age, African-American race, diabetes, and extensive tobacco use.[4,5] Although usually nonprogressive in patients without risk factors for severe infection, complications may include respiratory failure, chronic pneumonia,[5] and disseminated disease, for which treatment is needed.[85]

Table 6
Sensitivity and specificity of serologic tests in blastomycosis

Parameter	Test Method		
	EIA %	ID %	CF %
Sensitivity (N = 47)	77	28	9
Specificity (N = 89)	92	100	100

Data from Klein BS, Vergeront JM, Kaufman L, et al. Serological tests for blastomycosis: assessments during a large point-source outbreak in Wisconsin. J Infect Dis 1987;155: 262–8.

In acute coccidioidomycosis, cultures are infrequently positive, and, when positive, they require approximately 1 week for recognition of growth. Cultures were positive in only 6% to 11% of pneumonia cases and in 39% of those who had extrapulmonary disease in one study,[4] but in others, culture of respiratory specimens was positive in 86% to 100% of cases.[86,87]

Direct Examination

Rapid diagnosis is possible based on microscopic examination of respiratory specimens or tissues.[88] In a study of patients who had severe pneumonia,[86] examination of bronchial washings was positive in 64% of cases (**Table 7**). Lower rates between 15% and 35% have been reported in other studies.[62,87,89]

Antigen Detection

Detection of antigenemia has been reported several times dating back to the 1980s.[90–93] In 2007, detection of a cross-reactivity antigen was reported using the MVista *Histoplasma* antigen EIA.[62] Sensitivity was 59% in patients who had pneumonia (see **Table 7**). More recently, a specific MVista *Coccidioides* antigen EIA has been developed, with a sensitivity of 71% in patients who had underlying immunosuppression and moderately severe to severe coccidioidomycosis.[94] Specificity was 98%, but cross-reactivity occurred in approximately 10% of patients who had other endemic mycoses.

Serology

Serology is highly useful for diagnosis of coccidiodomycosis.[95] Using ID, CF, and EIA, the results of serology were positive in 82% of cases (Pollage CR, et al. Revisiting the sensitivity of serologic testing and culture-positive coccidioidomycosis. 106th Annual Meeting of the American Society of Microbiology, Orlando, FL, unpublished data). Immunosuppression may cause false-negative results, however.[96] The results of serology also may be negative during the first few months after acute infection.[97] A negative test result, even

Table 7
Sensitivity of diagnostic tests in coccidioidomycosis

Test	Pulmonary (N = 19)	Pulmonary (N = 14)	Pulmonary (N = 54)	Pulmonary or Disseminated
Immunosuppressed	63%	93%	NS, but 35% HIV-positive	0%
Antigen	58%–69%[94]	ND	ND	69%
Antibody	58%	54%	55%	90%
Cytology or histopathology	21%	64%	35%	17%
Culture	74%	86%	100%	23%
Reference	Kuberski[62]	Sarosi[86]	DiTomasso[87]	Santelli[89]

Abbreviations: N, population size; ND, not done.

when all three methods are used, does not exclude coccidioidomycosis.

Antibodies can be differentiated as IgG or IgM by ID or EIA. IgG antibodies react with a heat-labile chitinase, whereas IgM antibodies recognize a heat-stable glycopeptide (**Table 8**).[95] IgM antibodies appear earlier in the course of infection than do IgG antibodies,[98] but they are less specific. The ID and CF methods are more accurate than EIA.[99] Quantitation is possible by testing serial dilutions of the specimen.[99,100]

In healthy subjects, the sensitivity of the ID test was 73% compared with 75% for CF and 87% for EIA (see **Table 8**).[96] In immunocompromised subjects, sensitivity was higher by CF (67%) than by ID (53%). Others have reported the sensitivity of ID to be 50% to 60% in pulmonary coccidioidomycosis.[62,86,87] The sensitivity of ID may be improved by concentration of the specimen.[99] In an outbreak of acute coccidioidomycosis, antibodies were detected in unconcentrated serum in 10% of cases compared with 90% after concentration.[101]

EIA methods are popular because of ease of performance and ability to test large numbers of specimens. Although EIA results correlate with CF titers, the correlation is weak[102] and EIA is not as accurate as ID or CF. For example, using one EIA kit (Meridian Bioscience, Cincinnati, Ohio), the IgM assay was positive in only 54% and the IgG assay was positive in only 67% of CF-positive specimens.[102] Using another kit measuring IgM, IgA, or IgG anti-*Coccidioides* antibodies (Coccidioides Dx Select; Focus Diagnostics, Cyprus, California), the EIA was positive in only 71% of CF-positive specimens and was falsely positive in 12% of CF-negative specimens.

In the early studies, Smith and colleagues[103] noted that CF titers of 1:32 higher were more common in disseminated (61%) than in primary or chronic (~5%) pulmonary coccidiodomycosis. Considering that 16% of cases were disseminated in that study, titers of 1:32 or higher were 2.5 times more common with disseminated than nondisseminated disease. Similar studies have not been reported with the reagents and assay procedures currently used, however.

The CF test may be used to monitor therapy.[95] Its role for this purpose is controversial, however.[5] No association between changes in CF titers and

Table 8
Sensitivity of serologic tests in coccidioidomycosis

Category of Underlying Disease	EIA (IgM or IgG)	Test Method	
		ID (IDTP [IgM] or IDCF [IgG])	CF (IgG)
Healthy (N = 244)	87	73	75
Immunocompromised (N = 57)	67	53	67

Abbreviations: IDTP, immunodiffusion tube precipitation; IDCF, immunodiffusion complement fixation; N, population size.
Data from Blair JE, Coakley B, Santelli AC, et al. Serologic testing for symptomatic coccidioidomycosis in immunocompetent and immunosuppressed hosts. *Mycopathologia* 2006;162:317–24.

clinical outcome was noted in treated patients, and titers changed little during treatment.[104] If titers are monitored, current and prior specimens should be tested together to control for interassay variability, a service provided at the Pappagianis laboratory.[99]

Guideline for Diagnosis and Monitoring Therapy

Serology is recommended in all cases of suspected coccidioidomycosis, and antigen detection is recommended in the more severe cases. Both methods are recommended in suspected extrapulmonary coccidioidomycosis. In acute cases, serology should be repeated in 4 to 8 weeks if the initial specimen is negative. Respiratory secretions should be examined by fungal stain and culture, and if bronchoscopy is performed, bronchial secretions or BAL should also be submitted for antigen testing. Biopsy of extrapulmonary lesions should be considered if the tissues are readily accessible with low risk for complication, and the specimens should be examined by fungal stain and culture for fungus. If central nervous system involvement is suspected, CSF should be tested for antigen and antibody, in addition to cytology and culture. Of note is that the results of serology and antigen tests may be falsely negative in up to 20% of patients who have extrapulmonary coccidioidomycosis, supporting repeat testing and performance of microscopic examination and fungal culture. The role of antigen testing for monitoring therapy requires further investigation.

REFERENCES

1. Mandell LA, Wunderink RG, Anzueto A, et al. Infectious Diseases Society of America/American Thoracic Society consensus guidelines on the management of community-acquired pneumonia in adults. Clin Infect Dis 2007;44(Suppl 2):S27–72.
2. Alves dos Santos JW, Torres A, Michel GT, et al. Non-infectious and unusual infectious mimics of community-acquired pneumonia. Respir Med 2004;98(6):488–94.
3. Dworkin MS, Duckro AN, Proia L, et al. The epidemiology of blastomycosis in Illinois and factors associated with death. Clin Infect Dis 2005; 41(12):e107–11.
4. Rosenstein NE, Emery KW, Werner SB, et al. Risk factors for severe pulmonary and disseminated coccidioidomycosis: Kern County, California, 1995–1996. Clin Infect Dis 2001;32(5):708–15.
5. Anstead GM, Graybill JR. Coccidioidomycosis. Infect Dis Clin North Am 2006;20(3):621–43.
6. Winthrop KL, Yamashita S, Beekmann SE, et al. Mycobacterial and other serious infections in patients receiving anti-tumor necrosis factor and other newly approved biologic therapies: case finding through the Emerging Infections Network. Clin Infect Dis 2008;46(11):1738–40.
7. Wood KL, Hage CA, Knox KS, et al. Histoplasmosis after treatment with anti-TNF-α therapy. Am J Respir Crit Care Med 2003;167:1279–82.
8. Wheat LJ, Conces DJ Jr, Allen S, et al. Pulmonary histoplasmosis syndromes: recognition, diagnosis, and management. Semin Respir Crit Care Med 2004;25:129–44.
9. Kauffman CA. Histoplasmosis: a clinical and laboratory update. Clin Microbiol Rev 2007;20(1):115–32.
10. Hage CA, Wheat LJ, Loyd J, et al. Pulmonary histoplasmosis. Semin Respir Crit Care Med 2008;29(2): 151–65.
11. Johnson PC, Sarosi GA. Community-acquired fungal pneumonias. Semin Respir Infect 1989; 4(1):56–63.
12. Wheat LJ, Slama TG, Eitzen HE, et al. A large urban outbreak of histoplasmosis: clinical features. Ann Intern Med 1981;94(3):331–7.
13. Wheat LJ, Freifeld AG, Kleiman MB, et al. Clinical practice guidelines for the management of patients with histoplasmosis: 2007 update by the Infectious Diseases Society of America. Clin Infect Dis 2007; 45(7):807–25.
14. Rubin H, Lehan PH, Furcolow ML. Severe nonfatal histoplasmosis; report of a typical case, with comments on therapy. N Engl J Med 1957;257(13): 599–602.
15. Naylor BA. Low-dose amphotericin B therapy for acute pulmonary histoplasmosis. Chest 1977; 71(3):404–6.
16. Ferguson GT, Irvin CG, Cherniack RM. Effect of corticosteroids on diaphragm function and biochemistry in the rabbit. Am Rev Respir Dis 1990;141(1):156–63.
17. Salomon J, Flament SM, De Truchis P, et al. An outbreak of acute pulmonary histoplasmosis in members of a trekking trip in Martinique, French West Indies. J Travel Med 2003;10(2):87–93.
18. Meals LT, McKinney WP. Acute pulmonary histoplasmosis: progressive pneumonia resulting from high inoculum exposure. J Ky Med Assoc 1998; 96(7):258–60.
19. Murdock WT, Travis RE, Sutliff WD, et al. Acute pulmonary histoplasmosis after exposure to soil contaminated by starling excreta. JAMA 1962; 179:73–5.
20. Lottenberg R, Waldman RH, Ajello L, et al. Pulmonary histoplasmosis associated with exploration of a bat cave. Am J Epidemiol 1979;110(2):156–61.

21. Schoenberger CI, Weiner JH, Mayo FJ, et al. Acute pulmonary histoplasmosis outbreak following home renovation. Md Med J 1988;37(6):457–60.

22. Craven SA, Benatar SR. Histoplasmosis in the Cape Province. A report of the second known outbreak. S Afr Med J 1979;55(3):89–92.

23. Nasta P, Donisi A, Cattane A, et al. Acute histoplasmosis in spelunkers returning from Mato Grosso, Peru. J Travel Med 1997;4(4):176–8.

24. Packard JS, Finkelstein H, Turner WE. Acute pulmonary histoplasmosis; treatment with cortisone. AMA Arch Intern Med 1957;99(3):370–5.

25. Valselow NA, Winthrop ND, Bocobo FC. Acute pulmonary histoplasmosis in laboratory workers: report of 2 cases. J Lab Clin Med 1962;59(2):236–43.

26. Sacks JJ, Ajello L, Crockett LK. An outbreak and review of cave-associated Histoplasmosis capsulatii. J Med Vet Mycol 1986;24:313–27.

27. Pecanha Martins AC, Costa Neves ML, Lopes AA, et al. Histoplasmosis presenting as acute respiratory distress syndrome after exposure to bat feces in a home basement. Braz J Infect Dis 2000;4(2):103–6.

28. Jones TF, Swinger GL, Craig AS, et al. Acute pulmonary histoplasmosis in bridge workers: a persistent problem. Am J Med 1999;106(4):480–2.

29. Disalvo AF, Johnson WM. Histoplasmosis in South Carolina: support for the microfocus concept. Am J Epidemiol 1979;109:480–92.

30. Wilcox KR Jr, Waisbren BA, Martin J. The Walworth, Wisconsin, epidemic of histoplasmosis. Ann Intern Med 1958;49:388–418.

31. Reynolds RJI, Penn RL, Grafton WD, et al. Tissue morphology of Histoplasma capsulatum in acute histoplasmosis. Am Rev Respir Dis 1984;130:317–20.

32. Kataria YP, Campbell PB, Burlingham BT. Acute pulmonary histoplasmosis presenting as adult respiratory distress syndrome: effect of therapy on clinical and laboratory features. South Med J 1981;74:534–7.

33. Prior JA, Saslaw S, Cole CR. Experiences with histoplasmosis. Ann Intern Med 1954;40:221–44.

34. Wynne JW, Olsen GN. Acute histoplasmosis presenting as the adult respiratory distress syndrome. Chest 1974;66:158–61.

35. Ashford DA, Hajjeh RA, Kelley MF, et al. Outbreak of histoplasmosis among cavers attending the National Speleological Society Annual Convention, Texas, 1994. Am J Trop Med Hyg 1999;60(6):899–903.

36. Conrad FG, Saslaw S, Atwell RJ. The protean manifestations of histoplasmosis as illustrated in twenty-three cases. Arch Intern Med 1959;104:692–709.

37. Ramirez JR. Acute pulmonary histoplasmosis: newly recognized hazard of marijuana plant hunters. Am J Med 1992;88(suppl):5-60N–5-61N.

38. Polos PG. Hypoxic respiratory failure in a 30-year-old spelunker. Chest 1998;113(4):1125–6.

39. Sollod N. Acute fulminating disseminated histoplasmosis. J S C Med Assoc 1971;67:231–4.

40. Beatty OA, Zwick LS, Paisley CG. Epidemic histoplasmosis in Ohio with source in Kentucky. Ohio State Med J 1967;63:1470–3.

41. Rubin H, Furcolow ML, Yates JL, et al. The course and prognosis of histoplasmosis. Am J Med 1959;27:278–88.

42. Paya CV, Roberts GD, Cockerill FRI. Transient fungemia in acute pulmonary histoplasmosis: detection by new blood-culturing techniques. J Infect Dis 1987;156:313–5.

43. Cullen JH, Hazen E, Scholdager R. Two cases of histoplasmosis acquired in felling a decayed tree in the Mohawk Valley. N Y State J Med 1956;56:3507–10.

44. Wolff M. [Outbreak of acute histoplasmosis in Chilean travelers to the Ecuadorian jungle: an example of geographic medicine]. Rev Med Chil 1999;127(11):1359–64.

45. Hoenigl M, Schwetz I, Wurm R, et al. Pulmonary histoplasmosis in three Austrian travelers after a journey to Mexico. Infection 2007;36:282–4.

46. Straub M, Schwarz J. The healed primary complex in histoplasmosis. Am J Cardiovasc Pathol 1955;25:727–41.

47. Wheat LJ, Slama TG, Norton JA, et al. Risk factors for disseminated or fatal histoplasmosis. Analysis of a large urban outbreak. Ann Intern Med 1982;96(2):159–63.

48. Zerbe CS, Holland SM. Disseminated histoplasmosis in persons with interferon-gamma receptor 1 deficiency. Clin Infect Dis 2005;41(4):e38–41.

49. Duncan RA, Von Reyn CF, Alliegro GM, et al. Idiopathic CD4+ T-lymphocytopenia—four patients with opportunistic infections and no evidence of HIV infection. N Engl J Med 1993;328(6):393–8.

50. Wheat LJ, Connolly-Stringfield PA, Baker RL, et al. Disseminated histoplasmosis in the acquired immune deficiency syndrome: clinical findings, diagnosis and treatment, and review of the literature. Medicine (Baltimore) 1990;69(6):361–74.

51. Wheat LJ, Connolly-Stringfield P, Williams B, et al. Diagnosis of histoplasmosis in patients with the acquired immunodeficiency syndrome by detection of Histoplasma capsulatum polysaccharide antigen in bronchoalveolar lavage fluid. Am Rev Respir Dis 1992;145(6):1421–4.

52. Wheat LJ. Improvements in diagnosis of histoplasmosis. Expert Opin Biol Ther 2006;6(11):1207–21.

53. Williams B, Fojtasek M, Connolly-Stringfield P, et al. Diagnosis of histoplasmosis by antigen detection during an outbreak in Indianapolis, Ind. Arch Pathol Lab Med 1994;118(12):1205–8.

54. Wheat J, French ML, Kohler RB, et al. The diagnostic laboratory tests for histoplasmosis: analysis of experience in a large urban outbreak. Ann Intern Med 1982;97(5):680–5.

55. Wheat LJ, Witt J III, Durkin M, et al. Reduction in false antigenemia in the second generation Histoplasma antigen assay. Med Mycol 2007;45(2):169–71.

56. Connolly PA, Durkin MM, LeMonte AM, et al. Detection of histoplasma antigen by a quantitative enzyme immunoassay. Clin Vaccine Immunol 2007;14(12):1587–91.

57. LeMonte A, Egan L, Connolly P, et al. Evaluation of the IMMY ALPHA Histoplasma antigen enzyme immunoassay for diagnosis of histoplasmosis marked by antigenuria. Clin Vaccine Immunol 2007;14(6):802–3.

58. Cloud JL, Bauman SK, Neary BP, et al. Performance characteristics of a polyclonal enzyme immunoassay for the quantitation of histoplasma antigen in human urine samples. Am J Clin Pathol 2007;128(1):18–22.

59. Gutierrez ME, Canton A, Connolly P, et al. Detection of Histoplasma capsulatum antigen in Panamanian patients with disseminated histoplasmosis and AIDS. Clin Vaccine Immunol 2008;15(4):681–3.

60. Hage CA, Davis TE, Egan L, et al. Diagnosis of pulmonary histoplasmosis and blastomycosis by detection of antigen in bronchoalveolar lavage fluid using an improved second-generation enzyme-linked immunoassay. Respir Med 2007;101(1):43–7.

61. Wheat J, Wheat H, Connolly P, et al. Cross-reactivity in Histoplasma capsulatum variety capsulatum antigen assays of urine samples from patients with endemic mycoses. Clin Infect Dis 1997;24(6):1169–71.

62. Kuberski T, Myers R, Wheat LJ, et al. Diagnosis of coccidioidomycosis by antigen detection using cross-reaction with a Histoplasma antigen. Clin Infect Dis 2007;44(1):e50–4.

63. Wheat LJ, Hackett E, Durkin M, et al. Histoplasmosis-associated cross-reactivity in the BioRad Platelia Aspergillus enzyme immunoassay. Clin Vaccine Immunol 2007;14(5):638–40.

64. Zhuang D, Hage C, De Jesus M, et al. Cryptococcal glucoxylomannan does not exhibit cross-reactivity in the MVista Histoplasma antigen enzyme immunoassay (EIA). Clin Vaccine Immunol 2007;15:392–3.

65. Davies SF. Serodiagnosis of histoplasmosis. Semin Respir Infect 1986;1(1):9–15.

66. Wheat LJ. Histoplasmosis in Indianapolis. Clin Infect Dis 1992;14(Suppl 1):S91–9.

67. Wingard JR, Herbrecht R, Mauskopf J, et al. Resource use and cost of treatment with voriconazole or conventional amphotericin B for invasive aspergillosis. Transpl Infect Dis 2007;9(3):182–8.

68. Walter JE. The significance of antibodies in chronic histoplasmosis by immunoelectrophoretic and complement fixation tests. Am Rev Respir Dis 1969;99:50–8.

69. Wheat LJ, French MLV. The diagnostic approach in histoplasmosis. Immunol Allergy Pract V 1983;9:19–28.

70. Kauffman CA. Endemic mycoses: blastomycosis, histoplasmosis, and sporotrichosis. Infect Dis Clin North Am 2006;20(3):645–62, vii.

71. Bradsher RW. Therapy of blastomycosis. Semin Respir Infect 1997;12(3):263–7.

72. Recht LD, Philips JR, Eckman MR, et al. Self-limited blastomycosis: a report of thirteen cases. Am Rev Respir Dis 1979;120:1109–11.

73. Meyer KC, McManus EJ, Maki DG. Overwhelming pulmonary blastomycosis associated with the adult respiratory distress syndrome. N Engl J Med 1993;329:1231–6.

74. Lemos LB, Baliga M, Guo M. Acute respiratory distress syndrome and blastomycosis: presentation of nine cases and review of the literature. Ann Diagn Pathol 2001;5(1):1–9.

75. Vasquez J, Mehta JB, Agarwal R, et al. Blastomycosis in Northeast Tennessee. Chest 1998;114:436–43.

76. Lemos LB, Guo M, Baliga M. Blastomycosis: organ involvement and etiologic diagnosis. A review of 123 patients from Mississippi. Ann Diagn Pathol 2000;4(6):391–406.

77. Chapman SW, Dismukes WE, Proia LA, et al. Clinical practice guidelines for the management of blastomycosis: 2008 update by the Infectious Diseases Society of America. Clin Infect Dis 2008;46:1801–12.

78. Martynowicz MA, Prakash UBS. Pulmonary blastomycosis—an appraisal of diagnostic techniques. Chest 2002;121(3):768–73.

79. Durkin M, Witt J, LeMonte A, et al. Antigen assay with the potential to aid in diagnosis of blastomycosis. J Clin Microbiol 2004;42(10):4873–5.

80. Mongkolrattanothai K, Peev M, Wheat LJ, et al. Urine antigen detection of blastomycosis in pediatric patients. Pediatr Infect Dis J 2006;25(11):1076–8.

81. Klein BS, Vergeront JM, Kaufman L, et al. Serological tests for blastomycosis: assessments during a large point-source outbreak in Wisconsin. J Infect Dis 1987;155(2):262–8.

82. Klein BS, Kuritsky JN, Chappell WA, et al. Comparison of the enzyme immunoassay, immunodiffusion, and complement fixation tests in detecting antibody in human serum to the A antigen of Blastomyces dermatitidis. Am Rev Respir Dis 1986;133(1):144–8.

83. Klein BS, Hogan LH, Jones JM. Immunologic recognition of a 25-amino acid repeat arrayed in tandem on a major antigen of Blastomyces dermatitidis. J Clin Invest 1993;92(1):330–7.

84. Valdivia L, Nix D, Wright M, et al. Coccidioidomycosis as a common cause of community-acquired pneumonia. Emerg Infect Dis 2006; 12(6):958–62.

85. Galgiani JN, Ampel NM, Blair JE, et al. Coccidioidomycosis. Clin Infect Dis 2005;41(9):1217–23.

86. Sarosi GA, Lawrence JP, Smith DK, et al. Rapid diagnostic evaluation of bronchial washings in patients with suspected coccidioidomycosis. Semin Respir Infect 2001;16(4):238–41.

87. DiTomasso JP, Ampel NM, Sobonya RE, et al. Bronchoscopic diagnosis of pulmonary coccidioidomycosis. Comparison of cytology, culture, and transbronchial biopsy. Diagn Microbiol Infect Dis 1994;18(2):83–7.

88. Saubolle MA, McKellar PP, Sussland D. Epidemiologic, clinical, and diagnostic aspects of coccidioidomycosis. J Clin Microbiol 2007;45(1):26–30.

89. Santelli AC, Blair JE, Roust LR. Coccidioidomycosis in patients with diabetes mellitus. Am J Med 2006;119(11):964–9.

90. Weiner MH. Antigenemia detected in human coccidioidomycosis. J Clin Microbiol 1983;18(1):136–42.

91. Galgiani JN, Dugger KO, Ito JI, et al. Antigenemia in primary coccidioidomycosis. Am J Trop Med Hyg 1984;33(4):645–9.

92. Wack EE, Dugger KO, Galgiani JN. Enzyme-linked immunosorbent assay for antigens of Coccidioides immitis: human sera interference corrected by acidification-heat extraction. J Lab Clin Med 1988;111(5):560–5.

93. Galgiani JN, Grace GM, Lundergan LL. New serologic tests for early detection of coccidioidomycosis. J Infect Dis 1991;163(3):671–4.

94. Durkin M, Connolly P, Kuberski T, et al. Diagnosis of coccidioidomycosis with use of the Coccidioides antigen enzyme immunoassay. Clin Infect Dis 2008;47(8):e69–73.

95. Pappagianis D. Coccidioides immitis antigen. J Infect Dis 1999;180(1):243–4.

96. Blair JE, Coakley B, Santelli AC, et al. Serologic testing for symptomatic coccidioidomycosis in immunocompetent and immunosuppressed hosts. Mycopathologia 2006;162(5):317–24.

97. Smith CE, Saito MT. Serologic reactions in coccidioidomycosis. J Chronic Dis 1957;5(5):571–9.

98. Smith CE, Saito MT, Simons SA. Pattern of 39,500 serologic tests in coccidioidomycosis. JAMA 1956;160(7):546–52.

99. Pappagianis D, Zimmer BL. Serology of coccidioidomycosis. Clin Microbiol Rev 1990;3:247–68.

100. Wieden MA, Galgiani JN, Pappagianis D. Comparison of immunodiffusion techniques with standard complement fixation assay for quantitation of coccidioidal antibodies. J Clin Microbiol 1983;18(3): 529–34.

101. Petersen LR, Marshall SL, Barton-Dickson C, et al. Coccidioidomycosis among workers at an archeological site, northeastern Utah. Emerg Infect Dis 2004;10(4):637–42.

102. Martins TB, Jaskowski TD, Mouritsen CL, et al. Comparison of commercially available enzyme immunoassay with traditional serological tests for detection of antibodies to Coccidioides immitis. J Clin Microbiol 1995;33(4):940–3.

103. Smith CE, Saito MT, Beard RR, et al. Serological tests in the diagnosis and prognosis of coccidioidomycosis. The Am J Hyg 1950;52(1):1–21.

104. Graybill JR, Stevens DA, Galgiani JN, et al. Itraconazole treatment of coccidioidomycosis. NAIAD Mycoses Study Group. Am J Med 1990;89(3): 282–90.

Fungal Molecular Diagnostics

Nancy L. Wengenack, PhD*, Matthew J. Binnicker, PhD

KEYWORDS

• Fungi • Molecular • Diagnostics • Sequencing • PCR

The incidence of invasive fungal infections has increased in recent years, especially among transplant recipients, patients who have hematologic neoplasms, patients who have AIDS, and those on immunosuppressive therapy for other serious illnesses.[1] This trend includes a rise in the number of patients who have infections caused by opportunistic fungi, endemic mycoses, and emerging infections caused by environmental fungi. Because of the increased incidence of invasive fungal infections and the high morbidity and mortality rates associated with these infections in immunocompromised patients, a significant emphasis has been placed over the past several decades on improving the laboratory diagnosis of fungal diseases.

Historically, the detection and identification of fungi has relied on a combination of microscopy- and culture-based techniques. The microscopic examination of clinical specimens using histopathologic studies or direct fluorescent stains (eg, calcofluor white) allows for rapid detection; however, these methods lack sensitivity and specificity[2–4] and typically allow for a preliminary identification only. Definitive identification requires recovery of the organism in culture, and this is still considered the gold-standard method for the laboratory diagnosis of fungal infections today. Although cultures demonstrate excellent sensitivity and specificity, their growth may take days (eg, *Aspergillus* spp) to weeks (eg, *Histoplasma capsulatum*), thereby delaying the diagnosis and the initiation of appropriate therapy. In addition, the recovery and accurate identification of fungi in the clinical laboratory requires considerable expertise and can often represent a significant safety hazard to laboratory personnel.[5]

The introduction of molecular methods into the clinical microbiology laboratory has led to significant advances in the diagnosis of infectious diseases,[6–8] with recent applications available for the detection and identification of fungal pathogens. Fungal nucleic acid–based tests, which include the commercially available AccuProbes (Gen-Probe, Inc., San Diego, California), allow for the identification of the dimorphic fungi from culture with high sensitivity and specificity.[9–11] DNA sequencing chemistry is also becoming more routinely available in clinical laboratories for the accurate differentiation of culture isolates,[12] especially for those organisms that are not easily identified by conventional techniques.[13] Other nucleic acid tests, such as real-time polymerase chain reaction (PCR) tests, allow for the detection of fungi directly from clinical specimens[14,15] and, in some instances, provide a means for their quantification.[16–18] Molecular assays offer a promising alternative to routine methods by reducing the time to identification, increasing sensitivity, and enhancing laboratory safety. However, a lack of test standardization and limited validation data for many fungal nucleic acid tests has hindered their general acceptance and broad implementation into clinical laboratories.

This article highlights the common molecular methods that have been routinely used for the laboratory diagnosis of fungal infections and summarizes their key performance characteristics.

The primers and probes for *Coccidioides*, *Pneumocystis*, and Zygomycetes real-time polymerase chain reaction have been licensed to a commercial entity. The authors and the Mayo Clinic have received royalties of less than the federal threshold for significant financial interest from the licensing of this technology.
Division of Clinical Microbiology, Mayo Clinic, 200 First Street SW, Rochester, MN 55905, USA
* Corresponding author.
E-mail address: wengenack.nancy@mayo.edu (N.L. Wengenack).

Clin Chest Med 30 (2009) 391–408
doi:10.1016/j.ccm.2009.02.014

chestmed.theclinics.com

In addition, the advantages and limitations of current molecular testing methods are discussed. Finally, the authors comment on the future of molecular fungal diagnostics, including the potential role of multiplex detection assays, microarrays, and the molecular determination of antifungal resistance directly from clinical specimens.

NUCLEIC ACID HYBRIDIZATION PROBES

Commercially available nucleic acid hybridization probes, under the brand name AccuProbes, were introduced in 1992 by Gen-Probe, Inc. for use with a limited number of fungi.[19,20] Initially, AccuProbes were available for *Histoplasma capsulatum*, *Blastomyces dermatitidis*, *Coccidioides immitis*, and *Cryptococcus neoformans*;[9,10,21] however, the *C neoformans* probe was discontinued in the mid-1990s because of a lack of customer demand. With the exception of a single report of the direct use of the *H capsulatum* probe on excised cardiac valve tissue,[22] the hybridization probes require growth of the fungus in pure culture to achieve their reported sensitivities. Culture is required because there is no PCR step used that would amplify the target. A small amount of the organism is removed from a culture plate and subjected to a lysis step to kill the organism and release the nucleic acid. The test relies on the sequence-specific hybridization of a chemiluminescent, single-stranded DNA probe with complementary ribosomal RNA released from the target organism to form a stable DNA:RNA hybrid. The nonbound probe is removed, and the amount of labeled DNA:RNA hybrid remaining is measured in relative light units (RLUs) using a luminometer. A positive reaction for the fungal probes is one that gives a signal greater than 50,000 RLUs.

A number of groups have reported on the performance characteristics of the AccuProbes, and a summary of these characteristics is presented in **Table 1**. The *B dermatitidis* probe is known to cross-react with several other fungal organisms, including *Paracoccidioides brasiliensis*, *Gymnascella hyalinospora*, and *Emmonsia parva*.[11,23] *P brasiliensis* may be distinguished from *B dermatitidis* by examining the morphologic characteristics of the yeast phase. *B dermatitidis* is typically a thick-walled yeast producing a single bud, and *P brasiliensis* often, although not always, produces multiple buds from a single yeast cell. The travel history of the patient should also provide clues because *Blastomyces* is endemic to North America and *Paracoccidioides* is typically found in South America, although exceptions to this geographic distribution have been reported.[24] *G hyalinospora* is associated with reptile and rodent dung and is rarely clinically significant.[25] It produces spherical asci in dense groups that can be microscopically differentiated from those of *B dermatitidis*.[26] *E parva* can cause human infection, typically manifesting in the lung, but it produces large adiaconidia (200–400μm in diameter) and can easily be differentiated from *B dermatitidis* (8–15μm budding yeast cells) by using microscopic examination.[27] As previously mentioned in this article, microscopy can be used to confirm *B dermatitidis* probe results, but this may cause

---

Table 1
Sensitivity and specificity of the AccuProbe nucleic acid hybridization probes for identification of the dimorphic fungi from culture

Fungi Targeted by AccuProbes	% Sensitivity (Number Tested)	% Specificity (Number Tested)	Reference
Blastomyces dermatitidis	100 (72)	100 (28)	99
	87.8 (74)	100 (219)	10
	100 (74)	66[a] (30)	11
	98.1 (108)	99.7 (288)	23
Coccidioides immitis	99.2 (122)	100 (164)	10
	100 (72)	100 (27)	11
	98.8 (166)	100 (305)	100
Histoplasma capsulatum	100 (86)	100 (154)	10
	100 (105)[b]	100 (57)	101
	100 (41)	100 (54)	9
	98.2 (54)[c]	97.5 (40)[c]	28
	100 (114)	100 (167)	102

[a] The *Blastomyces* probe cross-reacted with 10 of the 17 *Paracoccidioides brasiliensis* isolates tested.
[b] Two isolates were identified only after repeat testing because of culture contamination with bacteria.
[c] One isolate of *Aspergillus niger* was AccuProbe positive for *Histoplasma capsulatum*.

a delay of several days while waiting for development of the characteristic structures in culture. It is also possible to confirm the specificity of the *Blastomyces* probe using DNA sequencing, but this can add considerable cost.

There have been two reports of false-positive results for *H capsulatum* probes because of cross-reactivity with single isolates of *Aspergillus niger* and *Chrysosporium* spp.[28,29] These reports underscore the importance of confirming that the morphologic characteristics of the culture isolate are consistent with the molecular result obtained. The converse is also true, however, because molecular methods, as in tests that use the AccuProbes, may be useful in identifying morphologic variants of an organism, as has been demonstrated in two reports for *H capsulatum*.[30,31]

A limitation of the *Coccidioides* AccuProbe is that it cannot be used to differentiate between the two recognized species, *C immitis* and *C posadasii*, but thus far, differentiation of these species does not appear to have clinical significance.[32] Because of the select agent status of *C immitis* and *C posadasii*, it is difficult for many laboratories to use the *Coccidioides* hybridization probe assay because it requires the use of a live *Coccidioides* culture for the positive control reaction. Cultures of *Coccidioides* spp represent a significant safety hazard for laboratory personnel, and in addition, government regulations require laboratories to destroy select agents within 7 days of identification or to transfer them to a registered select agent laboratory. The requirement to destroy *Coccidioides* cultures within 7 days of identification makes maintenance of the positive control strain for the AccuProbe test difficult. Formalin-killed cultures have been reported to produce false-negative results with the *Coccidioides* probe and, therefore, are not recommended[33] but heat-killed, frozen cultures have been reported to provide a stable, safe control material for the AccuProbe test.[34,35] In addition, a mutated strain of *C posadasii*, Δchs5, has been excluded from the select agent list (http://www.selectagents.gov/) and has been demonstrated to be a satisfactory quality-control isolate for the AccuProbe test.[36]

Currently, there are no commercial sources of fungal hybridization probes other than the AccuProbe system. Two groups[37,38] have reported the development of genus- and species-specific probes for a number of fungal organisms in addition to the dimorphic pathogens detected by the AccuProbe system. However, these probes are not commercially available and are not yet routinely used in most diagnostic laboratories.

REAL-TIME POLYMERASE CHAIN REACTION TESTING

The implementation of real-time PCR testing into the clinical laboratory has transformed the way in which a variety of infectious diseases are now diagnosed.[6–8] This technology combines nucleic acid target amplification using standard PCR chemistry and detection using fluorescent probes in a simultaneous, single-well reaction. A variety of testing platforms and probe-based detection systems (eg, 5′ nuclease, molecular beacons, and fluorescent resonance energy transfer [FRET] hybridization probes) have been used with real-time PCR assays, and these technologies have been reviewed in detail previously.[8]

Testing using real-time PCR offers several advantages over conventional methods. First, real-time PCR testing has demonstrated equivalent sensitivity and specificity to conventional PCR testing[39] and in many instances has been shown to be more sensitive than culture-based detection.[40,41] Second, real-time PCR testing decreases the turnaround time in comparison with conventional PCR testing by eliminating the necessity to perform postamplification processing and detection. Third, by combining target amplification and detection in a single, closed-reaction vessel, real-time PCR testing reduces the possibility for environmental contamination with amplified nucleic acids. This is particularly important for fungal diagnostics because of the ubiquitous presence of environmental fungi. Contamination of subsequent PCR reactions with "carry-over" amplified product is a significant limitation of conventional and nested PCR assays and has prevented the routine use of these methods in the clinical microbiology laboratory. Finally, real-time PCR assays can be adapted to provide quantitative results relating to the amount of target nucleic acid present in a clinical specimen. The quantitation of fungal nucleic acid by using real-time PCR testing may have important applications in predicting clinical progression in transplant patients, differentiating colonization and disease, and monitoring the efficacy of antifungal therapy. A summary of real-time PCR assays reported for the detection and identification of fungi is presented in **Table 2**.

Aspergillus spp

Of all the fungal genera, *Aspergillus* has been the one most extensively targeted in the development of real-time PCR assays. The rationale behind this effort is that the timely detection of *Aspergillus* spp may decrease the high morbidity and mortality

Table 2
Real-time polymerase chain reaction assays for the detection and identification of fungi

Disease	Reference	Specimen Type (Number Tested)	Technology	Assay Target	Conventional Method	Clinical Sensitivity	Clinical Specificity	Comments
Aspergillosis	103	Blood, plasma (323)	ABI 7700 TaqMan	18S rRNA	Culture, histopathology	79%	92%	Quantitative; compared with antigen detection
Aspergillosis	104	BAL (114), tissue biopsy (16)	LightCycler FRET HP	mtDNA	Culture, histopathology	73%	93%	Semiquantitative; positive in tissue from all patients who had IA
Aspergillosis	14	BAL (44)	iCycler TaqMan	18S rRNA	Culture, histopathology	90%	100%	Compared with antigen detection
Aspergillosis	105	BAL (32), blood (64)	LightCycler FRET HP	cyt B	Culture, histopathology	NR	NR	Quantitative
Aspergillosis	106	Serum (559)	ABI 7700 TaqMan	5.8S rRNA	Culture, histopathology	NR	NR	Quantitative
Aspergillosis	43	BAL (93)	ABI 7700 TaqMan	18S rRNA	Culture, histopathology	67%	100%	Compared with antigen detection
Aspergillosis	44	Serum (246)	ABI 7700 TaqMan	28S rRNA	Culture, histopathology	84.6%	100%	Compared with antigen detection
Aspergillosis	18	BAL (94)	ABI 7500 TaqMan	18S rRNA	Culture, histopathology	77%	88%	Quantitative
Aspergillosis	107	Blood (948)	LightCycler FRET HP	18S rRNA	Culture, histopathology	NR	NR	Analytic sensitivity of 60 fg
Aspergillosis	108	Serum (938)	ABI 7300 TaqMan	28S rRNA	Culture, histopathology	76.5%	96.7%	Sensitivity increased to 100% using large serum volume (1 ml)

Fungal Molecular Diagnostics   395

Disease	Ref	Sample (n)	Platform	Target	Reference standard	Sensitivity	Specificity	Comments
Candidiasis	109	Blood (122)	ABI 5700 TaqMan	5.8S/28S rDNA	Culture	100%	97%	Quantitative
Candidiasis	110	Blood (74)	LightCycler FRET HP	ITS2	Culture	100%	100%	Detects and differentiates six species with four probe sets
Candidiasis	111	Blood (472)	LightCycler SYBR	18S rRNA	Culture	NR	NR	Detects seven species
Candidiasis	112	Serum (8)	LightCycler SYBR	mp65	Culture, histopathology	NR	NR	Quantitative
Candidiasis	50	Blood (43)	ABI 7700 TaqMan	18S rRNA, ITS	Culture	100% (33/33)	100%	Differentiates FLC-sensitive and -resistant species
Candidiasis	113	Blood (20)	RotorGene 3000 TaqMan	rpr1	Culture	NR	NR	Detects eight species
Candidiasis	49	Serum (58)	LightCycler SYBR	18S/28S rDNA	Culture	92%	100%	Detects five species
Coccidioidomycosis	53	Culture isolates (120)	LightCycler FRET HP	Ag2/PRA	Culture, nucleic acid probe	NA	NA	Correctly identified all culture isolates
Coccidioidomycosis	54	Culture isolates (56)	ABI 7500 TaqMan	PRA	Culture, nucleic acid probe	NA	NA	Allowed for speciation using SNP analysis
Coccidioidomycosis	55	Respiratory (266), fresh tissue (66), paraffin-embedded tissue (148), culture isolates (40)	LightCycler FRET HP	ITS2	Culture, nucleic acid probe	100%	98%	93% and 73% sensitivity from fresh and paraffin-embedded tissue, respectively

(continued on next page)

Table 2 *(continued)*

Disease	Reference	Specimen Type (Number Tested)	Technology	Assay Target	Conventional Method	Clinical Sensitivity	Clinical Specificity	Comments
Dermatophytosis	52	Skin, nail, hair (132)	iCycler TaqMan	ITS	Culture, microscopy	100%	NR	Identified dermatophytes in seven specimens that produced negative results using culture/microscopy
Dermatophytosis	51	Skin (58)	LightCycler SYBR	rDNA/ITS	Culture, microscopy	84%	NR	Seven primer sets used; provided new diagnostic information in nine cases
Histoplasmosis	59	BAL (1), lung biopsy (1), bone marrow (2), blood (1), culture isolates (107)	LightCycler FRET HP	ITS	Culture, nucleic acid probe	NR	NR	100% sensitive and specific from culture isolates; tested five clinical specimens
Histoplasmosis	60	Serum (35)	LightCycler FRET HP	ITS1	Culture, nucleic acid probe	70%	100%	Tested 10 specimens from four patients who had AIDS-related histoplasmosis

								Compared with conventional PCR testing
Pneumocystis	39	Respiratory (28)	LightCycler SYBR	5S rDNA	Stains, microscopy	100%	100%	Quantitative
Pneumocystis	16	Respiratory (98)	LightCycler FRET HP	msg	Stains, microscopy	NR	NR	Quantitative
Pneumocystis	63	BAL (173)	LightCycler FRET HP	msg	Stains, microscopy	100%	84.9%	Quantitative
Pneumocystis	17	BAL (53)	ABI 5700 TaqMan	β-tubulin	Stains, microscopy	100%	64%	Quantitative
Pneumocystis	62	BAL (214)	LightCycler FRET HP	cdc2	Stains, microscopy	100%	97%	Qualitative
Pneumocystis	114	BAL (141)	ABI 7000 TaqMan	dhps	Stains, microscopy	94%	96%	Quantitative
Pneumocystis	64	BAL (129)	LightCycler TaqMan	dhfr2	Stains, microscopy	82%	97%	Quantitative
Pneumocystis	65	BAL (136)	RotorGene 3000 TaqMan	hsp70	Stains, microscopy	98%	96%	Quantitative
Pneumocystis	15	BAL (400)	LightCycler FRET HP	msg	Stains, microscopy	100%	91%	Specificity increased to 98% with $C_t \geq 28$
Zygomycosis	68	Paraffin-embedded tissue (81), fresh tissue (2), culture isolates (103)	LightCycler FRET HP	cyt b	Culture, histopathology	56% (fixed tissue), 100% (fresh tissue)	100%	100% sensitive and 92% specific from culture isolates

Abbreviations: Ag2/PRA, antigen 2/proline-rich antigen; BAL, bronchoalveolar lavage; C_t, cycle threshold; fg, femtogram; FLC, fluconazole; HP, hybridization probes; IA, invasive aspergillosis; ITS, internal transcribed spacer; NA, not applicable; NR, not reported; PRA, proline-rich antigen; SNP, single nucleotide polymorphism; SYBR, SYBR green.

Adapted from Espy MJ, Uhl JR, Sloan LM et al. Real-time PCR in clinical microbiology: applications for routine laboratory testing. Clin Microbiol Rev 2006;19:165–256; with permission.

rates associated with invasive aspergillosis (IA). The majority of *Aspergillus* real-time PCR methods described in the literature target *A fumigatus*, with the second most frequently targeted species being *A flavus*. In most studies, the number of specimens from patients with proven or probable IA is relatively low, making the determination of assay sensitivity and specificity difficult. Furthermore, a direct comparison of methods is complicated by the variety of nucleic acid targets, clinical specimens, extraction procedures, and amplification platforms used for the detection and identification of *Aspergillus* spp.

Several studies have compared the results of real-time PCR assays with a clinical diagnosis of IA that was based on recently published consensus criteria.[42] Khot and colleagues[18] developed a quantitative PCR (qPCR) assay targeting the *Aspergillus* 18S rRNA gene and tested bronchoalveolar lavage (BAL) fluid from 94 episodes of pneumonia, 13 of which were categorized as being proven or probable invasive pulmonary aspergillosis (IPA). The qPCR assay was positive in 10 of 13 (76.9%) episodes of proven or probable IPA. However, the assay was also positive in 8 of 81 (9.9%) episodes without proven or probable IPA, yielding a specificity of 90.1%. In comparison, culture and histology demonstrated sensitivities of 84.6 and 53.8%, respectively, and a specificity of 100%.

A number of other studies have compared the performance of real-time PCR assays with the galactomannan enzyme immunoassay (GM EIA) for *Aspergillus* antigen. Musher and colleagues[43] compared a qPCR assay targeting the *Aspergillus* 18S rRNA gene to the GM EIA (Platelia Aspergillus, Bio-Rad, Edmonds, Washington) using BAL samples from 49 patients who had proven or probable IPA and 50 control patients who did not have IPA. The sensitivity and specificity of the qPCR assay were determined to be 67 and 100%, respectively. In contrast, the sensitivity of the GM EIA was 61% using an index cutoff of 1.0 and 76% when the cutoff value was lowered to 0.5. The specificities of the GM EIA at cutoff values of 1.0 and 0.5 were 98 and 94%, respectively. Interestingly, when a positive test was defined as a positive result obtained using either the qPCR assay or the GM EIA, the sensitivity increased to 82% and the specificity was 96%.

In a similar study, Challier and colleagues[44] compared an *A fumigatus*-specific real-time PCR assay to the GM EIA using 207 serum samples from 41 immunocompromised patients. Among the 41 patients included in this study, 26 had proven or probable IA. The real-time PCR assay was positive in 22 (84.6%) patients, whereas the

GM EIA was positive in 20 (76.9%). Notably, tests for all 26 patients with proven or probable IA showed positive results using either real-time PCR assays or the GM EIA. These findings, as well as those from other studies comparing the GM EIA with the real-time PCR assay,[14,45] suggest that a combination of the two methods may provide improved diagnosis of IA.

Candida spp

Candida spp are the fourth leading cause of nosocomial bloodstream infections and are associated with a mortality rate of 40 to 50%.[46–48] Therefore, the development of rapid and sensitive methods for the detection of candidemia has been an area of significant interest in recent years. Dunyach and colleagues[49] developed a real-time PCR method for the detection of five *Candida* spp (*C. albicans*, *C. glabrata*, *C. krusei*, *C. parapsilosis* and *C. tropicalis*) in clinical serum specimens. Two separate primer sets were evaluated; the first set (internal transcribed spacer [ITS]) targeted a conserved region of the 18S and 28S rDNA, and the second set (L18) targeted a variable region within the 18S rDNA. The study analyzed 58 sera from 23 patients who had either proven (n = 13) or probable (n = 10) fungal bloodstream infection. The L18 real-time PCR assay detected *Candida* nucleic acid in 12 of 13 (92%) patients who had proven infection, whereas the ITS PCR assay was positive in 10 of 13 (76.9%) patients. For patients who had probable infection, the L18 and ITS assays demonstrated sensitivities of 30% (3/10) and 50% (5/10), respectively. Notably, the ITS real-time PCR assay allowed for the differentiation of the five *Candida* spp based on melting curve analyses.

The accurate discrimination of *Candida* species by real-time PCR assays may assist physicians in selecting the most appropriate antifungal regimen in a timely manner. Metwally and colleagues[50] developed a real-time PCR assay for the differentiation of species in which fluconazole resistance is a concern (eg, *C krusei* and *C glabrata*) from characteristically fluconazole-sensitive species (eg, *C albicans*, *C dubliniensis*, *C parapsilosis*, *C tropicalis*) directly from positive-blood-culture bottles. The PCR method was validated using blood-culture sets that were either positive (n = 33) or negative (n = 10) for yeast and demonstrated 100% agreement with the findings of conventional phenotypic identification. Furthermore, the PCR assay allowed for the identification of *C glabrata* and *C krusei* in less than 3 hours, compared with the approximately 72 hours required using routine, phenotypic techniques.

Dermatophytes

Several real-time PCR methods have been described for the diagnosis of dermatophyte infections, which remain among the most common communicable diseases worldwide. Gutzmer and colleagues[51] compared the results of culture-based tests and direct microscopy to a PCR method targeting the fungal rDNA and ITS regions. Clinical specimens were screened for the presence of fungal DNA using an initial primer set, followed by the discrimination of dermatophyte and nondermatophyte molds and the subclassification of yeasts using additional primer sets, melting curve analyses, or assessment of restriction-fragment-length polymorphism. Thirty-eight clinical samples (ie, skin scales and swabs) from patients who had dermatophytosis were tested, of which 32 results (84%) were positive using melting curve analysis. Interestingly, the real-time PCR assay provided additional diagnostic information (not provided by culture or direct microscopy) in 9 of 38 (23.7%) cases.

A report by Arabatzis and colleagues[52] described the development of a real-time PCR method for the detection and identification of dermatophytes in clinical samples. The method involved the performance of two separate assays, the first detecting the *Trichophyton mentagrophytes* complex, *T tonsurans* and *T violaceum*, and the second targeting the *T rubrum* complex, *Microsporum canis*, and *M. audouinii*. Ninety-two skin, nail, and hair specimens from 67 patients who had suspected dermatophytosis were tested using PCR, culture and direct microscopy. The results of real-time PCR assays were positive in 47 of 92 (51.1%) specimens, versus 40 (43.5%) being positive using microscopy or culture. In addition, 20 skin scale specimens from patients who had psoriasis or eczema and 20 nail specimens from healthy patients were tested as controls. The results for all control specimens were negative using culture and microscopy, whereas one specimen was found to be weakly positive for *T mentagrophytes* using the PCR assay. These findings suggest that molecular methods may allow for a more rapid and sensitive diagnosis of dermatophyte infections. However, further validation studies will be necessary to determine the clinical sensitivity, specificity, and cost of the real-time PCR assay compared with traditional techniques prior to its implementation as a routine diagnostic approach in cases of dermatophytosis.

Dimorphic Fungi

Routine detection of the dimorphic fungi (eg, *Coccidioides* spp., *H capsulatum*, *B dermatitidis*) has

been achieved using culture, with subsequent identification of culture isolates using DNA-probe technology (AccuProbes) or microscopic examination for characteristic morphologic features.[9–11] Although these methods demonstrate high sensitivity and specificity, recovery of the dimorphic fungi in the clinical laboratory may take days to weeks and represents a significant safety hazard to laboratory personnel.[5] Despite the need for more rapid methods of detecting the dimorphic fungi, very limited progress has been made in the development and validation of molecular assays targeting the endemic mycoses.

Several studies have assessed the ability of real-time PCR assays to identify *Coccidioides* spp from culture. Bialek and colleagues[53] designed a real-time PCR assay targeting the antigen 2/proline-rich antigen (Ag2/PRA) gene of *C posadasii*. This assay correctly identified 120 clinical strains of *C posadasii* that had been isolated from 114 patients who resided in an endemic region for coccidioidomycosis. Castañón-Oliveres and colleagues[54] analyzed 56 clinical isolates of *Coccidioides* spp using a real-time PCR assay targeting single nucleotide polymorphisms in four target sequences. This assay correctly identified all 56 isolates and was able to distinguish between the two known species of *Coccidioides, C posadasii* and *C immitis*.

In 2007, the authors and their laboratory associates developed a real-time PCR assay for the detection and identification of *Coccidioides* spp from culture isolates and clinical specimens.[55] This assay was designed to target the ITS2 region of *Coccidioides* spp, and it demonstrated 100% sensitivity and specificity using culture isolates ($n = 64$). In addition, an analysis of 266 respiratory specimens showed the assay to be 100% sensitive and 98.4% specific when compared with culture. The assay was also validated using fresh ($n = 66$) and paraffin-embedded tissue specimens ($n = 148$), yielding sensitivities of 92.9 and 73.4%, respectively. Additional studies are underway to determine the diagnostic sensitivity and specificity of this assay in the clinical setting.[56]

The diagnosis of histoplasmosis has historically been made using a combination of culture, serologic, histopathologic, and recently, urine antigen testing. The *Histoplasma* antigen assay is most useful for the rapid diagnosis of severe, disseminated disease.[57] A study by Tang and colleagues[58] compared a conventional PCR-ELISA (enzyme-linked immunosorbent assay) method with the use of culture and urine antigen detection. The study demonstrated the PCR assay to be less sensitive, detecting only 4 of 51 (7.8%) specimens positive for antigenuria. Despite these preliminary findings, further studies comparing the performance of the real-time PCR assay with the *Histoplasma* antigen assay are lacking. In 2003, Martagon-Villamil and colleagues[59] developed a real-time assay targeting the ITS rRNA gene complex of *H capsulatum*. The assay was validated using 34 culture isolates of *H capsulatum* and 73 isolates of other fungal genera, and it demonstrated 100% sensitivity and specificity for identification. In addition, a limited number of clinical specimens (n = 5) from three immunocompromised patients who had culture-proven histoplasmosis were tested, and using the real-time PCR assay, the results were positive for 4 (80%) of the patients.

Buitrago and colleagues[60] developed a real-time PCR assay targeting the ITS1 region of *H capsulatum* and tested 10 serum samples from four patients who were infected with HIV using proven histoplasmosis methods. The assay was positive in 7 of 10 (70%) serum specimens. Specificity was assessed by testing 10 sera from patients who had proven aspergillosis and 15 sera from healthy control subjects, the results of which were negative using the real-time PCR assay. A subsequent study by these investigators tested 22 clinical samples from 14 patients who had proven histoplasmosis. The PCR assay was positive in 17 of 22 (77.3%) clinical samples, with 100% sensitivity from respiratory secretions and bone marrow samples, but only 70% sensitivity from serum specimens.[61]

Pneumocystis

The laboratory diagnosis of *Pneumocystis jirovecii* (formerly *P. carinii* f sp *hominis*) has traditionally been accomplished using histopathologic examination, direct fluorescent antibody examination, or examination of clinical specimens using fluorescent (e.g., calcofluor white) smear microscopy. These methods have several disadvantages, including subjective interpretation and an overall lack of sensitivity. Because of these limitations, real-time PCR testing has received attention related to the enhanced sensitivity and objectivity of this method.

Numerous studies have compared the performance of real-time PCR assays with conventional methods for the detection of *P jirovecii* in respiratory specimens. These reports have almost uniformly demonstrated the increased sensitivity of PCR assays over direct microscopy.[17,62] In one example, Fillaux and colleagues[15] analyzed 400 BAL specimens using both direct fluorescent antibody and real-time PCR assays and found the PCR assays to produce positive results in 66

(16.5%) samples versus only 31 (7.8%) using direct fluorescent antibody. Similarly, Flori and colleagues[63] tested 173 BAL specimens using smear microscopy and real-time PCR assays, and determined the sensitivity of these methods to be 60 and 100%, respectively.

The role of qPCR assays has gained considerable interest in recent years because molecular methods may be used to identify *P jirovecii* nucleic acid in respiratory samples from patients who do not show clinical evidence of *Pneumocystis* pneumonia (PCP). Bandt and colleagues[64] developed a quantitative, real-time PCR assay targeting the dihydrofolate reductase (DHFR) gene of *P jirovecii*. The assay was used to evaluate 69 BAL specimens from 26 patients who had PCP, as well as 60 negative control specimens. The results of this study suggest that a fungal load of less than 10 copies per reaction indicates asymptomatic colonization with *P jirovecii*. The authors also proposed that results of more than 100 copies per reaction may be consistent with possible PCP, whereas results of more than 1000 copies suggest confirmed PCP. A study by Huggett and colleagues[65] analyzed the cases of 61 patients who had 62 episodes of PCP using a quantitative real-time PCR assay. Quantifiable *Pneumocystis* nucleic acid was detected in 61 of 62 (98.4%) cases of PCP (range, 13–18,608 copies per reaction; mean, 332 copies). Receiver-operator curve analysis demonstrated a clinical sensitivity and specificity of 98 and 96%, respectively, when a cutoff of less 10 copies per reaction was used to establish a diagnosis of PCP. These findings suggest that qPCR assays may assist in the differentiation of colonization and clinical infection; however, further studies are needed to more extensively validate and standardize the methods of quantification before defined cutoff levels can be established.

Zygomycetes

The incidence of opportunistic infections caused by Zygomycetes has increased over the past several decades, especially among transplant patients and those who have underlying metabolic acidosis.[66] Disease caused by Zygomycetes may demonstrate rapid progression in immunocompromised hosts, emphasizing the importance for a timely diagnosis and initiation of therapy. Histopathology and culture of tissue specimens are commonly used in determining the laboratory diagnosis of zygomycosis, but these methods have significant limitations. The histopathologic examination of infected tissue is subjective and lacks sensitivity, and identification of culture isolates is time consuming and requires considerable expertise. Furthermore, it is not uncommon to have negative fungal cultures, even when histopathology results suggest a zygomycotic infection, because the processing of tissue specimens prior to culturing may rupture the pauciseptate hyphae of the organism, thereby preventing growth.

Despite the need for rapid and sensitive methods to detect Zygomycetes in clinical specimens, the development of molecular methods targeting this group of fungi has been limited. Imhof and colleagues[67] described a real-time PCR assay that detected *Conidiobolus* spp in a single, facial, soft tissue specimen. The assay was designed to use a broad-range fungal primer set targeting a conserved sequence of the 18S rRNA gene with subsequent identification obtained using melting curve analysis and sequencing of the PCR amplicon. In 2008, a study by Hata and colleagues[68] evaluated a real-time PCR method targeting the multicopy zygomycete cytochrome *b* gene. This assay demonstrated sensitivity and specificity of 100% (39/39) and 92% (59/64), respectively, using culture isolates. In addition, a limited number of fresh tissue specimens (n = 2) were tested, and the sensitivity was determined to be 100%. The sensitivity and specificity observed using paraffin-embedded tissues was 56% (35/62) and 100% (19/19), respectively.

Considerations for Real-time Polymerase Chain Reaction Testing and Result Interpretation

Real-time PCR testing offers several significant advantages over conventional techniques, including reduced turnaround time and increased sensitivity. However, several limitations of real-time PCR testing should be considered as this method becomes used more routinely in the diagnosis of fungal infections. First, the high sensitivity of real-time PCR assays may allow for the detection of fungi (eg, *Aspergillus* sp, *Candida* sp, *Pneumocystis jirovecii*) that are colonizing or causing a subclinical infection. Further validation studies focusing on the role of qPCR assays in distinguishing colonization from disease are needed and may assist in the interpretation of results. Second, fungal PCR assays may be prone to false-positive results because of contamination with environmental fungi. Precautions should be taken during specimen collection, processing, and testing to reduce the potential for contamination events. Finally, growth in culture is still required if antifungal susceptibility testing is to be performed. Several studies have evaluated the ability of real-time PCR assays to detect fungal resistance markers using culture isolates and clinical specimens,[69,70] and this approach may represent a promising alternative in the future.

SEQUENCE-BASED IDENTIFICATION OF FUNGI

Within the past decade, the amplification and sequencing of specific fungal nucleic acid targets has evolved from being primarily a research application to become a valuable clinical diagnostic tool. The traditional DNA-sequencing techniques (ie, the Maxam-Gilbert chemical cleavage method[71] and the Sanger chain-terminator method[72]) have been reviewed in detail in previous publications.[71–73] When attempting to identify microorganisms using DNA sequencing, the gene targeted must contain highly conserved regions that can serve as primer binding sites, and these conserved regions should flank regions with enough sequence variability to allow for discrimination to the genus or species level. Furthermore, the target gene should be present at high copy numbers whenever possible to increase the sensitivity of the PCR amplification prior to sequence analysis. The general structure of the fungal eurkaryotic rRNA gene region is shown in **Fig. 1** and consists of four ribosomal genes (the 18S small subunit, the 5.8S subunit, the 25–28S large subunit, and the 5S subunit genes) separated by ITS regions. The Clinical Laboratory Standards Institute recently published a guidance document that provides information about recommended sequencing methods, gene targets, and suggested interpretive criteria[74] for the identification of microorganisms, including the fungi. The targets most commonly used for fungi are the ITS1 and ITS2 regions between the 18S and 28S ribosomal subunits and an ~600 base-pair region of the D1-D2 region of the 25–28S large ribosomal subunit. In some instances, these regions may not provide sufficient variability between fungal genera or species, and alternate targets have been used, such as the elongation factor-1α for *Fusarium* spp or β-tubulin for *Phaeoacremonium* spp.[75,76] Continuously changing fungal taxonomy, limitations of the currently available fungal sequence libraries, and lack of a consensus agreement on the percent identity score needed to identify specimens to the genus or species level make fungal identification using sequence analysis somewhat less robust at the present time than bacterial identification using this technique.[74,77,78]

A significant body of literature exists supporting the clinical utility of sequencing for the identification of medically important yeast.[79] Leaw and colleagues[80] performed sequence analysis of the ITS region for 373 strains (86 species) of clinically

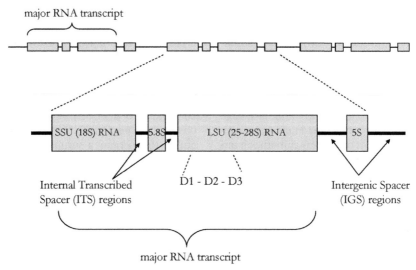

Fig. 1. Structural organization of the fungal ribosomal genes. SSU, small ribosomal subunit; LSU, large ribosomal subunit.

derived yeast and compared the results to those obtained using the API ID32C system (bioMerieux, Marcy l'Etoile, France). Sequencing of the ITS1 and ITS2 regions accurately identified 96.8% (361/373) and 99.7% (372/373) of isolates from isolated colonies within 24 hours, which represents a significant time savings compared with the 48 to 72 hour turnaround time required for the API ID32C system. In another study, Ciardo and colleagues[81] used sequencing of the ITS region to correctly identify 98% of 113 medically important yeast strains to the species level. These 113 yeast strains were selected because they failed to be identified by traditional methods using CHROMagar Candida (Becton Dickinson, Franklin Lakes, New Jersey) and morphology on rice agar. Further, the API ID32C system was able to correctly identify only 87% of these isolates, 7% of isolates could not be identified, and 6% were misidentified. Finally, Sugita and colleagues[82] demonstrated the utility of ITS1 and ITS2 region sequencing for the identification of *Trichosporon* species.

Sequencing of the D1-D2 region of the 25–28S rRNA gene has also been extensively investigated regarding the identification of yeast. Linton and colleagues[83] examined 3,033 clinical isolates of yeast submitted to the United Kingdom Mycology Reference Laboratory over a two-year period. The majority (>90%) could be identified using traditional methods, but sequencing of the D1-D2 region was useful for unambiguous identification of 153 isolates (5%) that exhibited atypical biochemical and phenotypic profiles using other methods. Hall and colleagues[84] reported on the

utility of a commercially available sequencing kit, the MicroSeq D2 large ribosomal subunit rDNA fungal kit (Applied Biosytems, Foster City, California), which they used for the identification of 131 yeast isolates recovered from clinical specimens at the Mayo Clinic, with 93.9% identified correctly to the genus and species level. They attributed most discrepancies to the lack of inclusion of the species sequence in the MicroSeq or API 20C AUX databases. Desnos-Ollivier and colleagues[85] demonstrated the utility of a combination of ITS and D1-D2 region sequencing to identify 36 isolates of yeast that had previously been incorrectly identified as *Debaromyces hansenii* (teleomorph of *C famata*) or *Pichia guilliermondii* (teleomorph of *C guilliermondii*) using morphology and carbon assimilation patterns alone. This work allowed the authors of this article to conclude that *D hansenii* and *P guilliermondii* may not be as common a cause of human fungemia as previously believed.

The utility of sequencing for the identification of medically important filamentous fungi (eg., *Aspergillus* sp, *Rhizopus* sp) has not been as extensively evaluated as it has for the yeast. Hall and colleagues[86] reported on the ability of the MicroSeq D2 large ribosomal subunit rDNA sequencing kit to identify 234 filamentous fungi previously identified using phenotypic methods, with 158 (67.5%) being correctly identified to the genus or genus and species level using sequencing. The most significant reason for failure to identify an isolate was a lack of sequence inclusion in the MicroSeq database (70/234, 29.9%). The utility of the MicroSeq D2 kit for identification of dermatophytes has been reported,[87] and this approach provides significant advantages over traditional phenotypic methods by reducing the turnaround time for dermatophyte identification by an average of 9 days (N.L. Wengenack, PhD, unpublished observation, 2008).

In addition to the traditional Sanger dideoxy-based sequencing method, several groups have used the more recently described Pyrosequencing technology for the identification of yeast and filamentous fungi.[88–90] Pyrosequencing is a proprietary technique marketed by Biotage AB (Uppsala, Sweden), and it is commonly referred to as "sequencing by synthesis." Pyrosequencing (**Fig. 2**) requires addition of a deoxynucleotide triphosphate (dNTP) molecule by DNA polymerase to a growing DNA strand. The addition of the dNTP releases a pyrophosphate molecule, which is subsequently converted by the enzyme ATP-sulfurylase into ATP. The newly generated ATP molecule is used as a substrate by a second enzyme, luciferase, to generate light, which is then quantitated. The four dNTP bases are added in a cyclic manner so that the identity of the incorporated base can be determined by measuring the light generated. The advantages of Pyrosequencing are that it is rapid (∼1 min/bp), technically simple to perform with little hands-on technologist intervention needed, and is reasonably priced (∼$1/ sample for reagent costs). Wiederhold and colleagues[91] recently demonstrated the utility of Pyrosequencing for detection of mutations in the *FKS1* gene that confer reduced susceptibility to

the echinocandin drugs (ie, anidulafungin, caspofungin, micafungin) in *C albicans*. Because in vitro susceptibility testing of the echinocandins can be challenging,[92,93] that study illustrates the potential of molecular methods for evaluation of drug susceptibility. Presently, Pyrosequencing is limited to the analysis of short templates with reads of ∼100 bp, and therefore sometimes lacks the ability to discriminate between closely related species,[89] but nevertheless, it represents a rapid, less expensive alternative to the use of conventional sequencing technology in the clinical laboratory.

FUTURE DIRECTIONS IN MOLECULAR FUNGAL DIAGNOSTICS

The introduction of the molecular methods described above into the clinical mycology laboratory has allowed for the sensitive, specific, and rapid detection of fungal pathogens. However, many fungi still require culture- and morphology-based identification, and therefore opportunities exist for continued advancement in the field of fungal molecular diagnostics. Future studies will likely be directed at adapting existing technologies, including liquid bead (Luminex)–based (Luminex Corporation, Austin, Texas) and microarray-based methods to further enhance the speed, throughput, and accuracy of fungal diagnostic testing. Luminex suspension assays and microarrays permit the detection and identification of multiple infectious agents in a single test and their use in the diagnosis of several fungal infections

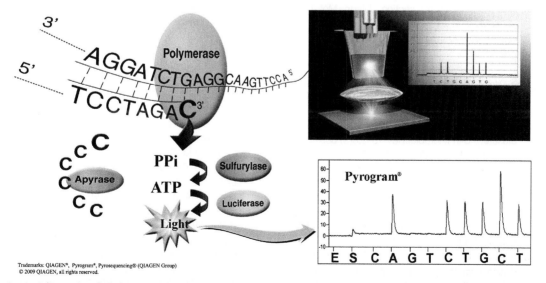

Fig. 2. Schematic of the Pyrosequencing reaction. Sequential incorporation of deoxynucleotide triphosphate molecules (dNTPs) into the growing DNA chain by DNA polymerase results in the release of inorganic phosphate (PPi) which in turn is converted to quantifiable light through the enzymatic activities of sulfurylase and luciferase. (*Courtesy of* Biotage AB, Uppsala, Sweden; with permission).

has recently been evaluated.[94–97] An oligonucleotide microarray developed by Huang and colleagues[98] was compared with conventional methods using 86 fungal culture isolates and a limited number (n = 16) of blood specimens. The microarray showed 100% agreement with conventional testing and was able to discriminate among 20 fungal species representing 8 genera in a rapid and high-throughput format. The ability to scan for multiple pathogens at one time represents a promising alternative to the current single-pathogen-targeted PCR assays, and the microarray may also be adapted to provide timely information on antifungal susceptibilities by using the targeted detection of resistance markers from culture isolates and clinical specimens. However, at the present time, array-based techniques require the manual manipulation of amplified DNA, which is undesirable in the clinical laboratory because of the potential for cross-contamination and false-positive results. Additional studies are needed to extensively validate and standardize these methods prior to their implementation for the routine laboratory diagnosis of fungal infections.

REFERENCES

1. Cuenca-Estrella M, Bernal-Martinez L, Buitrago MJ, et al. Update on the epidemiology and diagnosis of invasive fungal infection. Int J Antimicrob Agents 2008;32(Suppl 2):S143–7.

2. Hayden RT, Qian X, Roberts GD, et al. In situ hybridization for the identification of yeastlike organisms in tissue section. Diagn Mol Pathol 2001;10(1):15–23.

3. Kaufman L, Valero G, Padhye AA. Misleading manifestations of Coccidioides immitis in vivo. J Clin Microbiol 1998;36(12):3721–3.

4. Schwarz J. The diagnosis of deep mycoses by morphologic methods. Hum Pathol 1982;13(6): 519–33.

5. Sewell DL. Laboratory-associated infections and biosafety. Clin Microbiol Rev 1995;8(3):389–405.

6. Bankowski MJ, Anderson SM. Real-time nucleic acid amplification in clinical microbiology. Clin Microbiol Newsl 2004;26(2):9–15.

7. Cockerill FR III. Application of rapid-cycle real-time polymerase chain reaction for diagnostic testing in the clinical microbiology laboratory. Arch Pathol Lab Med 2003;127(9):1112–20.

8. Espy MJ, Uhl JR, Sloan LM, et al. Real-time PCR in clinical microbiology: applications for routine laboratory testing. Clin Microbiol Rev 2006;19(1): 165–256.

9. Huffnagle KE, Gander RM. Evaluation of Gen-Probe's Histoplasma capsulatum and Cryptococcus neoformans AccuProbes. J Clin Microbiol 1993;31(2):419–21.

10. Stockman L, Clark KA, Hunt JM, et al. Evaluation of commercially available acridinium ester-labeled chemiluminescent DNA probes for culture identification of Blastomyces dermatitidis, Coccidioides immitis, Cryptococcus neoformans, and Histoplasma capsulatum. J Clin Microbiol 1993;31(4): 845–50.

11. Padhye AA, Smith G, Standard PG, et al. Comparative evaluation of chemiluminescent DNA probe assays and exoantigen tests for rapid identification of Blastomyces dermatitidis and Coccidioides immitis. J Clin Microbiol 1994;32(4):867–70.

12. Pryce TM, Palladino S, Kay ID, et al. Rapid identification of fungi by sequencing the ITS1 and ITS2 regions using an automated capillary electrophoresis system. Med Mycol 2003;41(5):369–81.

13. Borman AM, Linton CJ, Miles SJ, et al. Molecular identification of pathogenic fungi. J Antimicrob Chemother 2008;61(Suppl 1):i7–12.

14. Sanguinetti M, Posteraro B, Pagano L, et al. Comparison of real-time PCR, conventional PCR, and galactomannan antigen detection by enzyme-linked immunosorbent assay using bronchoalveolar lavage fluid samples from hematology patients for diagnosis of invasive pulmonary aspergillosis. J Clin Microbiol 2003;41(8):3922–5.

15. Fillaux J, Malvy S, Alvarez M, et al. Accuracy of a routine real-time PCR assay for the diagnosis of Pneumocystis jirovecii pneumonia. J Microbiol Methods 2008;75(2):258–61.

16. Larsen HH, Masur H, Kovacs JA, et al. Development and evaluation of a quantitative, touchdown, real-time PCR assay for diagnosing Pneumocystis carinii pneumonia. J Clin Microbiol 2002;40(2):490–4.

17. Brancart F, Rodriguez-Villalobos H, Fonteyne PA, et al. Quantitative TaqMan PCR for detection of Pneumocystis jirovecii. J Microbiol Methods 2005; 61(3):381–7.

18. Khot PD, Ko DL, Hackman RC, et al. Development and optimization of quantitative PCR for the diagnosis of invasive aspergillosis with bronchoalveolar lavage fluid. BMC Infect Dis 2008;8:73.

19. Beard JS, Benson PM, Skillman L. Rapid diagnosis of coccidioidomycosis with a DNA probe to ribosomal RNA. Arch Dermatol 1993;129(12):1589–93.

20. Sandin RL, Hall GS, Longworth DL, et al. Unpredictability of commercially available exoantigen culture confirmation tests in confirming the identity of five Blastomyces dermatitidis isolates. Am J Clin Pathol 1993;99(5):542–5.

21. Kwon-Chung KJ, Wickes BL, Stockman L, et al. Virulence, serotype, and molecular characteristics of environmental strains of Cryptococcus neoformans var. gattii. Infect Immun 1992;60(5):1869–74.

22. Chemaly RF, Tomford JW, Hall GS, et al. Rapid diagnosis of *Histoplasma capsulatum* endocarditis using the AccuProbe on an excised valve. J Clin Microbiol 2001;39(7):2640–1.

23. Gen-Probe. AccuProbe Blastomyces dermatitidis culture identification test [product insert 102963-H]. 2005. Available at: http://www.gen-probe.com/products/culture_identification.aspx.

24. Perea S, Patterson T. Endemic mycoses. In: EJ A, McGinnis MR, MA P, editors. Clinical Mycology. Philadelphia: Elsevier Science; 2003. p. 352–69.

25. Iwen PC, Sigler L, Tarantolo S, et al. Pulmonary infection caused by *Gymnascella hyalinospora* in a patient with acute myelogenous leukemia. J Clin Microbiol 2000;38(1):375–81.

26. deHoog G, Guarro J, Figueras MJ. Atlas of clinical fungi. In: deHoog GA, Guarro J, Gene J, et al, editors. Spain: Centralbureau voor Schimmelcultures. 2nd edition. Universitate Rovira i Virgili; 2000.

27. Larone D. Medically important fungi. Washington, DC: ASM Press; 2002.

28. Hall GS, Pratt-Rippin K, Washington JA. Evaluation of a chemiluminescent probe assay for identification of *Histoplasma capsulatum* isolates. J Clin Microbiol 1992;30(11):3003–4.

29. Brandt ME, Gaunt D, Iqbal N, et al. False-positive *Histoplasma capsulatum* Gen-Probe chemiluminescent test result caused by a *Chrysosporium* species. J Clin Microbiol 2005;43(3):1456–8.

30. Sandin RL, Isada CM, Hall GS, et al. Aberrant *Histoplasma capsulatum*. Confirmation of identity by a chemiluminescence-labeled DNA probe. Diagn Microbiol Infect Dis 1993;17(3):235–8.

31. Sutton DA, Padhye AA, Standard PG, et al. An aberrant variant of *Histoplasma capsulatum* var. *capsulatum*. J Clin Microbiol 1997;35(3):734–5.

32. Saubolle MA. Laboratory aspects in the diagnosis of coccidioidomycosis. Ann N Y Acad Sci 2007; 1111:301–14.

33. Gromadzki SG, Chaturvedi V. Limitation of the AccuProbe *Coccidioides immitis* culture identification test: false-negative results with formaldehyde-killed cultures. J Clin Microbiol 2000;38(6): 2427–8.

34. Valesco M, Johnston K. Stability of hybridization activity of *Coccidioides immitis* in live and heat-killed frozen cultures tested by AccuProbe *Coccidioides immitis* culture identification test. J Clin Microbiol 1997;35(3):736–7.

35. Valesco M. Stability of frozen, heat-killed cultures of *Coccidioides immitis* as positive-control material in the Gen-Probe AccuProbe *Coccidioides immitis* culture identification test. J Clin Microbiol 2008; 46(4):1565.

36. McGinnis MR, Smith MB, Hinson E. Use of the *Coccidioides posadasii* Deltachs5 strain for quality control in the ACCUPROBE culture identification test for *Coccidioides immitis*. J Clin Microbiol 2006;44(11):4250–1.

37. Sandhu GS, Kline BC, Stockman L, et al. Molecular probes for diagnosis of fungal infections. J Clin Microbiol 1995;33(11):2913–9.

38. Lindsley MD, Hurst SF, Iqbal NJ, et al. Rapid identification of dimorphic and yeast-like fungal pathogens using specific DNA probes. J Clin Microbiol 2001;39(10):3505–11.

39. Palladino S, Kay I, Fonte R, et al. Use of real-time PCR and the LightCycler system for the rapid detection of *Pneumocystis carinii* in respiratory specimens. Diagn Microbiol Infect Dis 2001;39(4): 233–6.

40. Raggam RB, Leitner E, Muhlbauer G, et al. Qualitative detection of *Legionella* species in bronchoalveolar lavages and induced sputa by automated DNA extraction and real-time polymerase chain reaction. Med Microbiol Immunol 2002;191(2): 119–25.

41. Uhl JR, Adamson SC, Vetter EA, et al. Comparison of LightCycler PCR, rapid antigen immunoassay, and culture for detection of group a Streptococci from throat swabs. J Clin Microbiol 2003;41(1): 242–9.

42. Ascioglu S, Rex JH, de Pauw B, et al. Defining opportunistic invasive fungal infections in immunocompromised patients with cancer and hematopoietic stem cell transplants: an international consensus. Clin Infect Dis 2002;34(1):7–14.

43. Musher B, Fredricks D, Leisenring W, et al. *Aspergillus galactomannan* enzyme immunoassay and quantitative PCR for diagnosis of invasive aspergillosis with bronchoalveolar lavage fluid. J Clin Microbiol 2004;42(12):5517–22.

44. Challier S, Boyer S, Abachin E, et al. Development of a serum-based Taqman real-time PCR assay for diagnosis of invasive aspergillosis. J Clin Microbiol 2004;42(2):844–6.

45. Costa C, Costa JM, Desterke C, et al. Real-time PCR coupled with automated DNA extraction and detection of galactomannan antigen in serum by enzyme-linked immunosorbent assay for diagnosis of invasive aspergillosis. J Clin Microbiol 2002; 40(6):2224–7.

46. Edmond MB, Wallace SE, McClish DK, et al. Nosocomial bloodstream infections in United States hospitals: a three-year analysis. Clin Infect Dis 1999;29(2):239–44.

47. Gudlaugsson O, Gillespie S, Lee K, et al. Attributable mortality of nosocomial candidemia, revisited. Clin Infect Dis 2003;37(9):1172–7.

48. Pappas PG, Rex JH, Lee J, et al. A prospective observational study of candidemia: epidemiology, therapy, and influences on mortality in hospitalized adult and pediatric patients. Clin Infect Dis 2003; 37(5):634–43.

49. Dunyach C, Bertout S, Phelipeau C, et al. Detection and identification of *Candida* spp. in human serum by LightCycler real-time polymerase chain reaction. Diagn Microbiol Infect Dis 2008;60(3):263–71.

50. Metwally L, Hogg G, Coyle PV, et al. Rapid differentiation between fluconazole-sensitive and -resistant species of *Candida* directly from positive blood-culture bottles by real-time PCR. J Med Microbiol 2007;56(Pt 7):964–70.

51. Gutzmer R, Mommert S, Kuttler U, et al. Rapid identification and differentiation of fungal DNA in dermatological specimens by LightCycler PCR. J Med Microbiol 2004;53(Pt 12):1207–14.

52. Arabatzis M, Bruijnesteijn van Coppenraet LE, Kuijper EJ, et al. Diagnosis of common dermatophyte infections by a novel multiplex real-time polymerase chain reaction detection/identification scheme. Br J Dermatol 2007;157(4):681–9.

53. Bialek R, Kern J, Herrmann T, et al. PCR assays for identification of *Coccidioides posadasii* based on the nucleotide sequence of the antigen 2/proline-rich antigen. J Clin Microbiol 2004;42(2):778–83.

54. Castañón-Olivares LR, Güereña-Elizalde D, González-Martínez MR, et al. Molecular identification of *Coccidioides* isolates from Mexican patients. Ann N Y Acad Sci 2007;1111:326–35.

55. Binnicker MJ, Buckwalter SP, Eisberner JJ, et al. Detection of *Coccidioides* species in clinical specimens by real-time PCR. J Clin Microbiol 2007; 45(1):173–8.

56. Vucicevic D, Blair JE, Binnicker MJ, et al. The utility of *Coccidioides* PCR in the clinical setting. Paper presented at: Coccidioidomycosis Study Group, 52nd Annual Meeting; April 5, 2008; San Diego, CA.

57. Wheat LJ, Garringer T, Brizendine E, et al. Diagnosis of histoplasmosis by antigen detection based upon experience at the histoplasmosis reference laboratory. Diagn Microbiol Infect Dis 2002;43(1):29–37.

58. Tang YW, Li H, Durkin MM, et al. Urine polymerase chain reaction is not as sensitive as urine antigen for the diagnosis of disseminated histoplasmosis. Diagn Microbiol Infect Dis 2006;54(4):283–7.

59. Martagon-Villamil J, Shrestha N, Sholtis M, et al. Identification of *Histoplasma capsulatum* from culture extracts by real-time PCR. J Clin Microbiol 2003;41(3):1295–8.

60. Buitrago MJ, Berenguer J, Mellado E, et al. Detection of imported histoplasmosis in serum of HIV-infected patients using a real-time PCR-based assay. Eur J Clin Microbiol Infect Dis 2006;25(10):665–8.

61. Buitrago MJ, Gomez-Lopez A, Monzon A, et al. Assessment of a quantitative PCR method for clinical diagnosis of imported histoplasmosis. Enferm Infecc Microbiol Clin 2007;25(1):16–22.

62. Arcenas RC, Uhl JR, Buckwalter SP, et al. A real-time polymerase chain reaction assay for detection of *Pneumocystis* from bronchoalveolar lavage fluid. Diagn Microbiol Infect Dis 2006;54(3):169–75.

63. Flori P, Bellete B, Durand F, et al. Comparison between real-time PCR, conventional PCR, and different staining techniques for diagnosing *Pneumocystis jirovecii* pneumonia from bronchoalveolar lavage specimens. J Med Microbiol 2004;53(Pt 7):603–7.

64. Bandt D, Monecke S. Development and evaluation of a real-time PCR assay for detection of *Pneumocystis jirovecii*. Transpl Infect Dis 2007;9(3):196–202.

65. Huggett JF, Taylor MS, Kocjan G, et al. Development and evaluation of a real-time PCR assay for detection of *Pneumocystis jirovecii* DNA in bronchoalveolar lavage fluid of HIV-infected patients. Thorax 2008;63(2):154–9.

66. Husain S, Alexander BD, Munoz P, et al. Opportunistic mycelial fungal infections in organ transplant recipients: emerging importance of non-*Aspergillus* mycelial fungi. Clin Infect Dis 2003;37(2):221–9.

67. Imhof A, Schaer C, Schoedon G, et al. Rapid detection of pathogenic fungi from clinical specimens using LightCycler real-time fluorescence PCR. Eur J Clin Microbiol Infect Dis 2003;22(9):558–60.

68. Hata DJ, Buckwalter SP, Pritt BS, et al. Real-time PCR method for detection of Zygomycetes. J Clin Microbiol 2008;46(7):2353–8.

69. Kofla G, Ruhnke M. Development of a new real-time TaqMan PCR assay for quantitative analyses of *Candida albicans* resistance genes expression. J Microbiol Methods 2007;68(1):178–83.

70. Garcia-Effron G, Dilger A, Alcazar-Fuoli L, et al. Rapid detection of triazole antifungal resistance in *Aspergillus fumigatus*. J Clin Microbiol 2008; 46(4):1200–6.

71. Maxam AM, Gilbert W. A new method for sequencing DNA. Proc Natl Acad Sci U S A 1977;74(2):560–4.

72. Sanger F. Determination of nucleotide sequences in DNA. Science 1981;214(4526):1205–10.

73. Franca LT, Carrilho E, Kist TB. A review of DNA sequencing techniques. Q Rev Biophys 2002; 35(2):169–200.

74. CLSI. Interpretive criteria for microorganism identification by DNA target sequencing; approved guideline. CLSI document MM18. Wayne (PA): Clinical Laboratory Standards Institute; 2007.

75. O'Donnell K, Kistler HC, Cigelnik E, et al. Multiple evolutionary origins of the fungus causing Panama disease of banana: concordant evidence from nuclear and mitochondrial gene genealogies. Proc Natl Acad Sci U S A 1998;95(5):2044–9.

76. Mostert L, Groenewald JZ, Summerbell RC, et al. Species of *Phaeoacremonium* associated with infections in humans and environmental reservoirs in infected woody plants. J Clin Microbiol 2005; 43(4):1752–67.

77. Balajee SA, Sigler L, Brandt ME. DNA and the classical way: identification of medically important molds in the 21st century. Med Mycol 2007;45(6): 475–90.

78. Balajee SA, Borman AM, Brandt ME, et al. Sequence-based identification of *Aspergillus*, *Fusarium*, and *Mucorales* in the clinical mycology laboratory: where are we and where should we go from here? J Clin Microbiol 2008; [epub ahead of print].

79. Putignani L, Paglia MG, Bordi E, et al. Identification of clinically relevant yeast species by DNA sequence analysis of the D2 variable region of the 25-28S rRNA gene. Mycoses 2008;51(3): 209–27.

80. Leaw SN, Chang HC, Sun HF, et al. Identification of medically important yeast species by sequence analysis of the internal transcribed spacer regions. J Clin Microbiol 2006;44(3):693–9.

81. Ciardo DE, Schar G, Bottger EC, et al. Internal transcribed spacer sequencing versus biochemical profiling for identification of medically important yeasts. J Clin Microbiol 2006;44(1):77–84.

82. Sugita T, Nishikawa A, Ikeda R, et al. Identification of medically relevant *Trichosporon* species based on sequences of internal transcribed spacer regions and construction of a database for *Trichosporon* identification. J Clin Microbiol 1999;37(6): 1985–93.

83. Linton CJ, Borman AM, Cheung G, et al. Molecular identification of unusual pathogenic yeast isolates by large ribosomal subunit gene sequencing: 2 years of experience at the United Kingdom mycology reference laboratory. J Clin Microbiol 2007;45(4):1152–8.

84. Hall L, Wohlfiel S, Roberts GD. Experience with the MicroSeq D2 large-subunit ribosomal DNA sequencing kit for identification of commonly encountered, clinically important yeast species. J Clin Microbiol 2003;41(11):5099–102.

85. Desnos-Ollivier M, Ragon M, Robert V, et al. *Debaryomyces hansenii* (*Candida famata*), a rare human fungal pathogen often misidentified as *Pichia guilliermondii* (*Candida guilliermondii*). J Clin Microbiol 2008;46(10):3237–42.

86. Hall L, Wohlfiel S, Roberts GD. Experience with the MicroSeq D2 large-subunit ribosomal DNA sequencing kit for identification of filamentous fungi encountered in the clinical laboratory. J Clin Microbiol 2004;42(2):622–6.

87. Ninet B, Jan I, Bontems O, et al. Identification of dermatophyte species by 28S ribosomal DNA sequencing with a commercial kit. J Clin Microbiol 2003;41(2):826–30.

88. Boyanton BL Jr, Luna RA, Fasciano LR, et al. DNA Pyrosequencing-based identification of pathogenic *Candida* species by using the internal transcribed spacer 2 region. Arch Pathol Lab Med 2008; 132(4):667–74.

89. Montero CI, Shea YR, Jones PA, et al. Evaluation of Pyrosequencing technology for the identification of clinically relevant non-dematiaceous yeasts and related species. Eur J Clin Microbiol Infect Dis 2008;27(9):821–30.

90. Gharizadeh B, Norberg E, Loffler J, et al. Identification of medically important fungi by the Pyrosequencing technology. Mycoses 2004;47(1–2): 29–33.

91. Wiederhold NP, Grabinski JL, Garcia-Effron G, et al. Pyrosequencing to detect mutations in FKS1 that confer reduced echinocandin susceptibility in *Candida albicans*. Antimicrobial Agents Chemother 2008;52(11):4145–8.

92. Pfaller MA, Messer SA, Boyken L, et al. Further standardization of broth microdilution methodology for in vitro susceptibility testing of caspofungin against *Candida* species by use of an international collection of more than 3,000 clinical isolates. J Clin Microbiol 2004;42(7):3117–9.

93. Odds FC, Motyl M, Andrade R, et al. Interlaboratory comparison of results of susceptibility testing with caspofungin against *Candida* and *Aspergillus* species. J Clin Microbiol 2004;42(8):3475–82.

94. Diaz MR, Fell JW. Use of a suspension array for rapid identification of the varieties and genotypes of the *Cryptococcus neoformans* species complex. J Clin Microbiol 2005;43(8):3662–72.

95. Diaz MR, Boekhout T, Theelen B, et al. Microcoding and flow cytometry as a high-throughput fungal identification system for *Malassezia* species. J Med Microbiol 2006;55(Pt 9):1197–209.

96. Bovers M, Diaz MR, Hagen F, et al. Identification of genotypically diverse *Cryptococcus neoformans* and *Cryptococcus gattii* isolates by Luminex xMAP technology. J Clin Microbiol 2007;45(6): 1874–83.

97. Campa D, Tavanti A, Gemignani F, et al. DNA microarray based on arrayed-primer extension technique for identification of pathogenic fungi responsible for invasive and superficial mycoses. J Clin Microbiol 2008;46(3):909–15.

98. Huang A, Li JW, Shen ZQ, et al. High-throughput identification of clinical pathogenic fungi by hybridization to an oligonucleotide microarray. J Clin Microbiol 2006;44(9):3299–305.

99. Scalarone GM, Legendre AM, Clark KA, et al. Evaluation of a commercial DNA probe assay for the identification of clinical isolates of *Blastomyces dermatitidis* from dogs. J Med Vet Mycol 1992;30(1):43–9.

100. Gen-Probe. AccuProbe *Coccidioides immitis* culture identification test [product insert 102966, Rev. F. 2001]. Available at: http://www.gen-probe.com/products/culture_identification.aspx.

101. Padhye AA, Smith G, McLaughlin D, et al. Comparative evaluation of a chemiluminescent DNA probe and an exoantigen test for rapid identification of *Histoplasma capsulatum*. J Clin Microbiol 1992; 30(12):3108–11.

102. Gen-Probe. AccuProbe *Histoplasma capsulatum* culture identification test [product insert 102962-J.1. 2004]. Available at: http://www.gen-probe.com/products/culture_identification.aspx.

103. Kami M, Fukui T, Ogawa S, et al. Use of real-time PCR on blood samples for diagnosis of invasive aspergillosis. Clin Infect Dis 2001;33(9):1504–12.

104. Rantakokko-Jalava K, Laaksonen S, Issakainen J, et al. Semiquantitative detection by real-time PCR of *Aspergillus fumigatus* in bronchoalveolar lavage fluids and tissue biopsy specimens from patients with invasive aspergillosis. J Clin Microbiol 2003; 41(9):4304–11.

105. Spiess B, Buchheidt D, Baust C, et al. Development of a LightCycler PCR assay for detection and quantification of *Aspergillus fumigatus* DNA in clinical samples from neutropenic patients. J Clin Microbiol 2003;41(5):1811–8.

106. Pham AS, Tarrand JJ, May GS, et al. Diagnosis of invasive mold infection by real-time quantitative PCR. Am J Clin Pathol 2003;119(1):38–44.

107. Ramirez M, Castro C, Palomares JC, et al. Molecular detection and identification of *Aspergillus* spp. from clinical samples using real-time PCR. Mycoses 2008; [epub ahead of print].

108. Suarez F, Lortholary O, Buland S, et al. Detection of circulating *Aspergillus fumigatus* DNA by real-time PCR assay of large serum volumes improves early diagnosis of invasive aspergillosis in high-risk adult patients under hematologic surveillance. J Clin Microbiol 2008;46(11):3772–7.

109. Maaroufi Y, Heymans C, De Bruyne JM, et al. Rapid detection of *Candida albicans* in clinical blood samples by using a TaqMan-based PCR assay. J Clin Microbiol 2003;41(7):3293–8.

110. Selvarangan R, Bui U, Limaye AP, et al. Rapid identification of commonly encountered *Candida* species directly from blood culture bottles. J Clin Microbiol 2003;41(12):5660–4.

111. White PL, Shetty A, Barnes RA. Detection of seven *Candida* species using the Light-Cycler system. J Med Microbiol 2003;52(Pt 3):229–38.

112. Arancia S, Carattoli A, La Valle R, et al. Use of 65 kDa mannoprotein gene primers in Real-Time PCR identification of *Candida albicans* in biological samples. Mol Cell Probes 2006;20(5):263–8.

113. Innings A, Ullberg M, Johansson A, et al. Multiplex real-time PCR targeting the RNase P RNA gene for detection and identification of *Candida* species in blood. J Clin Microbiol 2007;45(3):874–80.

114. Alvarez-Martinez MJ, Miro JM, Valls ME, et al. Sensitivity and specificity of nested and real-time PCR for the detection of *Pneumocystis jirovecii* in clinical specimens. Diagn Microbiol Infect Dis 2006;56(2):153–60.

Index

Note: Page numbers of article titles are in **boldface** type.

Clin Chest Med 30 (2009) 409–413
doi:10.1016/S0272-5231(09)00038-0
0272-5231/09/$ – see front matter © 2009 Elsevier Inc. All rights reserved.

Moving?

Make sure your subscription moves with you!

To notify us of your new address, find your **Clinics Account Number** (located on your mailing label above your name), and contact customer service at:

E-mail: elspcs@elsevier.com

800-654-2452 (subscribers in the U.S. & Canada)
314-453-7041 (subscribers outside of the U.S. & Canada)

Fax number: 314-523-5170

Elsevier Periodicals Customer Service
11830 Westline Industrial Drive
St. Louis, MO 63146

*To ensure uninterrupted delivery of your subscription, please notify us at least 4 weeks in advance of move.